AMYLOIDOSIS - MECHANISMS AND PROSPECTS FOR THERAPY

Edited by **Svetlana Sarantseva**

Amyloidosis - Mechanisms and Prospects for Therapy
Edited by Svetlana Sarantseva

Published by InTech
Janeza Trdine 9, 51000 Rijeka, Croatia

Publishing Process Manager Petra Zobic

Technical Editor Teodora Smiljanic

Cover Designer InTech Design Team

Additional hard copies can be obtained from orders@intechopen.com

Amyloidosis - Mechanisms and Prospects for Therapy, Edited by Svetlana Sarantseva
p. cm.
978-953-307-253-1

For EU product safety concerns:
IN TECH d.o.o., Prolaz Marije Krucifikse Kozulić 3, 51000 Rijeka, Croatia,
info@intechopen.com or visit our website at intechopen.com.

Meet the editor

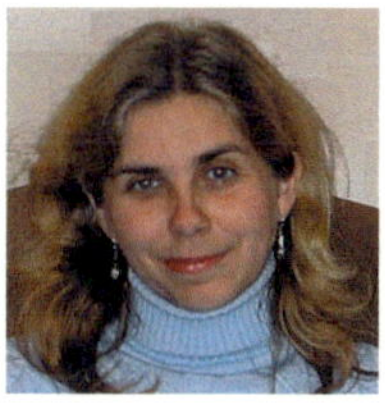

Dr. Sarantseva received M.S. (1989) and Ph.D (1999) in Genetics from the St. Petersburg State University. She did postdoctoral training in the Department of Molecular and Radiation Biophysics of Russian Academy of Sciences B.P. Konstantinov Petersburg Nuclear Physics Institute and spent several years in this Institute as a Head of research group studying different aspects of Drosophila Genetics. Presently Dr. Sarantseva is a head of Laboratory of Experimental and Applied Genetics at Russian Academy of Sciences in B.P.Konstantinov Petersburg Nuclear Physics Institute. The laboratory is actively using different genetic models of Alzheimer's disease and Parkinson's disease. The main focus is to discover cellular mechanisms of neurodegeneration and develop new therapeutics.

Contents

Preface

Amyloidoses are a heterogeneous group of diverse etiology diseases. They are characterized by an endogenous production of abnormal proteins called amyloid proteins, which are not hydrosoluble, form depots in various organs and tissue of animals and humans and cause dysfunctions. Twenty-seven such proteins have been identified as amyloid precursors in humans. However, the answer why these proteins form aggregates and cause disease is not still completely clear. At present, there is not an effective treatment to prevent protein misfolding in these amyloid diseases.

The aim of this book is to present an overview of different aspects of amyloidoses from basic mechanisms and diagnosis to latest advancements in treatment.

Chapters 1 to 3 provide description and clinical features as well as molecular and cellular mechanisms, and current strategies for treatment of AL amyloidosis and AA amyloidosis with rheumatoid arthritis. The next two chapters are focused on molecular mechanisms of amyloid formation. Chapter 4 elucidates influence of intrinsic and extrinsic factors on fibril deposition in Apolipoprotein A-I associated amyloidoses with particular emphasis on the role of the pathogenic polypeptide named [1–93]ApoA-I. Chapter 5 examines the role of synthetic glycopolymers mimicing glycosaminoglycans in aggregation of amyloid β-peptide, which is shown to play central role in the pathogenesis of Alzheimer's disease. Chapters 6 and 7 provide current methods for diagnosis and amyloid typing. More details are discussed on the advantages and limitations of the electron microscopy in the diagnosis of amyloidosis, particularly in early stage of disease. Chapter 8 covers the pathogenesis, lesions and clinical syndromes encompassing various forms of amyloidosis in animals.

Finally, Chapters 9 to 12 are focused on creating models of human amyloidosis in animals. Indeed, some animal models accurately reproduce one or several characteristics of the pathogenesis of amyloid diseases and could be useful for understanding the molecular and cellular mechanisms of amyloid formation and developing novel therapeutic strategies. Several animal models are presented in the final chapters of this book.

I would like to thank all the authors who have contributed to this book and I hope that this book will provide useful resource in study of amyloid disease pathogenesis and discovery of new therapeutic methods in the future.

Svetlana Sarantseva
Petersburg Nuclear Physics Institute, Russian Academy of Sciences
Russia

1

Current and New Perspectives on the Molecular and Cellular Mechanisms of Amyloid Formation and Toxicity in Light Chain Amyloidosis

Ara Celi Di Costanzo and Marina Ramirez-Alvarado
College of Medicine, Mayo Clinic. Rochester, USA

1. Introduction

Light chain (AL) amyloidosis is a protein misfolding disease characterized by the abnormal proliferation of monoclonal plasma cells that secrete free immunoglobulin light chains (LC) into circulation. These LCs misfold and aggregate as amyloid fibrils in vital organs. The process of amyloid formation causes organ failure, although the exact mechanism is unknown. The most frequently affected organs are the kidneys, heart, liver and peripheral nerves. AL amyloidosis is a devastating disease with a median survival of 12-40 months (Kumar et al., 2011; Wechalekar et al., 2008). The incidence of AL is 9 per million per year in the US, comparable to the incidence of Hodgkin's Lymphoma. Current treatments are harsh and not curative (chemotherapy and autologous stem cell transplantation), targeting the plasma cells producing the protein. There is currently no treatment that targets the misfolding process or the amyloid fibrils.

This chapter will discuss the latest developments in our understanding of the molecular mechanisms of AL amyloidosis including the role of mutations, cellular microenvironment, dimerization structures, different species populated in AL amyloid fibril formation, and light chain-associated cell and tissue toxicity. We will describe the challenges facing AL amyloidosis researchers to develop effective animal models of the disease and to find the best therapeutic strategies to treat this complex, devastating disease.

2. Light chain (AL) amyloidosis – Role of the protein in disease

A LC is composed of an N-terminal variable domain (V_L) and a C-terminal constant domain (C_L). The V_Ls are not uniformly variable throughout their lengths. Three small regions, the hypervariable regions or complementarity determining regions (CDR), show much more variability than the rest of the domain. These regions vary both in size and in sequence among different V_L germline isotypes; they determine the specificity of the antigen-antibody interactions. The remaining parts of the V_L, four framework regions (FRs), have quite similar amino acid sequences. The overall structure of the V_L is an immunoglobulin fold with 9 β-strands (A, B, C, C′, C″, D, E, F, and G) packed tightly against each other in two antiparallel β sheets joined together by a disulfide bridge in a form of a Greek key β-barrel. The N- and C- termini strands (A and G, respectively) are parallel (Branden & Tooze, 1999). The CDRs form three loops between amino acids 24-34, 50-56 and 89-95 that contain the sequence that will recognize the antigen.

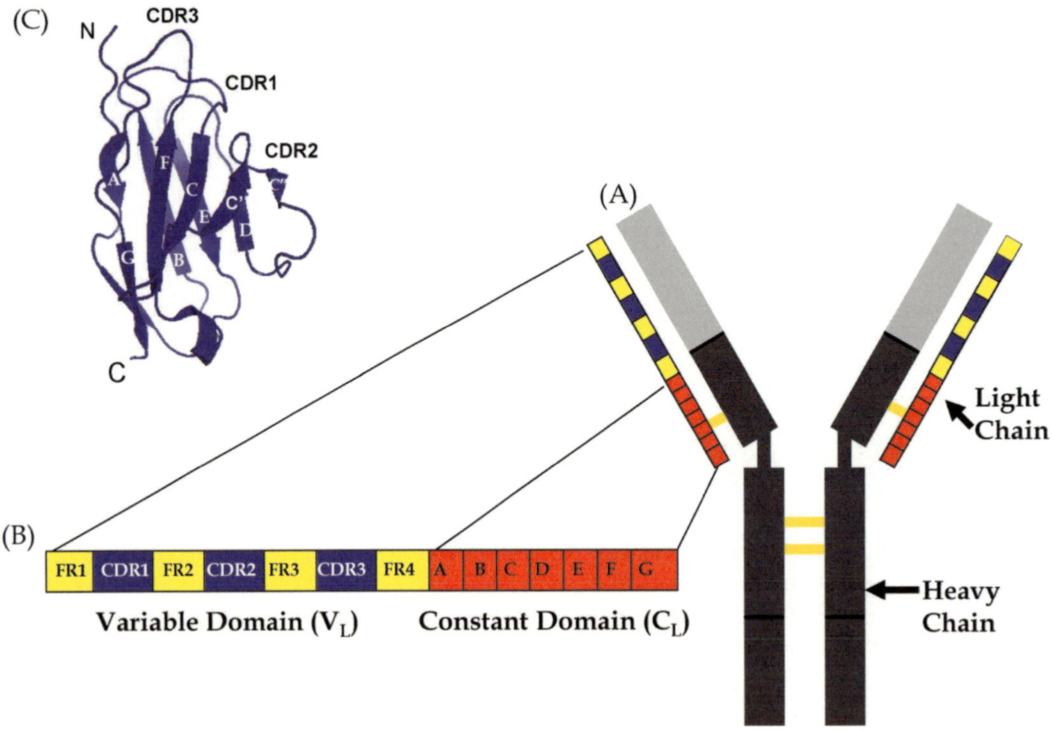

Fig. 1. (A) Immunoglobulin (IgG) structure showing heterotetramer of two light chains and two heavy chains linked by disulfide bonds (B) Schematic representation of a LC showing complementarity determining regions (CDR) and framework regions (FR) (C) V_L structure showing CDR regions, β strands C, C′, F, and G involved in heavy/light chain interface, and N and C termini (β strands A and G, respectively).

Immunoglobulin quaternary structure consists of a heterotetramer formed by the LC and the heavy chain (HC) linked together via disulfide bonds. The LC V_L domain interacts with the HC variable domain through β-strands C, C′, F and G. The source of sequence variability in LCs comes from combinatorial pairing of the V genes (discussed below) and the J genes (corresponding to strand G or FR4), making it possible to generate about 3000 different LC sequences. In addition, somatic mutations improve the antibody affinity for the antigen, leading to further sequence variation. LCs are secreted and are found in circulation and are sometimes referred to as Bence-Jones proteins. Heavy chains are unable to be secreted alone, so they are always present as part of an intact immunoglobulin molecule as shown in Figure 1.

There are 40 kappa and 33 lambda germline genes available to form a LC variable domain. In AL amyloidosis, there is an overrepresentation of specific germline genes: κI, λ1, λII, λIII, and λVI (Poshusta et al., 2009). The process of somatic hypermutation adds to the complexity of AL amyloidosis because it means that each patient possesses a unique amyloidogenic protein: a combination of different germline genes and different somatic mutations. These protein sequence differences could result in different propensities to form amyloid fibrils, and may be involved in the different organ involvement found in different AL patients as well as the different degrees of severity of the disease.

Most of the biochemical and biophysical studies reported in the literature have been conducted using the variable domain of AL proteins (Baden et al., 2009). This stems from the fact that variable domain fragments were found in AL amyloid deposits and for 20 years it was thought that the protein underwent limited proteolysis before or after becoming part of the amyloid fibril. However, a recent report describing the laser micro-dissection of amyloid deposits from biopsied tissue followed by mass spectrometry analysis determined that the full length immunoglobulin light chain is present in the amyloid deposits of these patients (Vrana et al., 2009), contradicting the previous assumption that only light chain variable domains are found in amyloid deposits.

2.1 What contributes to the amyloidogenicity of immunoglobulin light chains?

It is generally accepted that LCs from AL patients are prone to aggregation due to a number of factors: certain germline sequences are overrepresented and may be intrinsically more prone to aggregation (see section 2.1.1.); somatic mutations destabilize the protein and may promote conformations that are more favorable for amyloidogenesis (see section 2.1.2) or decrease thermodynamic stability (see section 2.1.3). Finally, the presence of co-factors and the cellular environment play an important role (section 2.1.4).

2.1.1 Sequence determinants of amyloidogenicity

In AL amyloidosis, λ is overrepresented (λ/κ=3:1) as compared to healthy individuals or multiple myeloma (MM, non amyloidogenic control) patients (λ/κ=1:2), especially the λ VI subtype (Kyle & Gertz, 1995). In addition, V_L germline donor gene usage in AL is biased (Abraham et al., 2003; Comenzo et al., 2001; Prokaeva et al., 2007). The Comenzo, Abraham and Prokaeva studies agree that AL V_L germline donor gene usage comprises Vλ I, Vλ II, Vλ III, Vλ VI, Vκ I, while there are slight differences in the sample size, sample selection and the frequency of use of each germline donor gene in each study. Comenzo and co-workers demonstrated that 30% of AL V_L genes used Vλ VI 6a germline donor (Comenzo et al., 2001). Abraham and co-workers found that most κ patients selected for their study used the Vκ I subgroup (77%) (Abraham et al., 2003); a similar observation was made by Prokaeva and co-workers (Prokaeva et al., 2007).

To determine if the germline sequences are prone to generating inherently more amyloidogenic AL proteins, two studies tested κ and λ germline proteins. Baden et al. compared AL-09, an amyloidogenic protein that has 7 somatic mutations, to its germline protein κI O18/O8 (Baden et al., 2008a). The germline protein was more thermodynamically stable than its amyloidogenic counterpart, and although it was able to form fibrils, its fibril formation kinetics were significantly slower than AL-09. Additionally, fibril formation of AL protein BIF and MM protein GAL (also of the κI O18/O8 germline) was compared at 37°C, but only BIF formed fibrils (Kim et al., 2000).

Because the λ6a germline is expressed almost exclusively in AL patients (it is one of the last germline genes screened in the process of selection) and is not expressed in the normal LC repertoire (Abraham et al., 2003; Comenzo et al., 2001; Prokaeva et al., 2007), del Pozo Yauner et al. hypothesized that this germline would be as unstable as AL proteins. However, experiments revealed that the λ6a germline protein was more stable than Wil, an amyloidogenic protein from that germline with 11 somatic mutations (Del Pozo Yauner et al., 2008). The λ6a germline also had significantly slower fibril formation kinetics than Wil. When compared to AL-09 and κI O18/O8, Wil and λ6a demonstrated a comparable increase in stability, but faster fibril formation kinetics (14 hours for λ6a compared to 216 hours for κI O18/O8 at 37°C). Additionally, λ6a was able to form fibrils in the absence of seeds, while κI O18/O8 required seeds for fibril formation. This may indicate an increase in fibrillogenic propensity for λ6a germline proteins. More studies are necessary to verify that AL-prone germline sequences are more amyloidogenic than normal Ig repertoire germline sequences.

The mutational diversity among AL proteins has been well documented. Several studies have compared amino acid sequences of AL proteins, searching for common mutations or mutational regions. In an analysis of 121 κI light chains (37 of which were amyloidogenic), Stevens found four structural features that render a LC protein more likely to be amyloidogenic (Stevens, 2000). All of these involved loss or gain of certain residues, including a mutation that introduces a glycosylation site, mutations of Arg61 or Ile27b and mutations of Pro residues in β-turns.

A more recent analysis of 141 κ and λ AL light chain sequences catalogued the non-conservative mutations in these proteins and modeled their positions onto known LC structures to correlate structural regions (β-strands or loops) with potentially destabilizing mutations (Poshusta et al., 2009). This study confirmed that the total number of non-conservative mutations may be less important than their location as an amyloidogenic determinant for LC proteins. Additionally, the patients' free light chain levels, an indicator of disease progression (Dispenzieri et al., 2008), were also assessed in a subset of the analyzed protein sequences. A correlation between non-conservative mutations in certain regions and free light chain (FLC) levels was revealed, suggesting that patients with initial low FLC levels acquired mutations in their LCs that rendered these proteins to be more amyloidogenic than LCs from patients with higher FLC levels. Analyzing the location of these mutations could further advance understanding of the mechanisms of amyloid formation and lead to a prognostic factor for AL disease progression.

2.1.2 Structural determinants of amyloidogenicity in light chain proteins

Structural studies have shown that most variable domains from AL amyloidosis patients crystallize as monomers or dimers with the expected antiparallel β-sheet immunoglobulin fold. The dimer observed is homologous to the conformation occurring between light and heavy chains in immunoglobulin molecules. The germline κI O18/O8 crystallizes as a canonical dimer while the amyloidogenic protein AL-09 adopts an altered dimer with a 90° rotation with respect to the canonical dimer structure (Baden et al., 2008a). Restorative mutational analysis showed that a single mutation in AL-09 (AL-09 H87Y) stabilized the protein, delayed amyloid formation, and changed its conformation from the altered dimer to the canonical dimer interface (Baden et al., 2008b). We have recently reported that the reciprocal mutant κI Y87H, in which we mutated the germline residue towards the residue found in AL-09, crystallized as a canonical dimer. However, using solution Nuclear Magnetic Resonance (NMR) spectroscopy, we showed that this protein adopts a different dimer interface rotated 180° from the canonical dimer interface and 90° from the AL-09 altered dimer interface (Peterson et al., 2010). The different dimer structures could be compared to the hands on a clock moving in intervals of 90° (Figure 2).

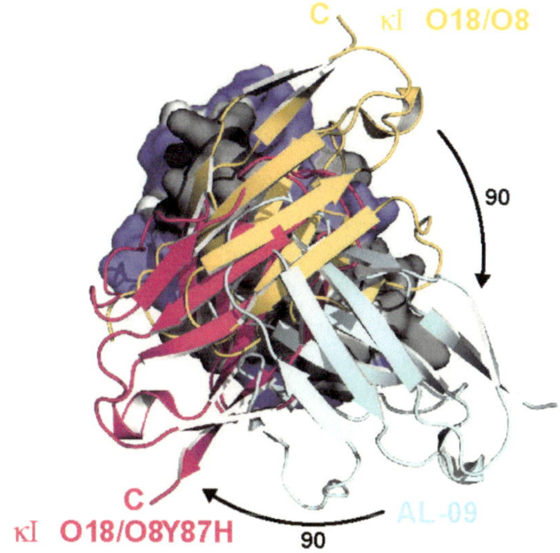

Fig. 2. Overlay of three different dimer orientations found in crystal structures of κI O18/O8, AL-09, and NMR structure of κI Y87H. (Figure adapted from (Peterson et al., 2010, Fig. 4), with permission of Elsevier. Copyright © 2010.)

Sequence alignments of the variable domains of 50 κ and 91 λ AL light chains revealed that non-conservative mutations on the dimer interface, especially Histidine mutations, are very common in AL proteins (Poshusta et al., 2009). Taken together with our structural analysis of AL-09, AL-09 H87Y and κI Y87H, our results suggest that dynamic dimerization could occur frequently in AL proteins. Our structural studies show that light chains are able to dimerize in different conformations; the residues in the dimer interface determine whether or not a dimer conformation will be favored or if the numerous interfaces will be populated at the same time.

2.1.3 Thermodynamic stability as a factor determining amyloidogenicity

Studies using variable domain proteins from AL patients have shown that mutations in the variable domain that reduce the thermodynamic stability are more prone to form amyloid fibrils (Hurle et al., 1994; Stevens et al., 1995; Wetzel, 1997). In an analysis linking mutations and stability, Hurle et al. analyzed 36 sequences (18 κ and 18 λ) in search of rare amino acid replacements that occurred in structurally significant regions of the proteins (Hurle et al., 1994). They then constructed single-point mutants incorporating the rare residues into a non-amyloidogenic Bence Jones LC protein to determine whether the amino acids destabilized the protein significantly enough to induce unfolding. Four of the six mutations were destabilizing, leading to the conclusion that some mutations are involved in amyloidogenicity.

To determine if a single mutation is enough to render a protein amyloidogenic, Davis et al. studied AL protein SMA and MM protein LEN. Only eight residues differ between these two proteins, and each SMA mutation was introduced into LEN to assess the individual effects on fibrillogenesis. Of the mutations tested only P40L, located in a loop region, was able to form Thioflavine T (ThT) positive fibrils in unseeded reactions (Davis 2000). Although stability data were not reported for these mutants, it is likely that the P40L mutant was less stable than wild-type LEN because Pro40 (very favorable for loops and turns) is conserved among 98% of all κ and λ germline sequences.

In vitro fibril formation studies have revealed that AL proteins form fibrils under a variety of solution conditions with varying kinetics and morphology of fibrils. AL-09 is unique because it forms amyloid fibrils with very similar kinetics across a wide variety of solution conditions (Martin & Ramirez-Alvarado, 2010). Additionally, AL-09's fibril formation kinetics are significantly faster than other AL proteins. We propose that the altered dimer interface populated by AL-09 facilitates the initial misfolding events that trigger amyloid formation, while the other proteins require stochastic conformational fluctuations to populate the appropriate misfolded intermediate that leads the amyloid formation reaction. Incubation of light chains from both κIV amyloidosis and multiple myeloma patients have shown that amyloid formation is enhanced at low pH while amorphous aggregation occurred around neutral pH; all of these reactions populated different partially folded intermediates (Ionescu-Zanetti et al., 1999; Khurana et al., 2001; Souillac et al., 2003; Souillac et al., 2002a,b; Souillac et al., 2002b).

Another link between thermodynamic stability and fibril formation is found in the recently analyzed κI O18/O8 and λ6a germline proteins. These proteins were significantly more stable than all AL amyloidogenic proteins that have been studied to date (Baden et al., 2008a; Del Pozo Yauner et al., 2008). The T_m values (melting temperatures, at which 50% of the proteins are unfolded) for the germline proteins were increased by 15°C and 11.6°C, respectively, over the corresponding AL proteins analyzed in each study. Both κI O18/O8 and λ6a germline proteins had slower fibril formation kinetics than their amyloidogenic counterparts.

Del Pozo Yauner and colleagues incorporated an R25G mutation into the λ6a germline protein (6aJL2-R25G), as this mutation is found in 25% of amyloidogenic λ6 LCs and presumably represents an allotypic variant (Ch'ang et al., 1994; del Pozo Yauner et al., 2006; Del Pozo Yauner et al., 2008). This mutation resulted in a 6°C decrease in T_m value for the mutated protein, and 6aJL2-R25G had a much shorter lag time and faster growth rate than the λ6a germline protein. The authors explain that the R25G mutation may affect the structure of complementarity determining region 1 (CDR1), resulting in an altered conformation and increased amyloidogenicity (del Pozo Yauner et al., 2006).

Further research on the κI O18/O8 germline protein and amyloidogenic AL-09 also connected thermodynamic stability to fibril formation. Baden et al. undertook a systematic restorative mutational analysis of the non-conservative mutations of AL-09, which are all located in the dimer interface (Baden et al., 2008b). Of the three non-conservative restorative mutations (I34N, Q42K and H87Y), restoring the His87 mutation to the Tyr87 residue found in the germline sequence increased the thermodynamic stability and decreased the fibril formation kinetics to the same levels as κI O18/O8. Significant structural alterations were also observed with this restorative mutant (discussed above, shown as a summary in Figure 2). Restoring the Asn34 residue had intermediate effects on stability and fibril formation propensity, while reintroducing Lys42 did not appear to alter the thermodynamics to any extent.

In complementary experiments introducing the His87 residue from the amyloidogenic protein into κI O18/O8, this protein was only destabilized half as much as AL-09. κI Y87H also had intermediate fibril formation kinetics between those measured for κI O18/O8 and AL-09, indicating that this mutation alone may not have been sufficient for the amyloidogenicity observed in AL-09. However, introducing a second mutation into κI O18/O8 (Ile34, in addition to His87) completely destabilized the protein and exhibited the same fast fibril kinetics as amyloidogenic AL-09. Thus, rather than a single mutation that causes amyloidogenesis, it is probable that a combination of destabilizing and compensatory mutations leads to fibrillogenicity among AL proteins.

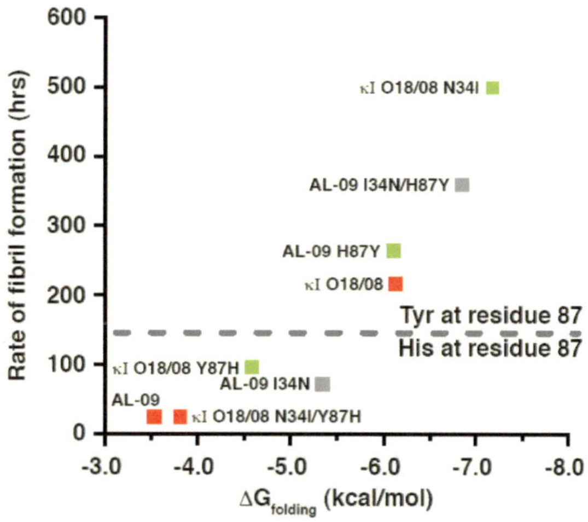

Fig. 3. In restorative AL-09 and reciprocal κI mutants, rates of fibril formation are inversely correlated with $\Delta G_{folding}$. Mutation of Tyrosine 87 to Histidine stabilizes an altered dimer interface and leads to faster fibril formation. HSQC Analysis was used to identify each protein as single-state (green) or promiscuous (red) dimers; others were not determined (grey). (Figure and legend adapted from (Peterson et al., 2010, Fig. 5), with permission of Elsevier. Copyright © 2010.)

Other groups have studied fibril formation using different AL and MM proteins. Jto, an MM protein, and Wil, an AL protein, are both light chain proteins from the λ6a germline that differ by 19 amino acids. Fibrils were formed with both Jto and Wil at 37°C, pH 7.5 (Wall et al., 1999). Jto fibrils appeared more rigid, were shorter and displayed slower kinetics than fibrils formed by Wil.

Certain ionic interactions may affect fibrillogenesis and be crucial to maintain the structure and stability of LC proteins. Wall et al. noted an ionic interaction between Asp29 and Arg68 in MM protein Jto, whereas AL protein Wil has neutral amino acids in these positions (Wall et al., 2004). To test the importance of this ionic interaction, mutations were made to Jto to introduce the neutral residues (from Wil) at these sites (JtoD29A, JtoR68S). The thermodynamic stabilities of these mutants were the same, and the rate of fibril formation for JtoD29A was the same as that for Jto. However, fibril formation kinetics were much faster for JtoR68S, and an X-ray crystal structure of this mutant revealed several side-chain differences compared to Jto and JtoD29A. These differences changed the electrostatic potential surface and increased the amount of solvent-exposed hydrophobic surface for the protein. These results highlight critical structural features such as ionic interactions that participate in the stability and fibrillogenicity of AL proteins.

Studies describing the properties of full length light chains from AL amyloidosis patients have been performed using both urine-derived proteins and recombinant full length constructs. The constant domain within the λ6a protein AL-01-095 (C_L belongs to LC3* 04) full length protein appears to confer great thermodynamic stability (Klimtchuk et al., 2011), while the kappa unique C_L does not play any role in the stability to the κI O18/O8 protein AL-09 (Olatoye, Levinson, and Ramirez-Alvarado, unpublished observations). Full length proteins isolated from urine samples from MM, Light Chain Deposition Disease (LCDD) and AL patients were studied to determine the type of aggregate formed by each type of protein. Fibril formation reactions were followed at the T_m for each protein for 72 hours. The results indicated that MM proteins formed spherical species, LCDD formed amorphous aggregates and AL proteins formed fibrils (Sikkink & Ramirez-Alvarado, 2008a). Amyloid formation reactions with full length AL-09 and κI O18/O8 show slow rates of amyloid formation with respect to variable domain AL-09 and κI O18/O8. The deposits found using electron microscopy show more disorder within the amyloid fibrils. These results suggest that the presence of the constant domain affects the misfolding pathway for these proteins.

Collectively, these results have shown how the differences between LCs from AL amyloidosis patients (from different germline sequences and with different mutations) can determine the LC thermodynamic stability and fibril formation propensity.

2.1.4 Effect of co-factors and protein modifications in amyloid formation reactions

Amyloid fibril formation is initiated by the accumulation of oligomers to form a critical nucleus during the lag phase. After nucleation, fibril growth occurs during the elongation phase. In addition to studying the characteristics that make a soluble LC protein more amyloidogenic, a tremendous amount of research has and is currently being done with respect to the factors that affect fibril formation *in vitro*. These factors include temperature, pH, ionic strength, agitation, protein concentration, and pressure, which all destabilize the protein in order to populate partially folded states that are prone to aggregation (Chiti et al., 1999). Each AL protein may be affected slightly differently by these co-factors (Figure 4).

2.1.4.1 pH

Experiments at various pH values showed differences between the AL and MM proteins. The rate of fibril formation for AL protein SMA was highly accelerated at pH 2 (Khurana et al., 2001). Both SMA and LEN formed fibrils at pH 2 with agitation, but SMA displayed faster kinetics (Khurana et al., 2003). Amorphous aggregation of SMA was observed in samples from pH 4 to 7, while fibrils were observed in samples at pH ≤3 implying that SMA formed different partially folded intermediates depending on the pH of the solution. At pH 4.5, 30 mM NaCl , SMA formed annular aggregates whereas at high ionic strength, fibrils and amorphous deposits were the predominant species (Zhu et al., 2004). At pH 7, the fibril formation kinetics of LEN was faster with lower protein concentrations and increased concentrations of urea (0 to 3 M) (Souillac et al., 2002a).

Dye binding studies such as Thioflavine T fluorescence are commonly used to monitor fibril formation. However, differentiating between different species formed during fibril formation is not possible with this method. Thus, atomic force microscopy imaging was used to observe the evolution of different fibrillar species during a fibril formation reaction of SMA at pH 2; different filament sizes were found at different time points during the fibrillation. A model was proposed where two filaments combine to form a protofibril and two protofibrils intertwine to form a type I fibril (Ionescu-Zanetti et al., 1999).

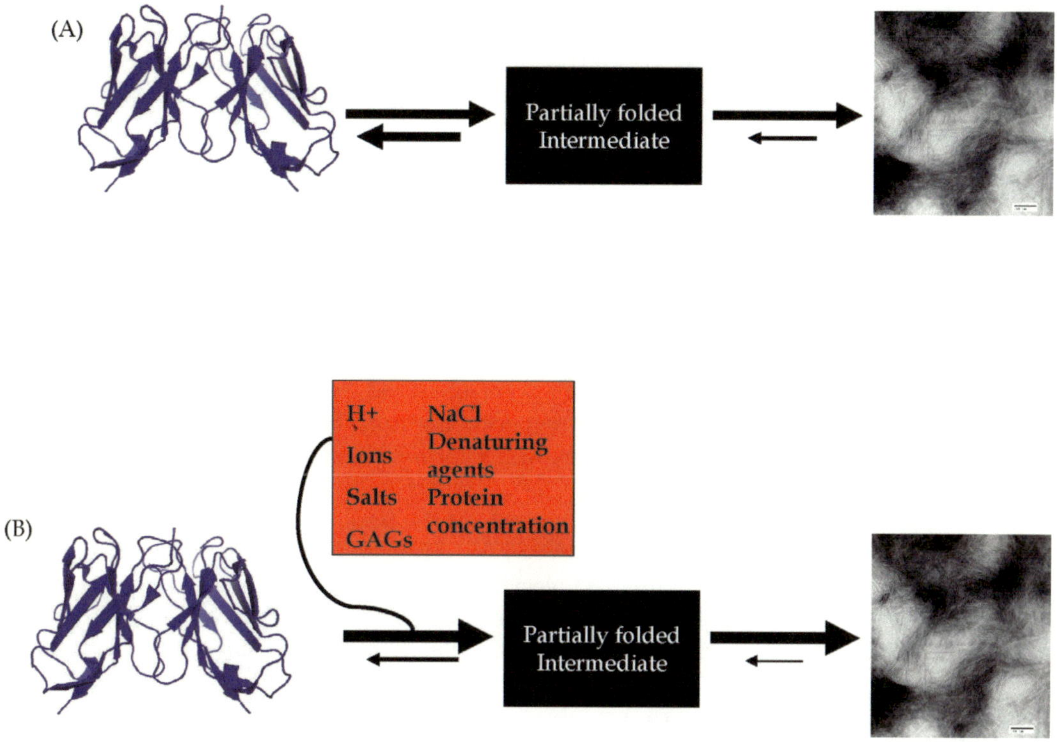

Fig. 4. The role of co-factors in amyloid formation: (A) amyloid formation reaction showing transition from native dimer structure to partially folded intermediate to amyloid fibrils (B) amyloid formation reaction accelerated by the presence of different co-factors. A common co-factor that accelerates fibril formation is low pH (high concentration of H+).

2.1.4.2 Effect of the microenvironment: renal solutes, denaturants, protein concentration, and surfaces

The use of renal solutes shed light onto the destabilizing and compensatory effects that different reagents can have on amyloid formation. Urea, a known protein denaturant, decreased the thermodynamic stability and the fibril formation kinetics of both SMA and LEN while betaine and sorbitol (organic osmolytes) had the opposite effect. A concentration of 1.5 M urea was enough to increase fibril formation of both SMA and LEN (Kim et al., 2001). Conversely, the presence of 0.5 M betaine or sorbitol partially inhibited SMA fibril formation showing the interplay between stabilizing and denaturing forces that may occur in physiological environments.

Other denaturant studies indicate that SMA fibril formation kinetics were dependent on the concentration of guanidine hydrochloride (GdHCl) (Qin et al., 2007). The reaction at 2 M GdHCl had the fastest amyloid formation kinetics and the presence of fibrils was confirmed by electron microscopy, whereas amorphous aggregates were formed at lower concentrations of GdHCl. Additionally, GdHCl affected the intermediate structures in fibril formation, determined by circular dichroism spectroscopy. At 1 M GdHCl, amorphous aggregates were formed by native-like intermediate structures, while at 2 M, amyloid fibrils were generated through an unfolded intermediate.

Protein concentration was another factor that influenced the fibril formation kinetics; low concentrations of LEN had faster kinetics of amyloid formation than higher concentrations (Souillac et al., 2002a,b). At high protein concentrations, LEN produced off-pathway oligomeric species before fibrils were formed (Souillac et al., 2003). At low protein concentrations, the off-pathway species were absent (Souillac et al., 2002b). Adding a "seed" of preformed fibrils to soluble protein solutions to trigger fibril growth also accelerated the kinetics of LEN fibril formation (Harper & Lansbury, 1997). The addition of 5% seeds in a SMA fibril formation reaction decreased the lag time by half when compared to an unseeded reaction (Davis et al., 2000).

Zhu et al. studied the effect of surfaces on SMA amyloid fibril formation. (Zhu et al., 2002). They found that on mica surfaces, the rate of fibrillation was faster and the amount of protein required for the reaction decreased. They also discovered different fibril growth mechanisms; on a mica surface, protofibrils were observed, while in solution, fibrils were present (Zhu et al., 2002). These surface experiments may be relevant *in vivo* since AL amyloid deposits are associated with the extracellular matrix in the basement membrane of tissues.

In an effort to understand the role of components of the basement membrane where fibrils deposit, the role of lipids in amyloid formation for AL was recently reported. The results indicated that a higher protein to lipid vesicles ratio slowed SMA amyloid formation kinetics (Meng et al., 2008). SMA fibrillation was affected by adding cholesterol to the lipid vesicles; specifically, cholesterol concentrations above 10% had an inhibitory effect. Additionally, in the presence of cholesterol and lipid vesicles, higher Ca^{2+} concentrations were shown to decrease SMA fibril formation kinetics The same effect was seen with Mg^{2+} and Zn^{2+} (Meng et al., 2008). This study suggests that amyloid deposition is influenced by the combined effects of cations and membrane surfaces.

2.1.4.3 Hofmeister series

One factor affecting fibril formation is the addition of salts or ions. The Hofmeister series is a tool to understand salt ionic effects that ranks ions according to their ability to stabilize or destabilize a protein (Cacace et al., 1997; Zhang et al., 2005). A proof of principle study was done with the amyloidogenic V_L protein AL-12 to determine the role of physiologically relevant anions and cations from the Hofmeister series on protein stability and amyloid fibril formation. The presence of various salts with AL-12 did not affect the secondary structure of the protein (Sikkink & Ramirez-Alvarado, 2008b), and all salts enhanced amyloid formation. Reactions with SO_4^{2-} and Mg^{2+} showed the largest enhancement of amyloid formation. In addition, we recently performed a systematic analysis of the effect of different concentrations of NaCl on amyloid formation using two similar amyloidogenic light chains. AL-09 readily formed fibrils across a wide range of salt concentrations; however, the amyloidogenic light chain AL-103 (90% sequence identity to AL-09) showed a roughly inverse dependence of the fibril formation rate on salt concentration (Martin & Ramirez-Alvarado, 2010). These studies with various AL proteins and salts will help determine how sulfate ions enhance amyloid formation and will shed light onto the role of glycosaminoglycan sulfation on fibril formation *in vivo*.

2.1.4.4 Glycosaminoglycans

Glycosaminoglycans (GAGs) are a component of the extracellular matrix (Bosman & Stamenkovic, 2003) and have been found extensively in amyloid deposits. They are long, unbranched, negatively charged heterogeneous polysaccharides formed by disaccharides of N-acetylglucosamine or N-acetylgalactosamine and uronic acid. Ohishi et al. found that GAGs are an integral part of AL amyloid fibrils and that the level of GAGs increased 10-fold in tissues from amyloidosis patients, suggesting that GAGs not only play a role interacting with amyloid fibrils but the presence of the fibrils affect GAG levels (Ohishi et al., 1990). *In vitro* studies using HPLC chromatography and sodium dodecyl sulfate-polyacrylamide gel electrophoresis (SDS-PAGE) showed an interaction between light chain proteins and various GAGs (Jiang et al., 1997). In another *in vitro* study, our laboratory showed that dermatan sulfate accelerated AL-09 amyloid fibril formation, whereas chondroitin sulfate A inhibited fibril formation and yielded a spherical intermediate (McLaughlin et al., 2006). More recently, we have found that GAGs enhance amyloid formation by a transient electrostatic interaction with an early intermediate of the amyloid formation reaction (Martin & Ramirez-Alvarado, 2011).

Further studies of GAG influence on AL fibrillogenesis via the multiple sulfate moieties or its possible crowding effect on the amyloid fibril reaction may reveal important clues about the mechanism of amyloidogenesis and the role that GAGs play in the *in vivo* extracellular matrix deposition.

2.1.4.5 Posttranslational modifications and oxidative stress

Posttranslational modifications (PTMs) are also implicated in amyloidogenicity. Of the amyloidogenic structural risk factors that Stevens identified in κI light chains, N-glycosylation was found in 22 of 121 samples, and 18 of those 22 samples were amyloidogenic (Stevens, 2000). None of the light chain germline genes encode a glycosylation site (N-x-S/T); thus, any putative glycosylation sites are introduced through somatic hypermutation. Of the 18 amyloidogenic glycosylated LCs in Stevens study, most of them (13/18) also had other PTMs (including S-cysteinylation, fragmentation, dimerization and S-sulfonation), so a definitive role for glycosylation is difficult to delineate.

Other studies also implicated glycosylation as an important characteristic among amyloidogenic proteins (Dwulet et al., 1986; Engvig et al., 1998; Foss et al., 1998; Omtvedt et al., 2000), and AL proteins were found to be glycosylated more frequently than circulating non-amyloidogenic free LCs (Holm et al., 1986; Omtvedt et al., 1997). Despite this evidence, the precise role of this PTM has yet to be determined.

A more recent study of nine κI light chains revealed several different PTMs in the full length LC proteins. Each of the proteins studied had at least one type of PTM, and the range of PTMs included N-glycosylation, disulfide-linked dimerization, S-cysteinylation, fragmentation, S-sulfonation, 3-chlorotyrosine formation, and conversion of aspartic acid to pyruvate (Connors et al., 2007). The exact relevance of these modifications to AL pathogenesis is unknown, but cysteinylation of other proteins was suggested to induce conformational changes (Chen et al., 1999; Watarai et al., 2000), which could play a role in misfolding. Additionally, chlorotyrosine residues were linked to oxidative damage (Mohiuddin et al., 2006).

Some PTMs found in AL proteins may actually have a protective role against amyloidogenesis. The two most heavily modified proteins in the aforementioned study (Connors et al., 2007) also included a methionine residue that had been oxidized to methionine sulfoxide. Methionine and cysteine are the most easily oxidized amino acids, and oxidation of a methionine residue could protect other critical residues from damage by reactive oxygen species (ROS) (Levine et al., 2000). A study of MM protein LEN showed that the methionine-oxidized form of the protein led to the formation of amorphous aggregates instead of fibrils (Hu et al., 2008). Thus, methionine oxidation may be part of a protective mechanism against amyloidogenic fibril formation for AL proteins. However, because methionine oxidation is a fluctuating process, its antioxidant effect could be overcome by a preponderance of other amyloidogenic factors.

Oxidation effects are particularly relevant to the study of AL proteins because oxidative stress has been linked both to amyloid fibril deposits and to the mechanism of cell death (Merlini & Westermark, 2004; Schubert et al., 1995). In a study by Ando and coworkers, AL amyloid deposits stained positively for 4-hydroxy-2-nonenal (HNE), a lipid peroxidation product indicative of oxidative injury (Ando et al., 1997). This result could not differentiate whether oxidative stress was involved in amyloid formation or if the fibrils triggered an oxidative stress reaction after deposition. However, a more recent study indicated that oxidative stress caused by soluble amyloidogenic AL proteins plays a role in cell death. Brenner et al. examined the effects of cardiac AL proteins on cardiomyocytes and found that the presence of the amyloidogenic proteins caused an increase in intracellular reactive oxygen species and upregulation of a redox-sensitive protein (heme oxygenase-1) (Brenner et al., 2004). In addition, the contractility and relaxation of the cardiomyocytes was impaired, directly linking these soluble light chain proteins to cardiomyopathy in AL patients.

Research is still being conducted to understand the mechanism of AL fibril formation and the role of co-factors and the cellular environment on amyloidogenicity. It is important to expand on the currently reported work with additional AL proteins to find commonalities and differences of fibril formation properties for the different AL proteins.

3. Tissue damage in AL amyloidosis-toxic effect of light chains

The most important aspect of AL amyloidosis pathophysiology is the tissue damage associated with the process of amyloid formation. AL amyloidosis is a systemic protein misfolding disease; the site of deposition is distant from the site of protein synthesis and secretion (in this case, bone marrow plasma cells). While there have been some advances in cellular and tissue studies on the effect of light chains in cellular and tissue viability, what happens to the protein while in circulation is unknown. This aspect of the pathophysiology could only be studied with appropriate animal models.

3.1 Cellular toxicity studies

One of the most important questions in amyloidosis research is to determine the most toxic species of the amyloid formation reaction. For years, researchers assumed that the amyloid fibril deposits were highly toxic to the cells near them by blocking the exchange of nutrients, creating a mechanical barrier around the cells, and by attracting macrophages that ultimately caused tissue damage. Later on, experiments conducted with soluble fractions from preparations of amyloid affected tissue showed that soluble species were as toxic as or more toxic than insoluble amyloid fibrils. Recent work done by our laboratory and others has shown that the presence of soluble AL proteins in cell culture induces apoptosis (Shi et al., 2010; Sikkink & Ramirez-Alvarado, 2010). In particular, we were able to demonstrate that the light chain species present in cell culture at the time of maximum apoptotic activity are primarily light chain monomer and dimers.

Internalization studies using immunoglobulin light chain proteins have shown that full length AL-09 internalizes into cardiomyocytes within 24 h, migrating into lysosomal compartments and in certain instances, the nucleus (Figure 5). Full length κI O18/O8 is delayed in this process. Single, restorative full length mutant AL-09 H87Y mimics the full length germline phenotype (Levinson, Olatoye, and Ramirez-Alvarado, unpublished observations). These studies are allowing us to fully characterize the biophysical, biochemical and cellular properties of amyloidogenic light chains to fully determine the role of somatic mutations in the disease process. These cellular internalization studies will reveal more details about the exact mechanism of toxicity by amyloidogenic light chains.

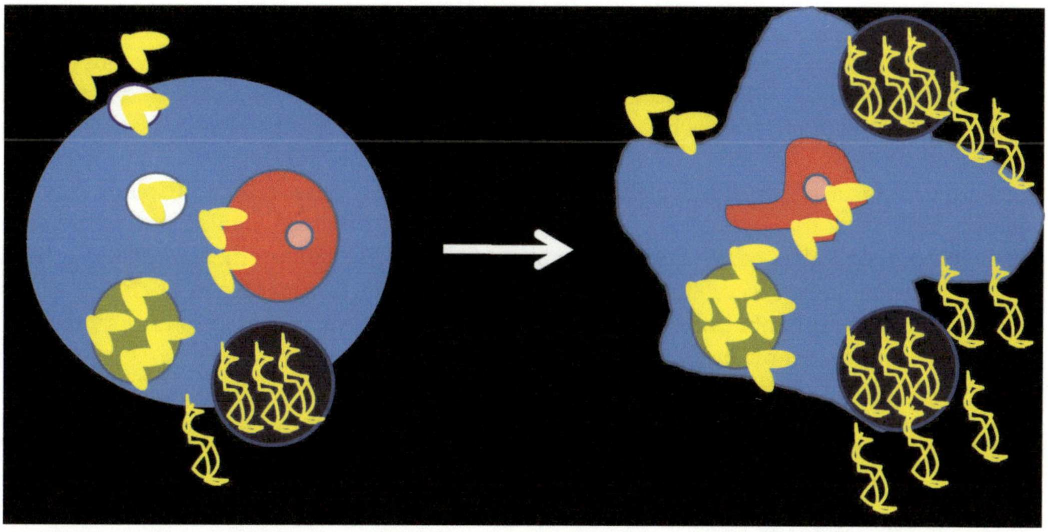

Fig. 5. Proposed model of LC internalization, aggregation, and apoptosis showing internalization through endosomes (light grey) to lysosome (green) and nucleus (red) and removal of amyloid fibrils by exocytosis (dark grey). Amyloid fibril formation may happen intracellularly and could be later excreted into extracellular compartments. Alternatively, the process of cell death may allow fibrils to move to the extracellular matrix.

3.2 Human tissue toxicity studies

The first tissues affected by AL protein deposition are the blood vessels. It was previously shown that AL amyloidosis patients present with early endothelial microcirculatory dysfunction (Berghoff et al., 2003), and that light chain amyloid infiltration in epicardial coronary arteries occurs in almost all of the AL amyloidosis patients analyzed (Wittich et al., 2007).

Another report showed that the presence of light chain is associated with histological evidence of myocardial ischemia (decrease in the blood supply) in the majority of AL patients studied (Neben-Wittich et al., 2005). These findings suggest that microvascular dysfunction is central to AL pathophysiology, yet its underlying mechanism is unknown. Migrino et al. recently reported an increase in protein oxidation in AL amyloidosis patients. When arterioles were exposed to amyloidogenic light chains, they observed higher levels of superoxide and impaired dilation to sodium nitroprusside (Migrino et al., 2010). Human arterioles are physiologically relevant to early AL pathophysiology and offer an important tissue system to study tissue dysfunction caused by AL light chains.

3.3 Model systems

Arendt and co-workers have established the first amyloidogenic human cell line system, ALMC-1 and ALMC-2 (Arendt et al., 2008). They used plasma cells from an AL patient isolated both pre- (ALMC-1) and post- (ALMC-2) stem cell transplant. These cell lines secrete a full length λ6a LC protein called ALMC. While there is some genetic variation between ALMC-1 and ALMC-2, the protein sequences from both cell lines are 100% identical. The protein secreted from these cell lines was fully folded with a β-sheet structure; it was as stable as other full length proteins (Sikkink & Ramirez-Alvarado, 2008a) and had the ability to form amyloid fibrils *in vitro*. These cell lines are a valuable tool because this is the only human-derived system that secretes a significant amount of protein for biophysical studies. We expect that future studies using these cell lines will advance our understanding of the cellular microenvironment and its possible role in the misfolding of light chain proteins.

Currently, there is no reported animal model for AL amyloidosis that displays the full pathophysiology of the disease. An animal model attempt involved cloning and expression of amyloidogenic light chains using the cytomegalovirus (CMV) promoter. SP2/O Ig null plasmacytoma cell lines were stably transfected with the amyloidogenic light chain vectors and were transplanted into Balb/c and RAG mice, where they grew as plasmacytomas that secrete the amyloidogenic light chains. 4-6 weeks post transplant of these cells, human amyloidogenic light chains were found in the urine of the transfected animals. Some protein casts and granular deposits were found in the tubules of the kidneys of some of the transfected animals. No Congo red staining (indicative of the presence of amyloid fibrils in tissues) was observed with these deposits. (Ward and coworkers abstract included in (Skinner et al., 2007))

Another animal model attempt involved creating a transgenic animal using the CMV promoter and bovine growth hormone polyadenylation signal. The expression of the transgenic protein was not ubiquitous, and the protein levels expressed were 1/10 of the levels found in the transplant model. Immunohistochemical analysis of different tissues showed the presence of the transgenic protein in the stomach gastric pit cells, the squamous epithelial cells of the bladder, the tubule cells in the kidney, in the cardiac cells and the pancreas. Congo red positive aggregation was observed in the lumen of the gastric glands of the stomach. The authors suggest that the low pH found in the stomach promoted amyloid formation of these amyloidogenic light chain after 4-6 months (Ward and coworkers abstract included in (Skinner et al., 2007)).

More recently, Shi and co-workers reported an animal model in which wild type and dominant negative p38α transgenic mice were initially injected with amyloidogenic light chains through the tail vein followed by systemic intravenous infusion via the use of an osmotic minipump for 7 days. Wild type animals with fully active p38α presented an increase in the Bax/Bcl2 ratio and a very modest increase in cellular apoptosis as determined by TUNEL staining (Shi et al., 2010).

Currently, none of the murine transgenic models of any of the systemic amyloidoses exhibit ideal characteristics to study the disease process. Buxbaum proposed that any future successful transgenic animal model of the extracellular amyloidoses should allow more precise understanding of the pathogenesis and the role of other proteins in facilitating or inhibiting amyloid generation and deposition. The use of worms (*Caenorhabditis elegans*) and flies (*Drosophila melanogaster*) to study amyloidoses has allowed the study of some disease processes, but Buxbaum argued that the relationship between the cellular and molecular phenotype and human disease may be problematic (Buxbaum, 2009).

4. How to ameliorate and eventually eliminate AL associated toxicity?

Current treatments for AL amyloidosis target the malignant plasma cell population in bone marrow. These treatments are somewhat successful, whilst they are poorly tolerated by some AL amyloidosis patients. New therapeutic strategies targeting the amyloidogenic light chains and the AL amyloid fibrils are currently in development and their efficacies are being studied.

4.1 Small molecules

Small molecules have been tested in search of fibril formation inhibitors. Congo red is a histological dye that binds to amyloid fibrils and presents a green birefringence under polarized light (Sipe & Cohen, 2000). AL-09 fibril formation was inhibited by Congo red at a 1:1 molar ratio (McLaughlin et al., 2006). In contrast, Congo red did not inhibit fibril formation of SMA suggesting some specificity in the role of Congo red as an inhibitor (Kim et al., 2003). More research is needed to find effective fibril inhibitors for a variety of AL proteins both *in vitro* and using cell culture systems.

4.2 Antibodies

A murine monoclonal antibody (mAB 11-1F4) that binds to light chain fibrils but not soluble proteins was generated and characterized by Solomon and co-workers (O'Nuallain et al., 2007; Solomon et al., 2003). Immunohistochemical analysis revealed that mAB 11-1F4 recognized light chain fibrils regardless of their V_L subgroup. The specificity of this antibody for AL fibrils (κI, κII, κIV, λ1, λ3, λ6, λ8) was shown by Europium-Linked Immunosorbant Assay (EuLISA) where an EC_{50} value (concentration of antibody at half maximum binding) for binding was ~130 ± 39 nM (O'Nuallain et al., 2007). The interaction of mAB 11-1F4 with native and fibrillar light chain LEN components was also checked by EuLISA and the antibody had similar avidity with both components. However, the fibrils had a ~2 fold reduction in signal (O'Nuallain et al., 2007). Peptide mapping was used to determine the cryptic epitope; it is located in the first 18 amino acids of the variable light chain domain and a prolyl residue at position 8 is necessary. A competition EuLISA was set up with mAB 11-1F4, and recombinant Wil fibrils were inhibited by a 50-fold molar excess of soluble LEN (1-22) peptide (O'Nuallain et al., 2007).

4.3 siRNA

A recent report has shown that small interference RNA (siRNA) can be used to reduce the amount of messenger RNA for amyloidogenic light chains. Phipps and co-workers transfected SP2/O mouse myeloma cells with a construct encoding the λ6 AL light chain Wil under control of the cytomegalovirus promoter, using the l2-producing myeloma cell line RPMI 8226 as a control. The siRNA were designed specifically to the V, J, or C portions of the molecules. Forty eight hrs after exposure to the siRNAs, the authors observed 40%

reduction in messenger RNA and LC production with a greater effect observed in the 8226 cells (Phipps et al., 2010).

5. Conclusion

Our knowledge of the molecular mechanisms of AL has greatly increased as a result of recent research about role of mutations, dimerization structures, different species populated in AL amyloid fibril formation, the cellular microenvironment, and light chain-associated cell and tissue toxicity. However, this complex disease is far from being understood, and each new discovery implicates other pathogenic factors, prompts additional questions, and reinforces the need for innovative research. In particular, the development of effective transgenic animal models and misfolding related therapeutic strategies, especially targeting light chain monomers and dimers, is necessary. A multidisciplinary research effort is required to analyze all aspects of the disease and provide a deeper understanding of its pathogenesis, ultimately leading to a successful therapeutic intervention.

6. Acknowledgments

The Ramirez-Alvarado team has been supported by the National Institutes of Health grants GM071514, CA111345, the American Heart Association grant AHA 06-30077N, the Mayo Foundation and the generous support of amyloidosis patients and their families. ACDC is supported by grant R25 GM 75148.

7. References

Abraham, R. S., Geyer, S. M., Price-Troska, T. L., Allmer, C., Kyle, R. A., Gertz, M. A. and Fonseca, R. (2003). Immunoglobulin light chain variable (V) region genes influence clinical presentation and outcome in light chain-associated amyloidosis (AL). *Blood* 101,10: 3801-08.

Ando, Y., Nyhlin, N., Suhr, O., Holmgren, G., Uchida, K., el Sahly, M., Yamashita, T., Terasaki, H., Nakamura, M., Uchino, M. and Ando, M. (1997). Oxidative stress is found in amyloid deposits in systemic amyloidosis. *Biochem Biophys Res Commun* 232,2: 497-502.

Arendt, B. K., Ramirez-Alvarado, M., Sikkink, L. A., Keats, J. J., Ahmann, G. J., Dispenzieri, A., Fonseca, R., Ketterling, R. P., Knudson, R. A., Mulvihill, E. M., Tschumper, R. C., Wu, X., Zeldenrust, S. R. and Jelinek, D. F. (2008). Biologic and genetic characterization of the novel amyloidogenic lambda light chain-secreting human cell lines, ALMC-1 and ALMC-2. *Blood* 112,5: 1931-41.

Baden, E. M., Owen, B. A., Peterson, F. C., Volkman, B. F., Ramirez-Alvarado, M. and Thompson, J. R. (2008). Altered dimer interface decreases stability in an amyloidogenic protein. *J Biol Chem* 283,23: 15853-60.

Baden, E. M., Randles, E. G., Aboagye, A. K., Thompson, J. R. and Ramirez-Alvarado, M. (2008). Structural insights into the role of mutations in amyloidogenesis. *J Biol Chem* 283,45: 30950-6.

Baden, E. M., Sikkink, L. A. and Ramirez-Alvarado, M. (2009). Light chain amyloidosis - current findings and future prospects. *Curr Protein Pept Sci* 10,5: 500-8.

Berghoff, M., Kathpal, M., Khan, F., Skinner, M., Falk, R. and Freeman, R. (2003). Endothelial dysfunction precedes C-fiber abnormalities in primary (AL) amyloidosis. *Ann Neurol* 53,6: 725-30.

Bosman, F. T. and Stamenkovic, I. (2003). Functional structure and composition of the extracellular matrix. *J Pathol* 200,4: 423-8.

Branden, C. and Tooze, J. (1999). *Introduction to Protein Structure* (2), Garland Publishing, 0-8153-2305-0, New York

Brenner, D. A., Jain, M., Pimentel, D. R., Wang, B., Connors, L. H., Skinner, M., Apstein, C. S. and Liao, R. (2004). Human amyloidogenic light chains directly impair cardiomyocyte function through an increase in cellular oxidant stress. *Circ Res* 94,8: 1008-10.

Buxbaum, J. N. (2009). Animal models of human amyloidoses: are transgenic mice worth the time and trouble? *FEBS Lett* 583,16: 2663-73.

Cacace, M. G., Landau, E. M. and Ramsden, J. J. (1997). The Hofmeister series: salt and solvent effects on interfacial phenomena. *Q Rev Biophys* 30,3: 241-77.

Ch'ang, L. Y., Yen, C. P., Besl, L., Schell, M. and Solomon, A. (1994). Identification and characterization of a functional human Ig V lambda VI germline gene. *Mol Immunol* 31,7: 531-6.

Chen, W., Yewdell, J. W., Levine, R. L. and Bennink, J. R. (1999). Modification of cysteine residues in vitro and in vivo affects the immunogenicity and antigenicity of major histocompatibility complex class I-restricted viral determinants. *J Exp Med* 189,11: 1757-64.

Chiti, F., Webster, P., Taddei, N., Clark, A., Stefani, M., Ramponi, G. and Dobson, C. M. (1999). Designing conditions for in vitro formation of amyloid protofilaments and fibrils. *Proc Natl Acad Sci U S A* 96,7: 3590-4.

Comenzo, R. L., Zhang, Y., Martinez, C., Osman, K. and Herrera, G. A. (2001). The tropism of organ involvement in primary systemic amyloidosis: contributions of Ig V(L) germ line gene use and clonal plasma cell burden. *Blood* 98,3: 714-20.

Connors, L. H., Jiang, Y., Budnik, M., Theberge, R., Prokaeva, T., Bodi, K. L., Seldin, D. C., Costello, C. E. and Skinner, M. (2007). Heterogeneity in primary structure, post-translational modifications, and germline gene usage of nine full-length amyloidogenic kappa1 immunoglobulin light chains. *Biochemistry* 46,49: 14259-71.

Davis, P. D., Raffen, R., Dul, L. J., Vogen, M. S., Williamson, K. E., Stevens, J. F. and Argon, Y. (2000). Inhibition of amyloid fiber assembly by both BiP and its target peptide. *Immunity* 13,4: 433-42.

del Pozo Yauner, L., Ortiz, E. and Becerril, B. (2006). The CDR1 of the human lambdaVI light chains adopts a new canonical structure. *Proteins* 62,1: 122-9.

Del Pozo Yauner, L., Ortiz, E., Sanchez, R., Sanchez-Lopez, R., Guereca, L., Murphy, C. L., Allen, A., Wall, J. S., Fernandez-Velasco, D. A., Solomon, A. and Becerril, B. (2008). Influence of the germline sequence on the thermodynamic stability and fibrillogenicity of human lambda 6 light chains. *Proteins* 72,2: 684-692.

Dispenzieri, A., Zhang, L., Katzmann, J. A., Snyder, M., Blood, E., Degoey, R., Henderson, K., Kyle, R. A., Oken, M. M., Bradwell, A. R. and Greipp, P. R. (2008). Appraisal of immunoglobulin free light chain as a marker of response. *Blood* 111,10: 4908-15.

Dwulet, F. E., O'Connor, T. P. and Benson, M. D. (1986). Polymorphism in a kappa I primary (AL) amyloid protein (BAN). *Mol Immunol* 23,1: 73-8.

Engvig, J. P., Olsen, K. E., Gislefoss, R. E., Sletten, K., Wahlstrom, O. and Westermark, P. (1998). Constant region of a kappa III immunoglobulin light chain as a major AL-amyloid protein. *Scand J Immunol* 48,1: 92-8.

Foss, G. S., Nilsen, R., Cornwell, G. C., 3rd, Husby, G. and Sletten, K. (1998). A glycosylated Bence Jones protein and its autologous amyloid light chain containing potentially amyloidogenic residues. *Scand J Immunol* 47,4: 348-54.

Harper, J. D. and Lansbury, P. T., Jr. (1997). Models of amyloid seeding in Alzheimer's disease and scrapie: mechanistic truths and physiological consequences of the time-dependent solubility of amyloid proteins. *Annu Rev Biochem* 66: 385-407.

Holm, E., Sletten, K. and Husby, G. (1986). Structural studies of a carbohydrate-containing immunoglobulin-lambda-light-chain amyloid-fibril protein (AL) of variable subgroup III. *Biochem J* 239,3: 545-51.

Hu, D., Qin, Z., Xue, B., Fink, A. L. and Uversky, V. N. (2008). Effect of methionine oxidation on the structural properties, conformational stability, and aggregation of immunoglobulin light chain LEN. *Biochemistry* 47,33: 8665-77.

Hurle, M. R., Helms, L. R., Li, L., Chan, W. and Wetzel, R. (1994). A role for destabilizing amino acid replacements in light-chain amyloidosis. *Proc Natl Acad Sci U S A* 91,12: 5446-50.

Ionescu-Zanetti, C., Khurana, R., Gillespie, J. R., Petrick, J. S., Trabachino, L. C., Minert, L. J., Carter, S. A. and Fink, A. L. (1999). Monitoring the assembly of Ig light-chain amyloid fibrils by atomic force microscopy. *Proc Natl Acad Sci U S A* 96,23: 13175-9.

Jiang, X., Myatt, E., Lykos, P. and Stevens, F. J. (1997). Interaction between glycosaminoglycans and immunoglobulin light chains. *Biochemistry* 36,43: 13187-94.

Khurana, R., Gillespie, J. R., Talapatra, A., Minert, L. J., Ionescu-Zanetti, C., Millett, I. and Fink, A. L. (2001). Partially folded intermediates as critical precursors of light chain amyloid fibrils and amorphous aggregates. *Biochemistry* 40,12: 3525-35.

Khurana, R., Souillac, P. O., Coats, A. C., Minert, L. J., Ionescu-Zanetti, C., Carter, S. A., Solomon, A. and Fink, A. L. (2003). A model for amyloid formation in immunoglobulin light chains based on comparison of amyloidogenic and benign proteins and specific antibody binding. *Amyloid* 10: 97-109.

Kim, Y., Wall, J. S., Meyer, J., Murphy, C., Randolph, T. W., Manning, M. C., Solomon, A. and Carpenter, J. F. (2000). Thermodynamic modulation of light chain amyloid fibril formation. *J Biol Chem* 275,3: 1570-4.

Kim, Y. S., Cape, S. P., Chi, E., Raffen, R., Wilkins-Stevens, P., Stevens, F. J., Manning, M. C., Randolph, T. W., Solomon, A. and Carpenter, J. F. (2001). Counteracting effects of renal solutes on amyloid fibril formation by immunoglobulin light chains. *J Biol Chem* 276,2: 1626-33.

Kim, Y. S., Randolph, T. W., Manning, M. C., Stevens, F. J. and Carpenter, J. F. (2003). Congo red populates partially unfolded states of an amyloidogenic protein to enhance aggregation and amyloid fibril formation. *J Biol Chem* 278,12: 10842-50.

Klimtchuk, E. S., Gursky, O., Patel, R. S., Laporte, K. L., Connors, L. H., Skinner, M. and Seldin, D. C. (2011). The critical role of the constant region in thermal stability and aggregation of amyloidogenic immunoglobulin light chain. *Biochemistry* 49,45: 9848-57.

Kumar, S. K., Gertz, M. A., Lacy, M. Q., Dingli, D., Hayman, S. R., Buadi, F. K., Short-Detweiler, K., Zeldenrust, S. R., Leung, N., Greipp, P. R., Lust, J. A., Russell, S. J., Kyle, R. A., Rajkumar, S. V. and Dispenzieri, A. (2011). Recent improvements in survival in primary systemic amyloidosis and the importance of an early mortality risk score. *Mayo Clin Proc* 86,1: 12-8.

Kyle, R. A. and Gertz, M. A. (1995). Primary systemic amyloidosis: clinical and laboratory features in 474 cases. *Semin Hematol* 32,1: 45-59.

Levine, R. L., Moskovitz, J. and Stadtman, E. R. (2000). Oxidation of methionine in proteins: roles in antioxidant defense and cellular regulation. *IUBMB Life* 50,4-5: 301-7.

Martin, D. J. and Ramirez-Alvarado, M. (2010). Comparison of amyloid fibril formation by two closely related immunoglobulin light chain variable domains. *Amyloid* 17,3-4: 129-36.

Martin, D. J. and Ramirez-Alvarado, M. (2011). Glycosaminoglycans promote fibril formation by amyloidogenic immunoglobulin light chains through a transient interaction. *Biophys Chem.* (158,1:81-9)

McLaughlin, R. W., De Stigter, J. K., Sikkink, L. A., Baden, E. M. and Ramirez-Alvarado, M. (2006). The effects of sodium sulfate, glycosaminoglycans, and Congo red on the structure, stability, and amyloid formation of an immunoglobulin light-chain protein. *Protein Sci* 15,7: 1710-22.

Meng, X., Fink, A. L. and Uversky, V. N. (2008). The effect of membranes on the in vitro fibrillation of an amyloidogenic light-chain variable-domain SMA. *J Mol Biol* 381,4: 989-99.

Merlini, G. and Westermark, P. (2004). The systemic amyloidoses: clearer understanding of the molecular mechanisms offers hope for more effective therapies. *J Intern Med* 255,2: 159-78.

Migrino, R. Q., Hari, P., Gutterman, D. D., Bright, M., Truran, S., Schlundt, B. and Phillips, S. A. (2010). Systemic and microvascular oxidative stress induced by light chain amyloidosis. *Int J Cardiol* 145,1: 67-8.

Mohiuddin, I., Chai, H., Lin, P. H., Lumsden, A. B., Yao, Q. and Chen, C. (2006). Nitrotyrosine and chlorotyrosine: clinical significance and biological functions in the vascular system. *J Surg Res* 133,2: 143-9.

Neben-Wittich, M. A., Wittich, C. M., Mueller, P. S., Larson, D. R., Gertz, M. A. and Edwards, W. D. (2005). Obstructive intramural coronary amyloidosis and myocardial ischemia are common in primary amyloidosis. *Am J Med* 118,11: 1287.

O'Nuallain, B., Allen, A., Kennel, S. J., Weiss, D. T., Solomon, A. and Wall, J. S. (2007). Localization of a conformational epitope common to non-native and fibrillar immunoglobulin light chains. *Biochemistry* 46,5: 1240-7.

Ohishi, H., Skinner, M., Sato-Araki, N., Okuyama, T., Gejyo, F., Kimura, A., Cohen, A. S. and Schmid, K. (1990). Glycosaminoglycans of the hemodialysis-associated carpal synovial amyloid and of amyloid-rich tissues and fibrils of heart, liver, and spleen. *Clin Chem* 36,1: 88-91.

Omtvedt, L. A., Bailey, D., Renouf, D. V., Davies, M. J., Paramonov, N. A., Haavik, S., Husby, G., Sletten, K. and Hounsell, E. F. (2000). Glycosylation of immunoglobulin light chains associated with amyloidosis. *Amyloid* 7,4: 227-44.

Omtvedt, L. A., Husby, G., Cornwell, G. G., 3rd, Kyle, R. A. and Sletten, K. (1997). The amino acid sequence of the glycosylated amyloid immunoglobulin light chain protein AL MS. *Scand J Immunol* 45,5: 551-6.

Peterson, F. C., Baden, E. M., Owen, B. A., Volkman, B. F. and Ramirez-Alvarado, M. (2010). A single mutation promotes amyloidogenicity through a highly promiscuous dimer interface. *Structure* 18,5: 563-70.

Phipps, J. E., Kestler, D. P., Foster, J. S., Kennel, S. J., Donnell, R., Weiss, D. T., Solomon, A. and Wall, J. S. (2010). Inhibition of pathologic immunoglobulin-free light chain production by small interfering RNA molecules. *Exp Hematol* 38,11: 1006-13.

Poshusta, T. L., Sikkink, L. A., Leung, N., Clark, R. J., Dispenzieri, A. and Ramirez-Alvarado, M. (2009). Mutations in specific structural regions of immunoglobulin light chains are associated with free light chain levels in patients with AL amyloidosis. *PLoS One* 4,4: e5169.

Prokaeva, T., Spencer, B., Kaut, M., Ozonoff, A., Doros, G., Connors, L. H., Skinner, M. and Seldin, D. C. (2007). Soft tissue, joint, and bone manifestations of AL amyloidosis: clinical presentation, molecular features, and survival. *Arthritis Rheum* 56,11: 3858-68.

Qin, Z., Hu, D., Zhu, M. and Fink, A. L. (2007). Structural characterization of the partially folded intermediates of an immunoglobulin light chain leading to amyloid fibrillation and amorphous aggregation. *Biochemistry* 46,11: 3521-31.

Schubert, D., Behl, C., Lesley, R., Brack, A., Dargusch, R., Sagara, Y. and Kimura, H. (1995). Amyloid peptides are toxic via a common oxidative mechanism. *Proc Natl Acad Sci U S A* 92,6: 1989-93.

Shi, J., Guan, J., Jiang, B., Brenner, D. A., Del Monte, F., Ward, J. E., Connors, L. H., Sawyer, D. B., Semigran, M. J., Macgillivray, T. E., Seldin, D. C., Falk, R. and Liao, R. (2010). Amyloidogenic light chains induce cardiomyocyte contractile dysfunction and apoptosis via a non-canonical p38alpha MAPK pathway. *Proc Natl Acad Sci U S A* 107,9: 4188-93.

Sikkink, L. A. and Ramirez-Alvarado, M. (2008). Biochemical and aggregation analysis of Bence Jones proteins from different light chain diseases. *Amyloid* 15,1: 29-39.

Sikkink, L. A. and Ramirez-Alvarado, M. (2008). Salts enhance both protein stability and amyloid formation of an immunoglobulin light chain. *Biophys Chem* 135,1-3: 25-31.

Sikkink, L. A. and Ramirez-Alvarado, M. (2010). Cytotoxicity of amyloidogenic immunoglobulin light chains in cell culture. *Cell Death and Disease* 1: e98.

Sipe, J. D. and Cohen, A. S. (2000). Review: history of the amyloid fibril. *J Struct Biol* 130,2-3: 88-98.

Skinner, M., Berk, J. L., Connors, L. H. and Seldin, D. C., Eds. (2007). XIth International Symposium on Amyloidosis. Boca Raton, FL, CRC Press

Taylor and Francis Group.

Solomon, A., Weiss, D. T. and Wall, J. S. (2003). Immunotherapy in systemic primary (AL) amyloidosis using amyloid-reactive monoclonal antibodies. *Cancer Biother Radiopharm* 18,6: 853-60.

Souillac, P. O., Uversky, V. N. and Fink, A. L. (2003). Structural transformations of oligomeric intermediates in the fibrillation of immunoglobulin light chain LEN. *Biochemistry* 42,26: 8094-104.

Souillac, P. O., Uversky, V. N., Millett, I. S., Khurana, R., Doniach, S. and Fink, A. L. (2002). Effect of association state and conformational stability on the kinetics of immunoglobulin light chain amyloid fibril formation at physiological pH. *J Biol Chem* 277,15: 12657-65.

Souillac, P. O., Uversky, V. N., Millett, I. S., Khurana, R., Doniach, S. and Fink, A. L. (2002). Elucidation of the molecular mechanism during the early events in immunoglobulin light chain amyloid fibrillation. Evidence for an off- pathway oligomer at acidic pH. *J Biol Chem* 277,15: 12666-79.

Stevens, F. J. (2000). Four structural risk factors identify most fibril-forming kappa light chains. *Amyloid* 7,3: 200-211.

Stevens, P. W., Raffen, R., Hanson, D. K., Deng, Y.-L., Berrios-Hammond, M., Westholm, F. A., Murphy, C., Eulitz, M., Wetzel, R., Solomon, A., Schiffer, M. and Stevens, F. J. (1995). Recombinant immunoglobulin variable domains generated from synthetic genes provide a system for in vitro characterization of light-chain amyloid proteins. *Protein Sci* 4: 421-32.

Vrana, J. A., Gamez, J. D., Madden, B. J., Theis, J. D., Bergen, H. R., 3rd and Dogan, A. (2009). Classification of amyloidosis by laser microdissection and mass spectrometry-based proteomic analysis in clinical biopsy specimens. *Blood* 114,24: 4957-9.

Wall, J., Schell, M., Murphy, C., Hrncic, R., Stevens, F. J. and Solomon, A. (1999). Thermodynamic instability of human lambda 6 light chains: correlation with fibrillogenicity. *Biochemistry* 38,42: 14101-8.

Wall, J. S., Gupta, V., Wilkerson, M., Schell, M., Loris, R., Adams, P., Solomon, A., Stevens, F. and Dealwis, C. (2004). Structural basis of light chain amyloidogenicity: comparison of the thermodynamic properties, fibrillogenic potential and tertiary structural features of four Vlambda6 proteins. *J Mol Recognit* 17,4: 323-31.

Watarai, H., Nozawa, R., Tokunaga, A., Yuyama, N., Tomas, M., Hinohara, A., Ishizaka, K. and Ishii, Y. (2000). Posttranslational modification of the glycosylation inhibiting factor (GIF) gene product generates bioactive GIF. *Proc Natl Acad Sci U S A* 97,24: 13251-6.

Wechalekar, A. D., Hawkins, P. N. and Gillmore, J. D. (2008). Perspectives in treatment of AL amyloidosis. *Br J Haematol* 140,4: 365-77.

Wetzel, R. (1997). Domain stability in immunoglobulin light chain deposition disorders. *Adv Protein Chem* 50: 183-242.

Wittich, C. M., Neben-Wittich, M. A., Mueller, P. S., Gertz, M. A. and Edwards, W. D. (2007). Deposition of amyloid proteins in the epicardial coronary arteries of 58 patients with primary systemic amyloidosis. *Cardiovasc Pathol* 16,2: 75-8.

Zhang, Y., Furyk, S., Bergbreiter, D. E. and Cremer, P. S. (2005). Specific ion effects on the water solubility of macromolecules: PNIPAM and the Hofmeister series. *J Am Chem Soc* 127,41: 14505-10.

Zhu, M., Han, S., Zhou, F., Carter, S. A. and Fink, A. L. (2004). Annular oligomeric amyloid intermediates observed by in situ atomic force microscopy. *J Biol Chem* 279,23: 24452-9.

Zhu, M., Souillac, P. O., Ionescu-Zanetti, C., Carter, S. A. and Fink, A. L. (2002). Surface-catalyzed amyloid fibril formation. *J Biol Chem* 277,52: 50914-22.

2

Amyloid A Amyloidosis Secondary to Rheumatoid Arthritis

Tadashi Nakamura
Kumamoto Center for Arthritis and Rheumatology, and Graduate School of Medical Sciences, Kumamoto University, Kumamoto, Japan

1. Introduction

Amyloids are insoluble fibrous protein aggregates sharing specific structural traits. Abnormal accumulation of amyloid in organs may lead to amyloidosis, and may play a role in various diseases. The name *amyloid* comes from the early mistaken identification of the substance as starch (*amylum* in Latin), based on crude iodine-staining techniques. For a period, it was debated whether or not amyloid deposits were fatty or carbohydrate deposits until it was finally found that they were, in fact, deposits of proteinaceous mass. The underlying molecular abnormalities may be either acquired or hereditary and more than 20 different proteins can form clinically or pathologically significant amyloid fibrils *in vivo*. Current nomenclature lists of amyloid fibril protein have been provided from the nomenclature committee of the International Society of Amyloidosis.
Amyloidosis is a disorder of protein conformation and metabolism that results in the deposition of insoluble amyloid fibrils in tissues, which causes organ dysfunction; systemic amyloidosis is characterized by failure of various organs and the presence of amyloid precursor protein in the serum. Reactive amyloid A (AA) amyloidosis is one of the most severe complications of several chronic disorders, particularly rheumatoid arthritis (RA), and indeed, most patients with reactive AA amyloidosis have an underlying rheumatic disease. An extra-articular complication of RA, AA amyloidosis is a serious, potentially life-threatening disorder caused by deposition in organs of AA amyloid fibrils, which derive from the circulatory acute-phase reactant, serum amyloid A protein (SAA). AA amyloidosis secondary to RA is thus one of the intractable conditions found in patients with collagen vascular diseases and is an uncommon yet important complication of RA.

2. Reactive systemic amyloid A (AA) amyloidosis

2.1 Associated conditions

Several chronic inflammatory disorders induce reactive systemic AA amyloidosis as one of the serious complications. Organ and tissue damage results from the extracellular aggregation of proteolytic fragments from SAA as insoluble AA amyloid fibrils. AA amyloidosis occurs in association with chronic inflammatory disorders, chronic local or systemic microbial infections, and occasionally malignant neoplasias. In Western countries, the most frequent predisposing conditions are rheumatic diseases. AA amyloidosis complicates about 6 % in patients with RA, although the reasons why the incidence is lower in the United States than in Europe and Japan are not clear. Tuberculosis and leprosy are important causes of AA amyloidosis where these infections are endemic. Chronic osteomyelitis, bronchiectasis, chronically infected burns, and decubitus ulcers as well as the chronic pyelonephritis of paraplegic patients are other well-recognized associations. Castleman's disease, Hodgkin's lymphoma and renal carcinoma, which often cause fever, other systemic symptoms, and a major acute phase response, are the malignancies most commonly associated with systemic AA amyloidosis.

Rheumatic disorders	Acne conglobata
Rheumatoid arthritis	Leprosy
Juvenile idiopathic arthritis	Chronic pyelonephritis in paraplegics
Ankylosing spondylitis	Whipple's disease
Psoriasis and psoriatic arthropathy	Decubitus ulcers
Reiter's syndrome	
Adult onset Still's disease	**Neoplasias**
Behçet's disease	Hepatocellular carcinoma
Crohn's disease	Renal carcinoma
Hereditary autoinflammatory syndrome	Lung adenocarcinoma
	Castleman's disease
Chronic infections	Hodgkin's lymphoma
Bronchietasis	Basal cell carcinoma
Tuberculosis	Hairy cell leukemia
Osteomyelitis	Gut carcinoma

Table 1. Conditions associated with reactive systemic amyloid A amyloidosis.

Persistent inflammation supported by chronic diseases, such as rheumatic disorders, chronic infections, and neoplasias, is associated with persistently increased release of proinflammatory cytokines. [Modified from Pepys, M.B. & Hawkins, P.N. (2003). Amyloidosis, In: *Oxford Textbook of Medicine*, Warrell, D.A., Cox, T.M., Firth J.D. & Benz E.J., (Eds), pp. 162-173, Oxford University Press, ISBN-10 0192629220, London, UK.]

2.2 Clinical features

AA amyloid fibril involves the viscera but may be widely disturbed without causing clinical symptoms. The most common presentation is renal, with non-selective proteinuria due to glomerular deposition, and nephrotic syndrome may develop before progression to endstage renal failure. The second most common is with organ enlargement, such as hepatosplenomegaly or thyroid goiter, with or without overt renal abnormality, but in any case AA amyloid fibril deposits are almost always wide spread at the time of presentation. Involvement of the heart and gastrointestinal (GI) tract is frequent, but rarely causes functional impairment.

AA amyloidosis may become clinically evident early in the course of associated disease, but the incidence increases with duration of the primary condition. For most patients the prognosis is closely related to the degree of renal involvement and the efficacy of treatment of the underlying inflammatory condition. Availability of chronic haemodialysis (HD) and transplantation prevents early death from uremia *per se*, but AA amyloid fibril deposition in extrarenal tissues is responsible for a less favorable prognosis than other causes of endstage renal failure.

3. Pathophysiology of AA amyloidosis secondary to RA

RA is a representative of collagen vascular diseases, a group of systemic chronic progressive inflammatory disorders based on immunological disharmonies. Typically, AA amyloidosis will occur in those patients, who have sustained long-standing active disease. Therefore, AA amyloidosis may not be suspected during the early course of a potential disease. In rare case, however, it may occur within a year of a clinically apparent inflammatory disease. AA amyloidosis does not occur in the absence of an acute-phase response or without elevated serum SAA levels. Thus, a sustained high concentration of SAA is a prerequisite for AA amyloidogenesis (Fig. 1). AA amyloidosis seems to develop in only a minority of patients with active, long-standing inflammatory diseases, which indicate that significant disease-modifying factors may help modulate the occurrence of AA amyloidosis, the rate of AA amyloid fibril deposition in tissues, or induction of tissue damage in this form of amyloidosis. The persistent inflammation caused by RA is associated with increased release of the proinflammatory cytokines interleukin (IL)-1, IL-6, and tumor necrosis factor (TNF) α. These cytokines induce a markedly increased synthesis of the acute-phase protein SAA by hepatocytes, the concentration of which can be 100 to 1000-fold higher than normal.

The progressive nature of AA amyloidosis largely reflects the persistent nature of the activity of the underlying conditions and, due to fluctuations of disease activity, not all patients show evidence of an acute-phase response at the very time of diagnosis. Although it is still unknown exactly how the pathophysiological functions of SAA are associated with the pathogenesis of AA amyloidosis, there appears a certain subset of patients, who are prone to process SAA into AA amyloid fibrils under different factors, such as proteases, proteoglycans, serum amyloid P component (SAP).

Human AA amyloid fibril deposits consist mostly of *N*-terminal fragments of SAA, which points to proteolytic cleavage of the precursor being a key event in pathogenesis. These AA amyloid fibril fragments almost exclusively derive from SAA1, which suggests that specific amino acid residues may contribute to a misfolding propensity or that differences in the catabolism exist. The fate of SAA depends largely on its interactions with cellular and extracellular tissue components. Mononuclear phagocytes are involved in SAA catabolism through endocytosis and trafficking to lysosomes, where SAA undergoes degradation.

A role of mononuclear phagocytes in initiating AA amyloid fibril formation was originally postulated because of the presence of AA amyloid fibrils in intracellular vesicles and close to cell membranes in amyloid-laden tissues. These phenomena were subsequently demonstrated in cell culture models. Studies of human monocyte cell lines showed the accumulation of newly formed AA amyloid fibrils in intracellular lysosomal compartments, which indicated that aberrant processing of SAA is relevant for the pathogenesis of AA amyloidosis. A role of monocytes in mediating prion-like transmissibility of AA amyoid fibrils acting as seeds was also suggested. Furthermore, SAA binds specifically to the heparan sulfate (HS)-

glycosaminoglycan complex, a common constituent of all kinds of amyloid deposits that was demonstrated to facilitate conformational conversion of a precursor to a β-plated sheet structure. Also, the SAA-HS interaction promotes AA fibrillogenesis by acting as a scaffold for fibril assembly. Both SAA and AA were reportedly biosynthesized by blood or tissue matrix metalloproteinases (MMPs) and cathepsin D, and this process may in part result in amyloidogenic peptide formation. AA amyloid fibrils would form within lysosomes in macrophages because of disturbed SAA processing. As another factor in amyloid metabolism, mannose-binding lectin (MBL) is a liver-derived protein involved in lectin-mediated complement activation, and lower serum MBL levels are thought to lead to reduced macrophage function. MBL-2 polymorphism determines the blood MBL level and is associated with the role of mononuclear phagocytes in amyloid metabolism. Susceptibility to AA amyloidosis has been linked to mononuclear phagocyte function, and SAA processing by monocytes under stimulation with IL-1 or interferon was reportedly disturbed in patients with AA amyloidosis, which suggests inflammation-induced abnormalities in monocyte function.

Although synthesis of AA amyloid fibrils may be closely related to abnormal processing of SAA and AA in macrophages, the affinity of AA amyloid fibrils for different organs largely accounts for the heterogeneity of such AA amyloid deposits, which still requires explanation. In addition, MMPs contribute to proteolytic remodeling of SAA, with production of amyloidogenic species. Tissue glycosaminoglycans facilitate formation and local deposition of AA amyloid fibrils, along with other amyloidogenic substances, which may be protected from clearance by interaction with the pentraxin SAP. The main target organ of deposition is the kidney, with resulting significant proteinuria and progression toward renal failure. In cases of GI AA amyloidosis, decreased GI motility causes bacterial overgrowth, bile acid deconjugation, and consequently diarrhea, steatorrhea, and severe malabsorption.

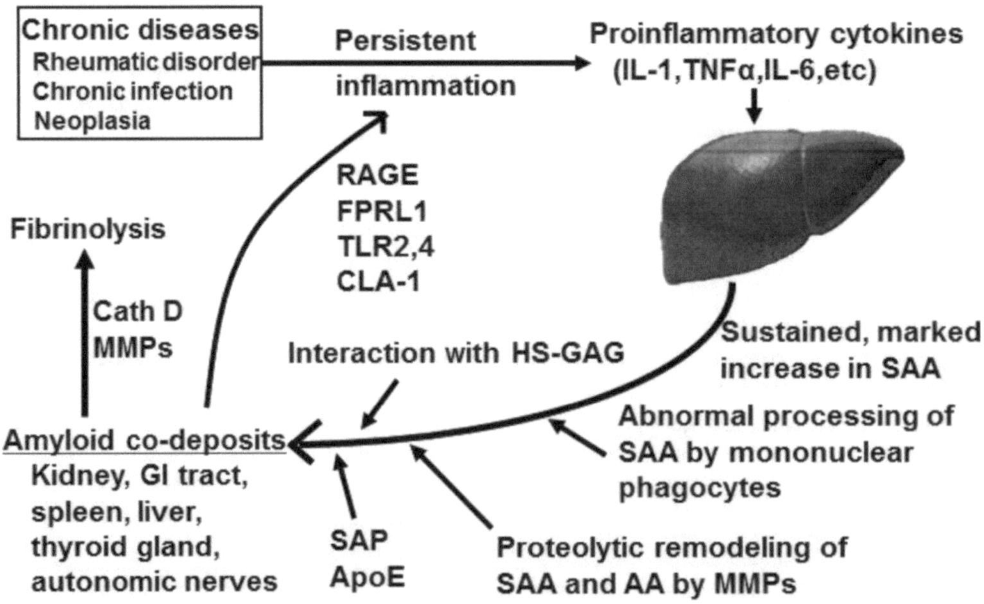

Fig. 1. Pathogenic events involved in amyloid A (AA) amyloidogenesis.

Persistent inflammation caused by chronic diseases is associated with a continuous increase in proinflammatory cytokines (IL-1: interleukin-1, TNFα: tumor necrosis factor α, IL-6: interleukin-6). These cytokines induce markedly increased synthesis of the acute phase-phase protein serum amyloid A protein (SAA). Abnormal processing of SAA by mononuclear phagocytes is thought to initiate amyloidogenic peptide production and formation of amyloid A (AA) amyloid fibrils in lysosomes. Matrix metalloproteinases (MMPs) and cathepsin D (Cath D) contribute to proteolytic remodeling of SAA, with production of amyloidogenic species. AA fibrils, plus serum amyloid P component (SAP) and apolipoprotein E (ApoE), and after interaction with haparan sulfate-glycosaminoglycans (HS-GAG), deposit in multiple organs. SAA and AA participate in inflammation through receptors on inflammatory cells. RAGE: receptor for advanced glycation end products; FPRL1: formyl peptide receptor-like 1; TLR2, 4: toll-like receptor 2 and 4; CLA-1: CD36 and LIMPII analogous-1, human orthologue of the scavenger receptor class B type I (SR-BI); GI: gastrointestinal. [From Nakamura, T. (2011). Amyloid A amyloidosis secondary to rheumatoid arthritis: pathophysiology and treatment. *Clinical and Experimental Rheumatology*, ISSN 0392-856X Accepted on March 8, 2011. (This article is now on process of publication.).]

4. SAA

SAA is produced primarily in the liver under proinflammatory cytokines stimulation; it is also a central acute-phase protein, like C-reactive protein (CRP). SAA complexes with a carrier protein, being transported into serum by high-density lipoprotein (HDL) in combination with apolipoprotein E, and plays an important role in enterohepatic cholesterol circulation. In obese individuals, the frequency of SAA mRNA expression and blood SAA level are both significantly high. Thus, the biologically versatile SAA has a significant relationship with lipid metabolism.

Human SAA composes 104 amino acids, and the four SAA-encoding genes are on chromosome 11p15.1. SAA contains three subtypes with different primary structures-SAA1, SAA2 and SAA4-which make up two groups. Those in the first group, SAA1 and SAA2, serve as acute-phase proteins. In the second group, SAA4 is expressed constitutively in plasma, is synthesized by different organs and tissues, and is not an acute-phase protein. Inflammation induces *SAA1* and *SAA2* genes and their expression but not expression of *SAA3* (a pseudogene) and *SAA4*. *SAA4* encodes a structural protein of HDL. Because of allele polymorphism, SAA1 has three isoforms (SAA1.1, SAA1.3, and SAA1.5) and SAA2 has two (SAA2.1 and SAA2.2), and the serum level of SAA is affected by SAA1 polymorphism. Expression of the SAA1.5 allele is associated with high blood SAA levels, and SAA1.5 has a high affinity for HDL. The primary structures of SAA1 and SAA2 have a 93% amino acid homology. SAA4 shows a 50% homology with the other SAA acute-phase proteins. Thus, acute-phase SAA has multiple patterns of protein polymorphism.

The normal functions of SAA are not known fully, although modulating effects on reverse cholesterol transport and on lipid functions in the microenvironment of inflammatory foci have been proposed. Other reports of potent cell regulatory functions of isolated denatured delipidated SAA have yet to be confirmed with physiological preparations of SAA-rich HDL. Regardless of its physiological role, the behaviour of SAA as an exquisitely sensitive acute phase protein with an enormous dynamic range makes it an extremely valuable empirical clinical marker. It can be used to monitor objectively the biological disease responses. Furthermore, routine monitoring of SAA should be an integral part of the management of all patients with AA amyloidosis or disorders predisposing to it, as control of the primary inflammatory process in order to reduce SAA production is essential if AA amyloidosis is to be halted, enable d to regress, or prevented.

4.1 SAA1.3 allele and genetic factors related to AA amyloidosis

Genetic factors seem to be involved in the prevalence and prognosis, and some factors would have an influence on the development and length of the latent period in AA amyloidosis secondary to RA. The frequency of SAA1 gene polymorphism and that of SAA1 alleles differ among races and regions worldwide. Three main SAA1 alleles-SAA1.1, SAA1.3, and SAA1.5- are defined by two single-nucleotide polymorphisms (SNPs) in exon 3, resulting in two amino acid differences at positions 52 and 57, respectively. In Japanese people, the three alleles occur at approximately the same rate. The association between AA amyloidosis and the SAA1 genotype was first observed in Japanese patients with RA, in whom homozygosity for the SAA1.3 allele proved to be a risk factor. The SAA1.3/1.3 genotype in Japanese patients with RA was associated with a shorter latency period before AA amyloidosis onset and more severe AA amyloidosis-related symptoms; it was also a univariate predictor of survival. Thus, the SAA1.3 allele was a risk factor for AA amyloidosis, had an association with clinical severity in this population, and served as an indicator of poor prognosis. Among Caucasians, AA amyloidosis was often observed in SAA1.1 homozygous individuals, and the SAA1.1 allele was thought to be a risk factor for AA amyloidosis.

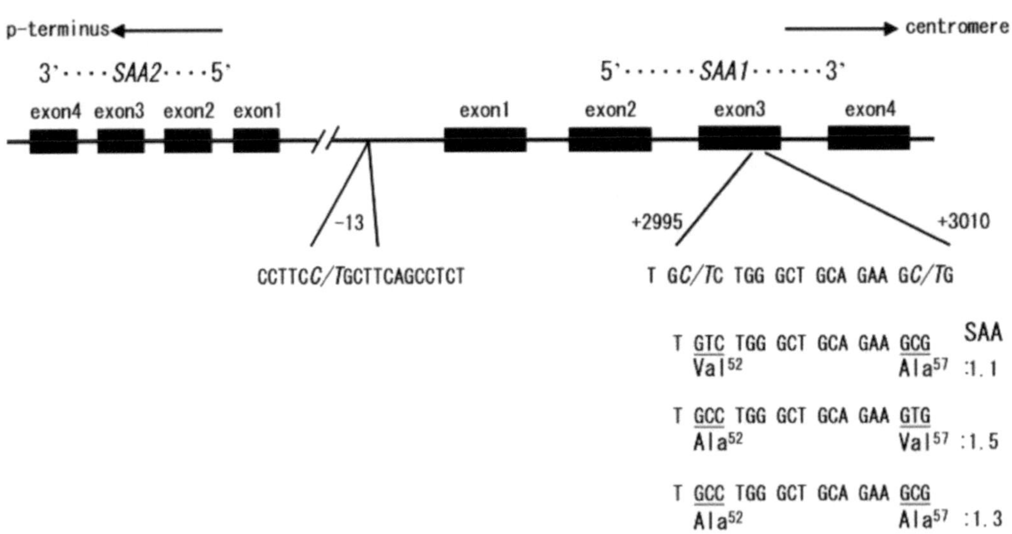

Fig. 2. Partial genomic structure and location of single nucleotide polymorphism (SNPs) in the *SAA1* gene. [From Nakamura, T. (2007). Amyloid A amyloidosis secondary to rheumatoid arthritis: an uncommon yet important complication. *Current Rheumatology Reviews*, Vol. 3, No. 3, (August 2007), pp. 231-241, ISSN 1573-3971.]

With regard to SNPs of the *SAA1* gene promoter region, -13T is a high-risk factor for AA amyloidosis in Japanese patients with RA, with -13T/T and -13T/C being closely associated with AA amyloidosis than is -13C/C. Because *SAA1* gene polymorphism affects both blood SAA levels and SAA transcriptional activity in hepatocytes, differences in SAA1 proteolysis by MMPs indicate a close association between *SAA1* gene polymorphism and onset of AA amyloidosis. However, the mechanism by which *SAA1* gene polymorphism is related to the onset of AA amyloidosis and the reason for ethnic differences in disease-susceptible SNPs are yet unknown.

The most extensively studied genetic marker in RA is *HLA-DRB1*. Several *HLA-DRB1* alleles share a common amino acid sequence, which is commonly called the shared epitope (SE), in the third hypervariable region of the molecule. Recently, it is reported that SE associates with not only the disease susceptibility of RA, but also the RA chronicity, severity, and extra-articular manifestations, in particular AA amyloidosis in RA patients. It is of particular importance that DRB1*04SE has an increased risk of AA amyloidosis in RA and a higher prevalence of double *04SE of *HLA-DR4* is demonstrated in patients with AA amyloidosis secondary to RA.

The *SAA2* gene is located in p-terminus side from the *SAA1* gene. Positions of nucleotides in the sequence of *SAA1* are numbered relative to transcription start site of exon 1. The site of SNPs at both 2995 and 3010 underlined, leading to the SAA1 protein polymorphism.

4.2 SAA receptors

Several SAA receptors have been described, including CD36 and LIMPII analogous-1 (CLA-1); lipoxin A1 receptor/formyl peptide receptor-like 1 (FPRL1); tanis, a hepatic receptor activated by glucose; and toll-like receptor (TLR) 4 and TLR2. SAA reportedly activated rheumatoid synovial fibroblasts by binding to receptors for advanced glycation end products (RAGE). Also, an HDL receptor, the scavenger receptor class B type I (SR-BI), is expressed in RA synovial tissue and is apparently involved in SAA-induced inflammation in arthritis, including production of SAA-induced reactive oxygen species (ROS) and proliferation of fibroblasts. Although RAGE is a receptor for signal transduction with biological stimuli, neither SAA nor AA is incorporated into cells via this receptor. SAA serves as a chemoattractant for neutrophils, T cells, and monocytes via FPRL1 and induces production of CCL2, which is a prototype of the CC chemokine subfamily that has the highest chemotactic activity for monocytes. Because cytotoxic drugs and cytokine inhibitors affect AA amyloid deposits via their ability to suppress SAA production, anticytokine therapies, by inhibiting expression of RAGE, have been proposed to reduce interactions between AA amyloid fibrils and RAGE and thereby prevent AA-mediated cell toxicity.

SAA reportedly exerts cytokine-like actions, stimulates fibroblast differentiation, and elevates ROS production in neutrophils and fibroblasts. Furthermore, not only does SAA induce synthesis of MMP-1 and MMP-3 in synoviocytes and chondrocytes and increase production of MMP-9, but it is also involved in innate immunity via TLR4. Additional studies must identify specific receptor(s) involved in SAA-induced biological phenomena in health and disease.

5. Clinical features and diagnosis of AA amyloidosis secondary to RA

Clinical features of overt AA amyloidosis include long-term psychological distress of RA, markedly high disease activity, and significant inflammatory states. Although a high level of blood SAA is an important factor associated with AA amyloidosis onset, this factor does not always lead to AA amyloidosis in all patients. Several important factors, including the genetic one, are believed to modify the onset of AA amyloidosis. The actual incidence of AA amyloidosis in RA is still undefined and probably underestimated, in that distinguishing clinical and subclinical phase is quite difficult. A cohort study of patients with RA showed that fat AA amyloid deposits were not uncommon-16.3%-so subclinical AA amyloidosis may indeed be common in RA. Prevalent values of AA amyloidosis in RA patients in recent series ranged from 7% to 26%. The prevalence of clinical amyloidosis is likely to be lower, however, as it probably reflects differences in RA treatments and in genetic backgrounds.

AA amyloid deposits primarily target the kidneys, liver, and spleen, and AA amyloidosis becomes clinically overt mainly when renal damage occurs, manifesting as proteinuria, nephrotic syndrome, or impaired renal function. Proteinuria is the clinical sign that most often leads to diagnosis of AA amyloidosis in RA patients. Diagnosis must be based on histological examination of tissue specimen, such as from upper GI or rectal biopsy. Although mucosal biopsy of the upper GI tract to screen for AA amyloid fibril deposition is an easy, simple diagnostic method, antiulcer drugs may mask amyloidotic signs and symptoms in the GI tract, which may delay diagnosis of AA amyloidosis in RA patients. Positive Congo-red staining, susceptibility to oxidation with potassium permanganate, and green birefringence by polarization microscopy after Congo-red staining can confirm the presence of AA amyloid fibrils, however.

5.1 Predictive and prognostic factor of SAA1.3 allele genotype

Whereas there is startling variation in the frequency of AA amyloidosis worldwide, differences also exist for AA amyloidosis complicating RA. The reasons, however, for the marked geographic differences are still unclear. A closer relationship between SAA1.3 allele and AA amyloidosis secondary to RA is known, that is considered to be one of the factors responsible for the lower incidence of AA amyloidosis among Western patients with RA.

Though AA amyloidosis usually develops more than 10 years after the onset of RA, one RA patient complicated by severe AA amyloidosis was encountered just one year after the onset of RA, who was proven to be an SAA1.3 homozygote. Subsequent statistical analysis of a large number of RA patients with AA amyloidosis carrying SAA1.3 allele revealed that the risk for association of AA amyloidosis was about 8 times higher for SAA1.3 homozygotes than for the control group, and that homozygotes can develop AA amyloidosis very early after the onset of RA. It was thus shown that SAA1.3 allele serves not only as a risk factor for the association with AA amyloidosis, but also as a poor prognostic factor in Japanese patients with AA amyloidosis secondary to RA (Fig.3). The generalization of the importance of SAA1.3 allele as both risk and poor prognostic factor may be limited for some reasons; the lack of wide-range control studies, the ethnic differences in SAA gene polymorphism, the relative small number of patients with AA amyloidosis, and the heterogeneity in RA and healthy controls. Although a crude agreement of the significance of SAA1.3 allele in AA amyloidosis in Japanese RA patients is recognized, careful and discreet attitude should be required when judging the utility in between SAA1.3 allele and AA amyloidosis.

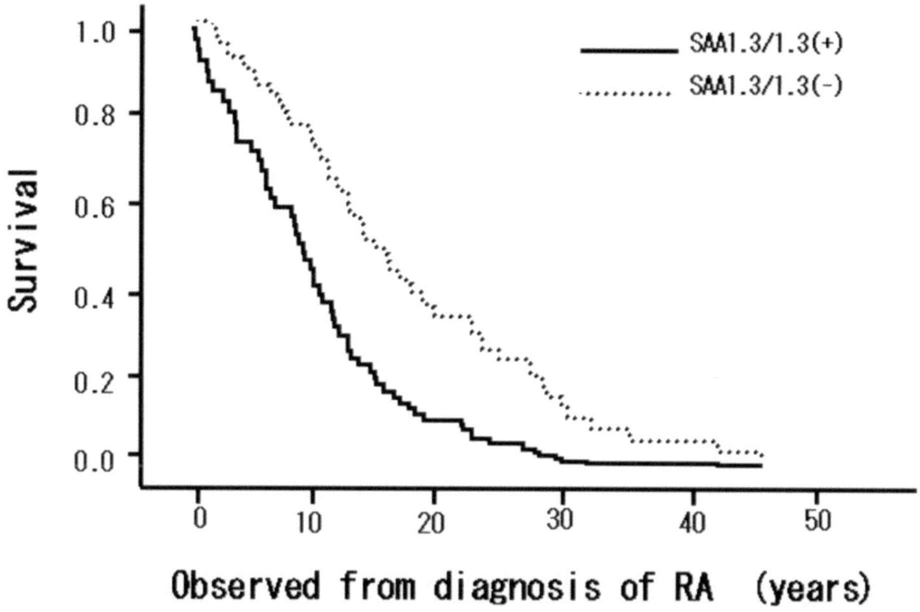

Fig. 3. Kaplan-Meier survival curve in RA disease course for RA patients with (continuous line) and without (dotted line) SAA1.3/1.3 (p=0.015, log-rank test). [From Nakamura, T., Higashi, S., Tomoda, K., Tsukano, M., Baba, S. & Shono, M. (2006). Significance of SAA1.3 allele genotype in Japanese patients with amyloidosis secondary to rheumatoid arthritis. *Rheumatology (Oxford)*, Vol. 45, No. 1, (January 2006), pp. 43-49, ISSN 1462-0324.]

5.2 Clinical diversity and severity

It is suggested that SAA1.3 allele genotype could be related with the symptomatic diversity and severity in patients with AA amyloidosis secondary to RA. Amyloidotic involvement of the urinary bladder is very rare but severe, which is often revealed massive macroscopic hematuria. Once massive hematuria occurs it would trend to be fatal. Secondary bladder AA amyloidosis should be considered as a possible cause of hematuria in patients with long-standing RA, especially carrying SAA1.3 allele, and as an important prognostic factor of RA.

5.3 Prevalence

Though subclinical phase of AA amyloidosis is defined by the formation of AA amyloid deposits in tissue without any clinical manifestation, it is very hard to distinguish clinical from subclinical phase. Obviously, it is difficult to evaluate the natural history of AA amyloid deposition and to know the length of this phase and its final outcome. The prevalence of clinical amyloidosis is likely to be lower. Taking the discordance between prevalence rates of clinical and subclinical AA amyloidosis into consideration, the wide variation in the prevalence of AA amyloidosis secondary to RA is due, in part, to the frequency for the marked geographic differences worldwide, possibly including genetic factors, and due to the lack of unified statistical studies for AA amyloidosis between races and districts. That seems to reach the notion AA amyloidosis would be complicated with RA more than so far estimated.

5.4 Outcome

The survival time after the diagnosis of AA amyloidosis secondary to RA seems to be 4-5 year. These are, of course, dependent on the time at which AA amyloidosis is verified, which may differ considerably among patients. This partly explains the great individual variation in survival time observed, that leads us the notion that an active diagnostic attitude towards AA amyloidosis in patients with RA is advisable. Although the relationship among the production of AA precursor protein, the turnover of AA amyloid fibrils, and amyloidotic organ function is complex, it has been proved that outcome is favorable in AA amyloidosis when SAA concentration is maintained below 10μg/ml. The clinical risk factors associated with a poor survival included female, older age, a reduced serum albumin, and an increased serum creatinine concentration upon diagnosis of AA amyloidosis (Fig. 4). Renal involvement has been considered to be the most critical problem in patients with AA amyloidosis, and dominates the clinical picture in AA amyloidosis

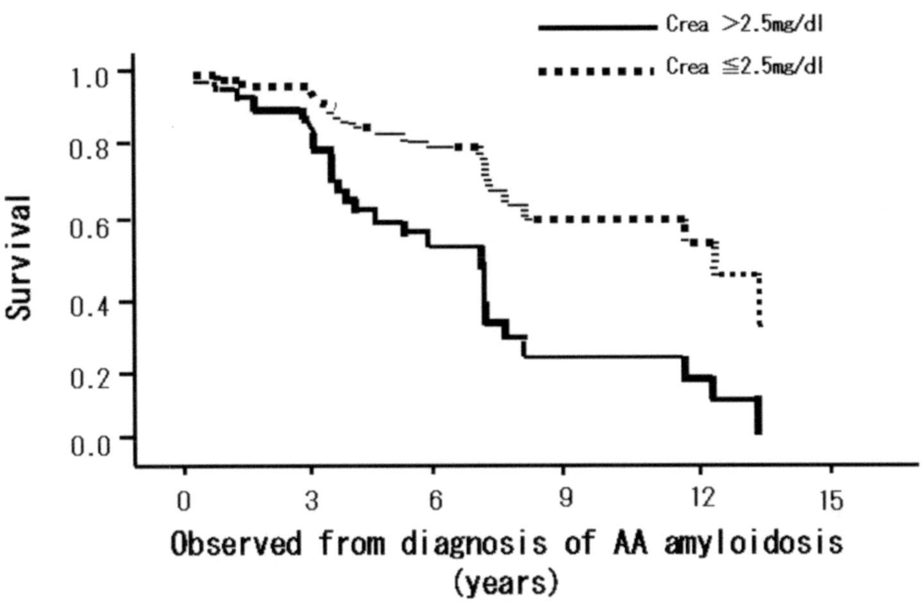

Fig. 4. Kaplan-Meier survival curve after diagnosis of AA amyloidosis for patients with serum creatinine >2.5 mg/dl (continuous line) and serum creatinine≦2.5 mg/dl (dotted line) (p=0.013, log-rank test). [From Nakamura, T., Higashi, S., Tomoda, K., Tsukano, M., Baba, S. & Shono, M. (2006). Significance of SAA1.3 allele genotype in Japanese patients with amyloidosis secondary to rheumatoid arthritis. *Rheumatology (Oxford)*, Vol. 45, No. 1, (January 2006), pp. 43-49, ISSN 1462-0324.]

Amyloidotic cardiac involvement has been revealed to trend to be a poor prognostic factor. Heart failure is likely to be directly responsible for death in only a minority of patients, however, patients with heart failure may be complicated by multiple organ failures in later phase of the RA disease course. It seems to be suggested that dysautonomia plays an important role in etiology of heart failure to some extent in patients with AA amyloidosis in addition to direct AA amyloid fibril deposits *in situ*. Although the number of reports published to date concerning AA amyloidosis and autonomic nerve dysfunction in patients with RA is extremely rare, taking an importance of cardiovascular symptoms into account of dysautonomia, which could induce sudden death in AA amyloidosis secondary to RA, autonomic nerve dysfunctions may serve as one of the clinical predictors of poor prognosis in RA. Dysautonomia like abnormal gustatory sweating or orthostatic hypotension seems to be one of the typical symptoms in endstage of the disease course in RA patients with AA amyloidosis.

5.5 Causes of death

Infection and renal failure are generally the commonest causes of death in RA patients with AA amyloidosis, and they comprised 42.3% and 19.2% of deaths, respectively. A higher risk of severe infections is a substantial problem in management of RA with AA amyloidosis. Also, the higher causal proportion of renal failure and GI diseases than RA patients without AA amyloidosis can be attributable to more AA amyloid fibril deposition in these organs.

6. Treatment of AA amyloidosis secondary to RA

The principal aim in treating RA patients with AA amyloidosis is to switch off SAA production, by controlling the RA inflammatory process. Anti-inflammatory treatment must be empirical but, as in all patients with AA amyloidosis, should be guided by frequent assessment of SAA concentrations in view of reported correlations between survival and this measure. Estimated survival at 10 years was 90% in AA amyloidosis patients whose median SAA concentration was below 10 μg/ml and was 40% among those whose median SAA exceeded this value, which were statistically significant results. Treatment of AA amyloidosis secondary to RA may involve the following strategies.

6.1 Suppression of SAA production

The efficacy of corticosteroid treatment on AA amyloidosis secondary to RA is still controversial. Corticosteroids are capable of reducing the magnitude of acute phase reaction including synthesis of CRP and SAA. In human hepatocyte cultures a stimulating effect of corticosteroids was seen on SAA but not on CRP production. Although corticosteroid suppresses both CRP and SAA levels in longitudinal studies of patients with RA, the effect is somewhat more pronounced for CRP than for SAA. Monitoring of SAA instead of CRP levels would be advisable particularly if corticosteroids are being used. It seems reasonable to treat patients with AA amyloidosis secondary to RA using cytostatic drugs either alone or in combination with prednisolone. As the effect of cytostatics may take weeks or months to appear, it is recommended to give steroids in addition in order to ensure an immediate reduction of the acute phase response and in particular the synthesis of SAA.

Traditional management of AA amyloidosis has been to target RA disease process behind the inflammation. Although there is no evidence that disease-modifying anti-rheumatic drugs (DMARDs) have a specific effect on amyloidogenesis and AA amyloidosis in RA, there have been encouraging reports evaluating alkylating agents as beneficial in clinical trials in RA patients with AA amyloidosis. It is suggested that the use of immunosuppressive agents can improve prognosis, and cyclophosphamide (CYC) has been proved to be superior to methotrexate (MTX) in treatment with RA patients with AA amyloidosis (Fig.5). The possibility that CYC would be more effective predominantly in patients with SAA1.3/1.3 homozygosity than heterozygosity, suggesting SAA1.3/1.3 homozygosity as a CYC treatment-susceptible factor.

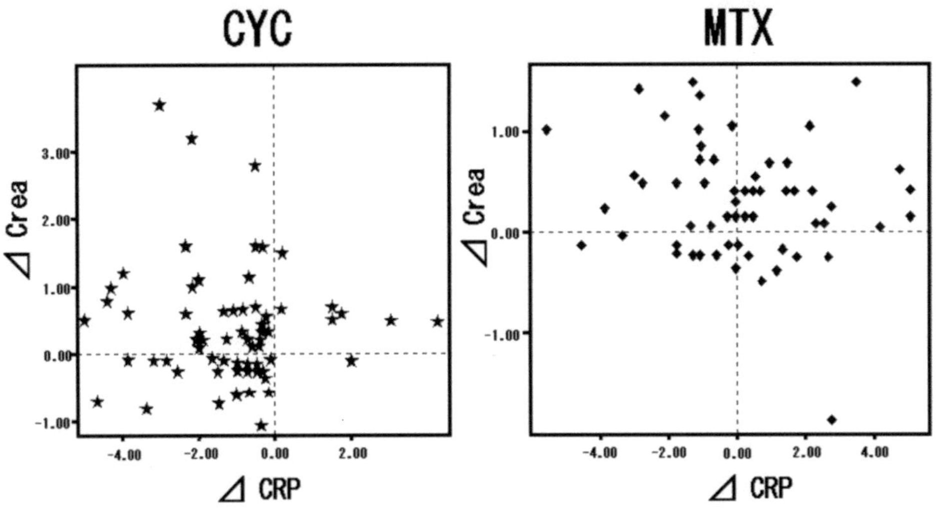

Fig. 5. Differences between CYC and MTX treatments for RA patients with AA amyloidosis. The deducted value (placed in figures) was calculated by subtracting the starting value of CRP and/or serum creatinine from the endpoint value in each treatment. [From Nakamura, T., Higashi, S., Tomoda, K., Tsukano, M., Baba, S. & Shono, M. (2006). Significance of SAA1.3 allele genotype in Japanese patients with amyloidosis secondary to rheumatoid arthritis. *Rheumatology (Oxford)*, Vol. 45, No. 1, (January 2006), pp. 43-49, ISSN 1462-0324.]

For AA amyloidosis in patients with RA, treatment has centered on using cytotoxic agents and biologics. Although case reports and studies of small series of patients showed that these agents can reverse nephrotic syndrome and even lead to complete resolution of proteinuria, anticytokine agents have recently been proposed as therapeutic options (Table 2). Anti-proinflammatory cytokine therapy is expected to show efficacy against systemic inflammation and against local inflammation mediated by macrophage differentiation or activation in glomeruli, such as in renal AA amyloidosis secondary to RA. The strategy of these treatments focuses on tight control of underlying RA disease activity. Requirements include diagnosis of RA as early as possible and treatment with DMARDs, including MTX as the anchor drug. Achieving low disease activity via DMARDs early in the disease course has a strong positive outcome on disease progression. However, although MTX is the most common and effective drug for RA, management of patients with AA amyloidosis secondary to RA and renal involvement is too complex to limit the discussion to MTX.

In RA treatment, tight control of RA is emphasized to obtain clinical remission or lower disease activity; this control is possible through periodic evaluations of RA disease activity and aggressive pursuit of other more effective treatments. Together with this strategy, the genetic predisposition allele SAA1.3, which is a known risk factor for AA amyloidosis in Japanese RA patients, should be evaluated when treating both RA and AA amyloidosis.

For TNFα antagonists	E: etanercept/ I: infliximab
Elkayam O, *et al*: Arthritis Rheum 2002; 46: 2571-3	I
Gottenberg J-E, *et al*: Arthritis Rheum 2003; 48: 2019-24	E/I
Ortiz-Santamaria V, *et al*: Rheumatology 2003; 42: 1425-6	E/I
Smith GR, *et al*: Intern Med J 2004; 34: 570-2	E
Ravindran J, *et al*: Rheumatology 2004; 43: 669-72	E/I
Fernandes-Nebro A, *et al*: Am J Med 2005; 118: 552-6	E/I
Nakamura T, *et al*: Clin Exp Rheumatol 2007; 25: 518-22	E
Kuroda T, *et al*: Rheumatol Int 2008; 28: 1155-9	I
Kuroda T, *et al*: J Rheumatol 2009; 36: 2409-15	E/I
Nakamura T, *et al*: Clin Rheumatol 2010; 29: 1395-401	E
Nobre CA, *et al*: Rev Bras Reumatol 2010; 50: 205-10	E
Ishii W, *et al*: Rheumatol Int 2011; 31: 247-50	E
For the IL-6 receptor antagonist	
Okuda Y, *et al*: Arthritis Rheum 2006; 54: 2997-3000	
Sato H, *et al*: Clin Rheumatol 2009; 28: 1113-6	
Inoue D, *et al*: Clin Rheumatol 2010; 29: 1195-7	

Table 2. Selected references to biologics for treatment of AA amyloidosis secondary to RA. [Modified from Nakamura, T. (2011). Amyloid A amyloidosis secondary to rheumatoid arthritis: pathophysiology and treatment. *Clinical and Experimental Rheumatology*, ISSN 0392-856X Accepted on March 8, 2011 (This article is now on process of publication.).]

Etanercept and infliximab, both TNFα antagonists, can reduce serum SAA levels in RA patients with AA amyloidosis, which improves rheumatoid inflammation, reduces swollen and tender joint counts, lowers or normalizes proteinuria, and ameliorates renal function. Despite the small number of series of patients with AA amyloidosis secondary to RA who had etanercept treatment, this drug did benefit both RA inflammation and AA amyloidosis, as measured via the surrogate markers DAS28-ESR, CRP, SAA, and proteinuria, in SAA1.3 allele-carrying RA patients. Also, serum creatinine levels significantly improved in patients with mild RA disease and renal dysfunction. This result suggests that the earlier the intervention with biologics, the better the outcome for patients. Etanercept alone may therefore be efficacious, without MTX.

Tocilizumab, an IL-6 receptor antagonist, also demonstrates excellent suppression of SAA levels and may have potential as a therapeutic agent for AA amyloidosis. Circulating SAA normally reflects changes in CRP, and levels of both acute-phase reactants usually increase simultaneously, but some differences can occur. SAA and CRP seem to be partly influenced by different cytokines. IL-6-blocking therapy has shown promise in normalizing serum SAA levels in RA patients. Moreover, blocking IL-6 alone, but not IL-1 or TNFα, completely prevented SAA mRNA expression in human hepatocytes during triple cytokine stimulation. For signal transduction, IL-6 binds to membrane-bound IL-6 receptor gp80, and then the IL-6-gp80 dimer interacts with gp130. Formation of gp130-

containing complexes leads to activation of Janus kinases (JAKs), which stimulates signal transducers and activators of transcription (STATs). Certain evidence suggests that STAT3 is the key transcription factor responsible for IL-6 activation of SAA gene transcription. Therefore, the function of JAK inhibition in the IL-6 signaling pathway will be one target of RA treatments. Suppressing IL-6-mediated proinflammatory signaling pathways via JAK inhibitors may be a novel anti-inflammatory therapeutic strategy for RA and AA amyloidosis. Another agent, tacrolimus, may inhibit T-cell function in pathogenesis of AA amyloidosis.

6.2 Inhibition of AA amyloid fibril deposits

Eprodisate, a small sulfonated molecule with structural similarity to heparan sulfate, which can cause regression of amyloidosis by destabilizing the glycoasaminoglycan backbone of amyloid deposits, delayed progression of renal disease associated with AA amyloidosis. In a trial for AA amyloidosis, eprodisate had a beneficial effect on the rate of deterioration of renal function but no effect on urinary protein excretion . That eprodisate did not affect SAA levels and preserved kidney function but had no effect on proteinuria raises the interesting possibility that it is the precursors of mature amyloid fibrils are responsible for proteinuria in amyloidosis.

6.3 Removal of deposited AA amyloid fibrils

The normal plasma protein SAP binds to all types of amyloid fibrils and contributes to amyloidosis pathogenesis. A pyrrolidine carboxylic acid derivative, which is a competitive inhibitor of SAP binding to amyloid fibrils, can intervene in this process and affect SAP levels. This compound cross-linked and dimerized SAP molecules, which led to extremely rapid clearance by the liver, and thus produced marked depletion of circulating human SAP. This drug action thus removed SAP from human amyloid deposits in tissues and may have a favorable effect on amyloidosis.

Another compound, dimethyl sulfoxide (DMSO), is a hydrogen-bond disrupter, cell-differentiating agent, hydroxyl radical scavenger, cryoprotectant, and solubilizing agent that is used as a compound for preparation of samples for electron microscopy, as an intracellular low-density lipoprotein-derived cholesterol-mobilizing antidote to extravasation of vesicant anticancer agents, and as a topical analgesic. A notable DMSO side effect is garlic-like breath odor and taste in the mouth because of pulmonary excretion of a small amount of DMSO as dimethyl sulfide. Oral DMSO was effective against AA amyloidosis, especially GI involvement and early renal dysfunction, but using it would not likely be feasible in current clinical practice.

6.4 Treatment of organ failure

The predominant feature of AA amyloidosis is proteinuria with or without renal failure. If conservative treatment of renal failure is not sufficient, renal replacement therapy including renal transplantation, continuous ambulatory peritoneal dialysis, or HD should be considered. Even in RA patients with AA amyloidosis who undergo HD, anti-TNFα blockers can demonstrate efficacy. HD reportedly had no effect on plasma etanercept concentration, and etanercept pharmacokinetics in patients undergoing HD for chronic renal failure were similar to those with normal renal function. Administration of etanercept to HD patients would therefore appear reasonable.

For RA patients complaining severe diarrhea due to AA amyloidosis, corticosteroid, codeine phosphate, and lactate bacteriae are useful. In remarkable protein losing enteropathy with intractable diarrhea due to AA amyloidosis, a successful treatment combined with somatostatin analogue octreotide and corticosteroid has been reported.

7. Biological diversity and significance of SAA

The life expectancy of patients with RA has been estimated to be 1.2 to 1.7 times worse than that of the general population. Complications involving AA amyloidosis may further reduce life expectancy in such patients. Treatment-related clinical remission in RA may lead to structural and functional remissions, which will result in a better quality of life. SAA has biologically diverse and significant roles in health and disease (Fig. 6). Thus, SAA may modify progression of disease-either AA amyloidosis (high-grade inflammation) or metabolic syndrome (low-grade inflammation)-via its biological actions. Alleviated inflammation and improved nutritional metabolism would lead to suppression of cardiovascular events and would reduce the incidence of AA amyloidosis in RA. Elucidation of the biological diversity and significance of SAA should enhance understanding of the pathophysiology of AA amyloidosis secondary to RA.

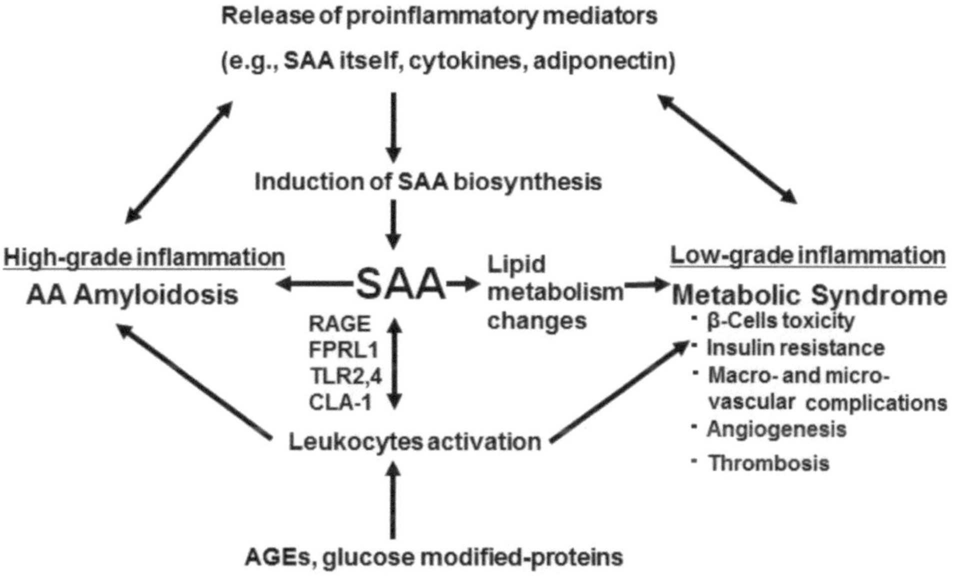

Fig. 6. Biological versatility of serum amyloid A protein (SAA).

SAA plays important roles in both high-grade inflammation and low-grade inflammation. It acts, as cytokines do, via autocrine, endocrine, and paracrine mechanisms. As a precursor protein of amyloid A (AA) fibrils, SAA induces AA amyloidosis. SAA also affects metabolic syndrome via various modes of action. These humoral and cellular inflammatory events interact, with SAA being a key player. RAGE: receptor for advanced glycation end products; FPRL1: formyl peptide receptor-like 1; TLR2, 4: toll-like receptor 2 and 4; CLA-1: CD36 and

LIMPII analogous-1, human orthologue of the scavenger receptor class B type I (SR-BI); AGEs: advanced glycation end products. [From Nakamura, T. (2011). Amyloid A amyloidosis secondary to rheumatoid arthritis: pathophysiology and treatment. *Clinical and Experimental Rheumatology*, ISSN 0392-856X Accepted on March 8, 2011 (This article is now on process of publication.).]

8. Issues that require further perspective

Important issues of future interest that are related to AA amyloidosis secondary to RA include the following: i) tight control of inflammation occurring with underlying RA; ii) factors associated with the risk of AA amyloidosis, such as SAA1.3 allele, which indicates a genetic predisposition to the disease; and iii) screening tools for AA amyloidosis for use even during the subclinical phase. The mechanisms of AA amyloid fibril formation are complicated pathways involving multiple factors, as Figure 1 shows, and elucidation of mechanisms on both deposition and turnover of AA amyloid fibrils should allow development of novel therapeutic options. Reducing the supply of amyloidogenic precursors is usually associated with reabsorption of AA amyloid deposits and perhaps recovery of target organ function. Because AA amyloid fibril shows heterogeneity in organ deposition, clarification of the affinity of AA amyloid fibrils to various organs is needed. Addressing the involvement of various organs and systems- renal, GI, cardiac, thyroid, and autonomic nervous-may permit development of therapeutic countermeasures against complications.

9. Conclusion

Although significant advances have been made in understanding of the pathology, pathogenesis, and clinical treatment of AA amyloidosis secondary to RA, the disease is still an important complication that warrants investigation. The SAA1.3 allele serves not only as a risk factor for AA amyloidosis but also as a factor related to poor prognosis and shortened survival of Japanese patients with RA, and understanding both disorders would benefit from investigation of the SAA1.3 allele. AA amyloidosis secondary to RA is now clearly influenced by many variables, and clinical pictures differ among patients. The pathological process in RA patients with AA amyloidosis seems to be more complicated and subtle than previously realized. Clarification of the formation and degeneration or turnover of AA amyloid fibrils and elucidation of the biological contributions of SAA in health and disease are indispensable prerequisites to the management of AA amyloidosis secondary to RA.

The introduction of biological therapies targeting specific inflammatory mediators revolutionized the treatment of RA. Targeting key components of the immune system allows efficient suppression of the pathologic inflammatory cascade that gives rise to RA symptoms and subsequent joint destruction. Reactive AA amyloidosis is one of the most severe complications of RA, and is a serious, potentially life-threatening disorder caused by deposition in multiple organs of AA amyloid fibrils. The AA amyloid fibrils are derived from the circulatory acute-phase reactant, SAA, and likely subject to control. With newly developed biologics, AA amyloidosis secondary to RA seems to become a treatable and even controllable disorder. The pathophysiological understanding and clinical factors including the genetic predisposition require that rheumatologists need to take these into account when diagnosing and treating patients with AA amyloidosis secondary to RA. Based on previous works as to AA amyloidosis secondary to RA, the critical overview in terms of AA amyloidosis is discussed with special reference to therapeutic importance of biologic agents.

10. Acknowledgments

The author would like to thank his colleagues, Syu-ichi Higashi, MD, PhD, Hironori Kudoh, MD, PhD, Kunihiko Tomoda, MD, PhD, Michishi Tsukano, MD, PhD, Satoshi Baba, MD, PhD, and Masahiro Shono, MD, PhD, for their collaborations and contributions to the work. This work was supported in part by a Grant-in-Aid for scientific research from the Japanese Ministry of Health, Labor, and Welfare and the Amyloidosis Research Committee for Intractable Diseases, Epochal Diagnosis, and Treatment in Japan.

11. References

Baba, S., Masago, S.A., Takahashi, T., Kasama, T., Sugimura, H., Tsugane, S., Tsutsui, Y. & Shirasawa, H. (1995). A novel allelic variant of serum amyloid A, SAA1γ: genomic evidence, evolution, frequency, and implication as a risk factor for reactive systemic AA-amyloidosis. *Human Molecular Genetics,* Vol. 4, No. 6, (June 1995), pp. 1083-1087, ISSN 0964-6906

Bergesio, F., Ciciani, A.M., Manganaro, M., Palladini, G., Santostefano, M., Brugnano, R., Di Palma, A.M., Gallo, M., Rosati, A., Tosi, P.L., Salvadori, M. & Immunopathology Group of the Italian Society of Nephrology (2008). Renal involvement in systemic amyloidosis: an Italian collaborative study on survival and renal outcome. *Nephrology and Dialysis Transplantation,* Vol. 23, No. 3, (March 2008), pp. 941-951, ISSN 1460-2385

Dember, L.M. (2009). Modern treatment of amyloidosis: unresolved questions. *Journal of American Society of Nephrology,* Vol. 20, No. 3, (March 2009), pp. 469-472, ISSN 1533-3450

Enqvist, S., Sletten, K. & Westermark, P. (2009). Fibril protein fragmentation pattern in systemic AL-amyloidosis. *Journal of Pathology,* Vol. 219, No. 4, (December 2009), pp. 473-480, ISSN 1096-9896

Gillmore, J.D., Lovat, L.B., Persey, M.R., Pepys, M.B. & Hawkins, P.N. (2001). Amyloid load and clinical outcome in AA amyloidosis in relation to circulating concentration of serum amyloid A protein. *Lancet,* Vol. 358, No. 9275, (July 2001), pp. 24-29, ISSN 0140-6736

Gómez-Casanovas, E., Sanmartí, R., Solé, M., Cañate, J.D. & Muñoz-Gómez, J. (2001). The clinical significance of amyloid fat deposits in rheumatoid arthritis: A systematic long-term followup study using abdominal fat aspiration. *Arthritis and Rheumatism,* Vol. 44, No. 1, (January 2001), pp. 66-72, ISSN 0004-3591

Gonzalez-Alvaro, I., Carmona, L., Balsa, A., Sanmarti, R., Belmonte, M.A., Tena, X. & EMECAR Study Group (2003). Patterns of disease modifying antirheumatic drug use in a Spanish cohort of patients with rheumatoid arthritis. *Journal of Rheumatology,* Vol. 30, No. 4, (April 2003), pp. 697-704, ISSN 0315-162X

Hagihara, K., Nishikawa, T., Sugamata, Y., Song, J., Isobe, T., Taga, T. & Yoshizaki, K. (2005). Essential role of STAT3 in cytokine-driven NF-κB-mediated serum amyloid A gene expression. *Genes to Cells,* Vol. 10, No. 11, (November 2005), pp. 1051-1063, ISSN 1356-9597

Hatanaka, E., Furlaneto, C.J., Ribeiro, F.P., Souza, G.M. & Campa, A. (2004). Serum amyloid A-induced mRNA expression and release of tumor necrosis factor-alpha (TNF-alpha) in human neutrophils. *Immunology Letters,* Vol. 91, No. 1, (January 2004), pp. 33-37, ISSN 0165-2478

He, R.L., Zhou, J., Hanson, C.Z., Chen, J., Cheng, N. & Ye, R.D. (2009). Serum amyloid A induces G-CSF expression and neutrophilia via Toll-like receptor 2. *Blood* , Vol. 113, No. 2, (January 2009), pp. 429-437, ISSN 1528-0020

Koivuniemi, R., Paimela, L., Suomalainen, R. & Leirisalo-Repo, M. (2008). Amyloidosis as a cause of death in patients with rheumatoid arthritis. *Clinical and Experimental Rheumatology,* Vol. 26, No. 3, (May-June 2008), pp. 408-413, ISSN 0392-856X

Koivuniemi, R., Paimela, L., Suomalinen, R., Tornroth, T. & Leirisalo-Repo, M. (2008). Amyloidosis is frequently undetected in patients with rheumatoid arthritis. *Amyloid,* Vol. 15, No. 4, (December 2007), pp. 262-268, ISSN 1744-2818

Kuroda, T., Wada, Y., Kobayashi, D., Murakami, S., Sakai, T., Hirose, S., Tanabe, N., Saeki, T., Nakano, M. & Narita, I. (2009). Effective anti-TNF-α therapy can induce rapid resolution and sustained decrease of gastrointestinal mucosal amyloid deposits in reactive amyloidosis associated with rheumatoid arthritis. *Journal of Rheumatology,* Vol. 36, No. 11, (November 2009), pp. 2409-2415, ISSN 0315-162X

Lachmann, H.J., Goodman, H.J., Gilbertson, J.A., Gallimore, J.R., Sabin, C.A., Gillmore, J.D. & Hawkins, P.N. (2007). Natural history and outcome in systemic AA amyloidosis. *New England Journal of Medicine,* Vol. 356, No. 23, (June 2007), pp. 2361-2371, ISSN 1533-4406

Lundmark, K., Westermark, G.T., Nyström, S., Murphy, C.L., Solomon, A. & Westermark, P. (2002). Transmissibility of systemic amyloidosis by a prion-like mechanism. *Proceedings of National Academy of Sciences (USA),* Vol. 99, No. 10, (May 2002), pp. 6979-6984, ISSN 0027-8424

Lundmark, K., Westermark, G.T., Olsén, A. & Westermark, P. (2005). Protein fibrils in nature can enhance amyloid protein A amyloidosis in mice: cross-seeding as a disease mechanism. *Proceedings of National Academy of Sciences (USA),* Vol. 102, No. 17, (April 2005), pp. 6098-6102, ISSN 0027-8424

Magy, N., Benson, M.D., Liepnieks, J.J. & Kluve-Beckerman, B. (2007). Cellular events associated with the initial phase of AA amyloidogenesis: insights from a human monocyte model. *Amyloid,* Vol. 14, No. 1, (March 2007), pp. 51-63, ISSN 1350-6129

Sanmartí R., Gómez-Casanovas E., Solé M., Cañete J., Gratacós J., Carmona L., Gonzalez Alvaro I. & Muñoz-Gómez, J. (2004). Prevalence of silent amyloidosis in RA and its clinical significance. *Journal of Rheumatology,* Vol. 31, No. 5, (May 2004), pp. 1013-1014, ISSN 0315-162X

Moriguchi, M., Kaneko, H., Terai, C., Koseki, Y., Kajiyama, H., Inada, S., Kitamura, Y. & Kamatani, M. (2005). Relative transcriptional activities of SAA1 promoters polymorphic at position -13(T/C): potential association between increased transcription and amyloidosis. *Amyloid,* Vol. 12, No. 1, (March 2005), pp. 26-32, ISSN 1350-6129

Nakamura, T., Higashi, S., Tomoda, K., Tsukano, M., Baba, S. & Shono, M. (2006). Significance of SAA1.3 allele genotype in Japanese patients with amyloidosis secondary to rheumatoid arthritis. *Rheumatology (Oxford),* Vol. 45, No. 1, (January 2006), pp. 43-49, ISSN 1462-0324

Nakamura, T. (2007). Amyloid A amyloidosis secondary to rheumatoid arthritis: an uncommon yet important complication. *Current Rheumatology Reviews*, Vol. 3, No. 3, (August 2007), pp. 231-241, ISSN 1573-3971

Nakamura, T., Higashi, S., Tomoda, K., Tsukano, M., & Baba, S. (2007). Efficacy of etanercept in patients with AA amyloidosis secondary to rheumatoid arthritis. *Clinical and Experimental Rheumatology*, Vol. 25, No. 4, (July-August 2007), pp. 518-522, ISSN 0392-856X

Nakamura, T. (2008). Clinical strategies for amyloid A amyloidosis secondary to rheumatoid arthritis. *Modern Rheumatology*, Vol. 18, No. 2, (March 2008), pp. 109-118, ISSN 1439-7595

Nakamura, T., Higashi, S., Tomoda, K., Tsukano, M. & Shono, M. (2010). Etanercept can induce resolution of renal deterioration in patients with amyloid A amyloidosis secondary to rheumatoid arthritis. *Clinical Rheumatology*, Vol. 29, No. 12, (December 2010), pp. 1395-1401, ISSN 1434-9949

Nakamura, T. (2011). Amyloid A amyloidosis secondary to rheumatoid arthritis: pathophysiology and treatment. *Clinical and Experimental Rheumatology*, ISSN 0392-856X Accepted on March 8, 2011 (This article is now on process of publication.)

Obici, L., Raimondi, S., Lavatelli, F., Bellotti, V. & Merlini, G. (2009). Susceptibility to AA amyloidosis in rheumatic diseases: a critical overview. *Arthritis and Rheumatism (Arthritis Care & Research)*, Vol. 61, No. 10, (October 2009), pp. 1435-1440, ISSN 0004-3591

Okuda, Y. & Takasugi, K. (2006). Successful use of a humanized anti-interleukin-6 receptor antibody, tocilizumab, to treat amyloid A amyloidosis complicating juvenile idiopathic arthritis. *Arthritis and Rheumatism*, Vol. 54, No. 9, (September 2006), pp. 2997-3000, ISSN 0004-3591

Perfetto, F., Moggi-Pignone, A., Livi, R., Tempestini, A., Bergesio, F. & Matucci-Cerinic, M. (2010). Systemic amyloidosis: a challenge for the rheumatologist. *Nature Reviews. Rheumatology*, Vol. 6, No. 7, (July 2010), pp. 417-429, ISSN 1759-4804

Pepys, M.B., Herbert, J., Hutchinson, WL., Tennent, G.A., Lachmann, H.J., Gallimore, J.R., Lovat, L.B., Bartfai, T., Alanine, A., Hertel, C., Hoffmann, T., Jakob-Roetne, R., Norcross, R.D., Kemp, J.A., Yamamura, K., Suzuki, M., Taylor, G.W., Murray, S., Thompson, D., Purvis, A., Kolstoe, S., Wood, S.P. & Hawkins, P.N. (2002). Targeted pharmacological depletion of serum amyloid P component for treatment of human amyloidosis. *Nature*, Vol. 417, No. 6886, (May 2002), pp. 254-259, ISSN 0028-0836

Pepys, M.B. & Hawkins, P.N. (2003). Amyloidosis, In: *Oxford Textbook of Medicine*, Warrell, D.A., Cox, T.M., Firth J.D. & Benz E.J., (Eds), pp. 162-173, Oxford University Press, ISBN-10 0192629220, London, UK

Pettersson, T., Konttinen, Y.T. & Maury, C.P.J. (2008). Treatment strategies for amyloid A amyloidosis. *Expert Opinion Pharmacotherapy*, Vol. 9, No. 12, (August 2008), pp. 2117-2128, ISSN 1744-7666

Röcken, C., Kientsch-Engel, R., Mansfeld, S., Stix, B., Stubenrauch, K., Weigle, B., Bühling, F., Schwan, M. & Saeger, W. (2003). Advanced glycation end products and receptor for advanced glycation end products in AA amyloidosis. *American Journal of Pathology*, Vol. 162, No. 4, (April 2003), pp. 1213-1220, ISSN 0002-9440

Sokka, T., Abelson, B. & Pincus, T. (2008). Mortality in rheumatoid arthritis: 2008 update. *Clinical and Experimental Rheumatology,* Vol. 26, No. 5, Supple 51 (September-October 2008), pp. S35-S61, ISSN 0392-856X

Sattar, N., McCarey, D.W., Capell, H. & McInnes, I.B. (2003). Explaining how "high-grade" systemic inflammation accelerates vascular risk in rheumatoid arthritis. *Circulation,* Vol. 108, No. 24, (December 2003), pp. 2957-2963, ISSN 1524-4539

Sipe, J.D., Benson, M.D., Buxbaum, J.N., Ikeda, S., Merlini, G., Saraiva, M.J. & Westermark, P. (2010). Amyloid fibril protein nomenclature: 2010 recommendations from the nomenclature committee of the International Society of Amyloidosis. *Amyloid,* Vol.17, No. 3-4, (September 2010), pp. 101-104, ISSN 1744-2818

Ueda, M., Ando, Y., Nakamura, M., Yamashita, T., Himeno, S., Kim, J., Sun, X., Saito, S., Tateishi, T., Bergström, J. & Uchino, M. (2006). FK506 inhibits murine AA amyloidosis: possible involvement of T cells in amyloidogenesis. *Journal of Rheumatology,* Vol. 33, No. 11, (November 2006), pp. 2260-2270, ISSN 0315-162X

van der Hilst, J.C., Yamada, T., Op den Camp, H.J., van der Meer, J.W., Drenth, J.P. & Simon, A. (2008). Increased susceptibility of serum amyloid A 1.1 to degradation by MMP-1: potential explanation for higher risk of type AA amyloidosis. *Rheumatology (Oxford),* Vol. 47, No. 11, (November 2008), pp. 1651-1654, ISSN 1462-0332

van der Hilst, J.C.., Kluve-Beckerman, B., van der Meer, J.W. & Simon, A. (2009). Cathepsin D activity protects against development of type AA amyloid fibrils. *European Journal of Clinical Investigation,* Vol. 39, No. 5, (May 2009), pp. 412-416, ISSN 1365-2362

Westermark, G.T. & Westermark, P. (2009). Serum amyloid A and protein AA: molecular mechanisms of a transmissible amyloidosis. *Federation of European Biochemical Societies Letters,* Vol. 583, No. 16, (August 2009), pp. 2685-2690, ISSN 1873-3468

Yamada, T., Sato, J. & Okuda, Y. (2009). Differential affinity of serum amyloid A1 isotypes for high-density lipoprotein. *Amyloid,* Vol. 16, No. 4, (December 2009), pp. 196-200, ISSN 1744-2818

3

Diagnosis and Treatment of AA Amyloidosis with Rheumatoid Arthritis: State of the Art

Takeshi Kuroda[1], Yoko Wada[1] and Masaaki Nakano[2]
[1]*Division of Clinical Nephrology and Rheumatology, Niigata University Graduate School of Medical and Dental Sciences, Chuo-ku, Niigata City,*
[2]*Department of Medical Technology, School of Health Sciences, Faculty of Medicine, Niigata University, Chuo-ku, Niigata City,*
Japan

1. Introduction

Amyloidosis is a term applied to a heterogeneous group of rare diseases characterized by extracellular deposition of amyloid, causing target-organ dysfunction and a wide range of clinical symptoms [1]. These symptoms depend on the organ involved, and include nephrotic syndrome, hepatosplenomegaly, congestive heart failure, carpal tunnel syndrome, gastrointestinal (GI) symptoms and macroglossia [2]. Amyloidosis is clinically classified into several types depending on the precursor of the amyloid fibril. The disease involves amyloid fibrils formed in vivo by 27 different types of protein [3] (Table 1). Reactive amyloid A (AA) amyloidosis is the representative systemic condition that develops in patients with chronic inflammatory diseases such as rheumatoid arthritis (RA), juvenile idiopathic arthritis, ankylosing spondylitis, inflammatory bowel disease, familial periodic fever syndrome, and chronic infections [4,5,6,7]. In some parts of the world, heredofamilial causes and infections are responsible for a larger proportion of cases of AA amyloidosis. In Turkey, familial Mediterranean fever (FMF) is the cause of more than 60 percent of cases [8]. Other conditions that may be associated with AA amyloidosis include neoplasms, particularly renal cell carcinoma [9], non-Hodgkin lymphoma [10], Castleman's disease [11], and cystic fibrosis [12]. Recently, therapy with biologic agents including anti-tumor necrosis factor (anti-TNF) and anti-interleukin-6 (IL-6) is now employed routinely for the management of RA in patients for whom traditional disease-modifying anti-rheumatic drugs (DMARDs) have failed. In parallel with this shift of treatment strategy, the treatment of amyloidosis has also changed. This article discusses current concepts of AA amyloidosis that is mainly secondary to RA, and addresses various strategies for prophylaxis, diagnosis, and therapy of this important complication in the light of changes in clinical management, especially hemodialysis (HD).

2. Prevalence

Epidemiological data for AA amyloidosis, extrapolated from autopsy records in Western nations, has indicated that the prevalence varies from about 0.5% to 0.86% according to environmental risk factors and geographic clustering [13,14]. The incidence of AA amyloidosis in RA is still undefined, and is considered to be underestimated. In Europe, 5-20% of patients with RA develop amyloidosis, with the highest incidence in Finland [15], where reevaluation of autopsy materials for the period 1952-1991 yielded a 30% incidence of AA amyloidosis compared with 18% detected by routine testing, indicating that a significant proportion of cases may not be detected by standard histologic analysis [16]. Japanese autopsy reports have revealed that about 30% of autopsied RA patients have amyloid deposits [17]. Some Japanese medical centers have reported the incidence of amyloidosis in consecutive patients undergoing GI biopsy. The frequency of amyloidosis in RA has been reported to vary between 5% and 13.3% in cases confirmed by biopsy, and from 14% to 26% in cases confirmed at autopsy [18,19,20,21].

Amyloid protein	Precursor	Systemic (S) or localized, organ restricted (L)	Syndrome or involved tissues
AL	Immunoglobulin light chain	S, L	Primary Myeloma-associated
AH	Immunoglobulin heavy chain	S, L	Primary Myeloma-associated
Aβ_2M	β_2-microglobulin	S L?	Hemodialysis-associated Joints
ATTR	Transthyretin	S L?	Familial Senile systemic Tenosynovium
AA	(Apo)serumAA	S	Secondary, reactive
AApoAI	Apolipoprotein AI	S L	Familial Aorta, meniscus
AApoAII	Apolipoprotein AII	S	Familial
AApoAIV	Apolipoprotein AIV	S	Sporadic, associated with aging
AGel	Gelsolin	S	Familial (Finnish)
ALys	Lysozyme	S	Familial
AFib	Fibrinogen α-chain	S	Familial
ACys	Cystatin C	S	Familial
ABri	ABriPP	S	Familial dementia, British
ALect2	Leukocyte chemotactic factor 2	S	Mainly kidney
ADan*	ADanPP	L	Familial dementia, Danish
Aβ	Aβ protein precursor (AβPP)	L	Alzheimer's disease, aging
APrP	Prion protein	L	Spongioform encephalopathies
ACal	(Pro) calcitonin	L	C-cell thyroid tumors
AIAPP	Islet amyloid polypeptide**	L	Islets of Langerhans Insulinomas
AANF	Atrial natriuretic factor	L	Cardiac atria
APro	Prolactin	L	Aging pituitary Prolactinomas
Ains	Insulin	L	Iatrogenic
AMed	Lactadherin	L	Senile aortic, media
AKer	Kerato-epithelin	L	Cornea, familial
ALac	Lactoferrin	L	Cornea
AOaap	Odontogenic ameloblast-associated protein	L	Odontogenic tumors
ASemI	Semenogelin I	L	Vesicula seminalis

*Proteins are listed, when possible, according to relationship. Thus, apolipoproteins are grouped together, as are polypeptide hormones.
*ADan comes from the same gene as ABri. **Also called 'amylin'.

Table 1. Amyloid fibril proteins and their precursors in humans.*

Although the subclinical phase of AA amyloidosis is defined by the formation of amyloid deposits in tissue without any clinical manifestation, it is very difficult to distinguish between the clinical and subclinical phases. Obviously, it is difficult to evaluate the natural history of amyloid deposition and to know the length of this phase and its final outcome. In contrast, the prevalence of clinical amyloidosis is likely to be lower; at least half of amyloidosis patients have subclinical disease, and AA amyloidosis is clinically overt in only 25-50%, even after longer periods of follow-up sampling. Considering this discrepancy between the prevalence rates of clinical and subclinical AA amyloidosis, the wide variation in the prevalence of AA amyloidosis secondary to RA is due partly to marked geographic differences worldwide, possibly including genetic factors, and to the lack of unified statistical studies of AA amyloidosis among races and districts. In view of these factors, the prevalence of AA amyloidosis associated with RA is probably higher than that estimated so far.

3. Pathogenesis of amyloid fibril formation and genetic background

Precise details of the mechanism of amyloid fibril formation are unknown, and may differ among the various types of amyloid [22, 23]. Factors that contribute to fibrillogenesis include a variant or unstable protein structure, extensive β-conformation of the precursor protein, association with components of the serum or extracellular matrix, and physical properties including the pH of the tissue site. Extracellular matrix components include the amyloid P component, amyloid enhancing factor (AEF), apolipoprotein E, and glycosaminoglycans (GAG). Amyloidosis is classified clinically into several types according to the precursor of the amyloid fibril and the type of amyloid fibril protein. Any complete definition of amyloidosis includes the amyloid fibril protein precursor, the protein type or variant, and the clininal setting at diagnosis [3]. Table 1 shows the types of amyloid protein, precursor proteins, localization and syndrome, or the involved tissues. Reactive systemic AA (secondary) amyloidosis complicates many chronic inflammatory diseases and has been studied most widely in experimental animal models. AA amyloid also occurs spontaneously in various animal species, and can be induced by chronic inflammatory stimuli. The best-known model of this disease is amyloid induction by injection of casein/azocasein in certain genetically susceptible strains of mice. AA fibril formation can be accelerated by an AEF in murine models present at high concentraiton in the spleen, by basement membrane heparan sulfate proteoglycan, or by seeding with AA or heterologous fibrils [24,25]. (AEF has not yet been detected in humans.) Therefore, sustained overproduction of SAA is a prerequisite for the development of AA amyloidosis. The mechanism of amyloidosis is initiated by overproduction of SAA as a consequence of acute and chronic inflammation. Next, SAA is internalized by macrophages, followed by intracellular proteolysis, and subsequent release of amyloidogenic peptides into the extracellular space, apparently preceding fibril formation [26]. AA amyloidosis is caused by organ deposition of AA fibrils, which are formed from an N-terminal cleavage fragment of SAA [27]. SAA is a 104-amino-acid protein produced in the liver under transcriptional regulation by proinflammatory cytokines, and transported by a high-density lipoprotein (HDL), HDL3, in plasma [28,29,30,31]. SAA is encoded by a family of SAA genes, which are responsive to proinflammatory cytokines [32,33]. A major factor responsible for the development of AA amyloidosis is increased synthesis and subsequent degeneration of SAA under conditions of chronic inflammation. AA amyloidosis is a rare but serious complication of diseases that stimulate a sustained and substantial acute-phase response, and foremost of which is RA. In RA, there is increased synthesis of SAA accompanied by inflammation, which may be due to elevated levels of proinflammatory cytokines. The increased cytokine levels are correlated with synovitis, which may stimulate synoviocytes to produce SAA [26,34,35] (Figure 1). These mechanisms lead to elevated levels of SAA in joint fluid relative to serum [35], sometimes reaching up to 1,000 times the baseline level [36], thus facilitating the development of AA amyloidosis.

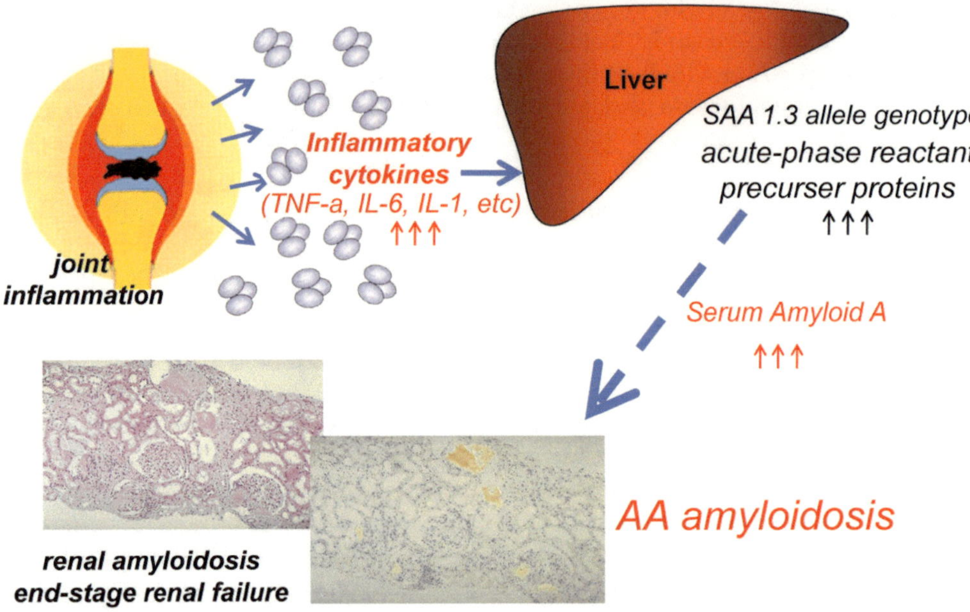

RA begins with joint synovitis, and serum amyloid A protein (SAA) is synthesized in the liver chiefly as a result of stimulation with proinflammatory cytokines. Genetic background factors such as the SAA 1.3 allele genotype are a risk factor for amyloidosis. Amyloid fibrils are deposited in tissues of various organs, leading to organ failure. TNF-α: tumor necrosis factor-α, IL-6: interleukin-6, IL-1: interleukin-1, SAA1.3: one of the SAA1 gene polymorphisms.

Fig. 1. Pathogenesis of AA amyloidosis secondary to RA

However, a high concentration of SAA alone is not sufficient for development of amyloidosis. Several genetic factors have been evaluated. Recent studies have focused on SAA polymorphism as a genetic background factor linked to amyloidogenesis. Allelic variants include acute phase SAAs (SAA1 and SAA2) and SAA4, and post-translational modifications of these gene products. SAA3 is a pseudogene with no product, and the serum concentration of SAA4 does not change during an acute-phase response [29]. The acute-phase proteins SAA1 and SAA2 are apolipoproteins, primarily associated with specific high-density lipoprotein (HDL), and are expressed extrahepatically in the absence of HDL [37]. SAA1 and SAA2 are inducible by interleukin (IL)-1, IL-6, tumor necrosis factor (TNF)- α, lipopolysaccharide (LPS), and several transcription factors, notably SAA activating factor (SAF-1) [38,39]. Both SAA1 and SAA2 are polymorphic proteins, and amyloid fibrils are considered to be formed in tissues from both SAAs1 and 2, but predominantly from SAA1 in humans [40]. Synthesis of amyloid protein from SAAs1 and 2 is strongly induced by inflammatory cytokines such as IL-6 in the liver, in parallel with the disease activity of RA [41]. SAA1 is the most important precursor for tissue AA deposition, because this isotype is predominant in plasma, and AA proteins are derived largely from it. SAA1 has three alleles, designated SAA1.1, SAA1.3, and SAA1.5, defined by amino acid substitutions at positions 52 and 57 of the molecule [3]. SAA2 has two alleles, SAA2.1 and 2.2. The frequency of these alleles varies among populations, and may be associated with the occurrence of AA amyloidosis in diseases such as RA, and also with the level of SAA in blood, efficacy of clearance, susceptibility to proteolytic cleavage by specific metalloproteinases, disease severity, and response to treatment [42]. The SAA1 alleles 1.1 and 1.3 have been proposed as positive risk factors in Caucasian and Japanese patients, respectively [43,44,45,46,47,48,49,50].

While the SAA1.1 allele was found to have a negative association with amyloidosis in Japanese subjects, it showed a positive association in Caucasians. Similarly, SAA1.3 showed an inverse association between Japanese and Caucasians. Recent new data have indicated that the -13T/C single nucleotide polymorphism in the 50-flanking region of SAA1 is a better marker of AA amyloidosis than the exon-3-based haplotype in both Japanese and American Caucasian populations [48,51,52].

Polymorphism of apolipoprotein E has been investigated as a potentially relevant genetic background factor, as this molecule is generally involved in the process of amyloid deposition [28]. According to several recent reports, apolipoprotein E4 is positively related to the development of AA amyloidosis in patients with RA [53]. Amyloid fibrils associate with other moieties, including GAG, serum amyloid P component (SAP) and apoprotein A-II of which are related to the onset of amyloidosis [30, 54]. The fibrils bind Congo red and exhibit green birefringence when viewed by polarization light microscopy, although the deposits can also be recognized in hematoxylin and eosin-stained sections [55, 56]. Electron microscopy demonstrates deposits of amyloid fibril protein in tissues as rigid, non-branching fibrils approximately 8 to 10 nm wide and of varying length, with a 2.5 to 3.5 nm filamentous subunit arranged with a slow twist along the long axis of the fibril [57]. When isolated and analysed by X-ray diffraction, the fibrils exhibit a characteristically abnormal β-sheet pattern [58]. Typing of amyloid deposits can be done by conventional immunohistochemical staining.

4. Diagnosis

A cohort study of patients with RA has shown that deposits of fat AA fibrils are not uncommon (16.3%) [59]. Any patient with long-standing active inflammatory disease, such as RA, who develops proteinuria or intractable diarrhea must first be investigated for AA amyloidosis. No blood test is specially diagnostic for amyloidosis. Results of tests confirming the presence of chronic inflammatory disease, such as increased levels of erythrocyte sedimentation rate (ESR), C-reactive protein (CRP), and SAA, are not necessarily discriminatory, because most patients with chronic inflammation do not develop amyloidosis. The next step for diagnosis is to perform a biopsy and histopathological examination. In order to begin intensive treatment as early as possible before organ function worsens, it is important to choose a high-sensitivity biopsy site and employ a safe technique. In general, subcutaneous fat, spleen, adrenal gland, liver, labial salivary gland, and sites in the alimentary canal ranging from the tongue and gingiva to the rectum, are frequent sites of AA amyloid deposition [60,61,62,63,64,65,66,67,68,69]. Many non-invasive techniques are useful for assessing organ involvement, but cannot establish whether the findings are related to amyloid. The definitive diagnostic test is biopsy of either an accessible tissue expected to contain amyloid, or a clinically affected organ. GI, rectal and subcutaneous fat biopsies are the procedures of choice, because the methodology is simple [18,70,71,72]. Aspiration biopsy of abdominal fat is recommended for screening in outpatient clinics because it is easy to perform in that setting, requires no specialty consultation or technical experience, has a high yield, and results in only minimal side effects [59]. As experience has shown that the amount of amyloid in fat tissue is low, the operator should aspirate as large a sample as possible. If possible, GI and rectal biopsies are also recommended because their sensitivity is high and they can also be performed at hospitals in an outpatient setting. Generally, in AA amyloidosis, the GI is a more sensitive site for biopsy than subcutaneous fat aspiration [18,61]. The detection rate is higher in the duodenal bulb and second portion of the small intestine than in the stomach. Additionally, the incidence of amyloidosis in GI biopsies is highly correlated with that in renal biopsies [19]. If GI biopsy reveals amyloid deposition, the presence of renal amyloidosis should be considered [19]. However, a more recent study has revealed that the amounts of amyloid deposition in GI and renal biopsies are not correlated. GI amyloid-positive areas are larger than renal amyloid-positive areas [73]. If a fat biopsy proves negative, biopsy of the clinically involved site is suggested for patients with a limited number of affected organs. More organ-specific biopsies, such as heart, kidney and liver, are recommended, and it is useful to determine the type of amyloidosis. However, such biopsy sites carry a relatively higher risk than GI, rectal or subcutaneous fat biopsies. In such cases, clinicians should weigh the risks and benefits of biopsy. In Japan, however, GI biopsy is commonly performed for screening, rather than fat biopsy. If amyloidosis is strongly suspected clinically in association with marked inflammation, annual screening biopsy is recommended. The many reports of renal biopsy results for RA patients have suggested that renal amyloidosis is the most serious complication. In RA patients, renal biopsy can sometimes be hazardous, because of difficulties in maintaining a fixed body position, osteoporosis, or advanced age [74]. Renal involvement tends to determine the clinical course in such patients. Renal biopsy can also reveal underlying renal disorder such as mesangial proliferative glomerulonephritis (MesPGN), membranous nephropathy (MN), and thin basement membrane disease (TBMD). Pathological information on such underlying conditions is sometimes very important for the treatment of concomitant amyloidosis. Amyloid cardiomyopathy and autonomic neuropathy have been extremely rare in previously reported series [66], but should be keep in mind when interpreting biopsy results. The third step is histological diagnosis of amyloidosis, which can be established by light microscopy using special staining for amyloid. Alkaline Congo red has long been the standard method of staining for amyloid [55,56,63]. Deposits of amyloid bind Congo red and exhibit apple-green birefringence when viewed by polarization light microscopy. This provides definitive diagnosis of amyloidosis. However, Dylon stain is more sensitive, and is therefore more useful for the detection of small amounts of amyloid [68, 69]. The use of Dylon stain, also known as direct fast scarlet, has recently become more popular. However, it requires more careful observation because of a tendency for over-staining (Figure 2). Thioflavin T is also more sensitive than Congo red, but less specific [75,76,77]. Although it yields a more intense fluorescent reaction, over-staining often hinders accurate diagnosis. If biopsy samples show a positive reaction, the type of amyloidosis should then be determined. Immunohistochemistry with fluorescent antibodies specific for precursor proteins, such as light chain j, k, SAA, etc., is a reliable diagnostic complement. Additional testing of serum and urine samples for monoclonal immunoglobulins, and of serum for free light chains, should be performed to exclude AL amyloidosis. Amino acid sequencing and mass spectroscopy of amyloid deposits have been utilitized to identify the precursor protein in some cases, but these techniques are not used routinely. Electron microscopy demonstrates straight, unbranched amyloid fibrils 8 to10 nm in width. Scintigraphy using radio-labeled SAP can identify the distribution of amyloid, and provide an estimate of the total body burden of fibrillar deposits [78]. However, the value of SAP scintigraphy is limited because

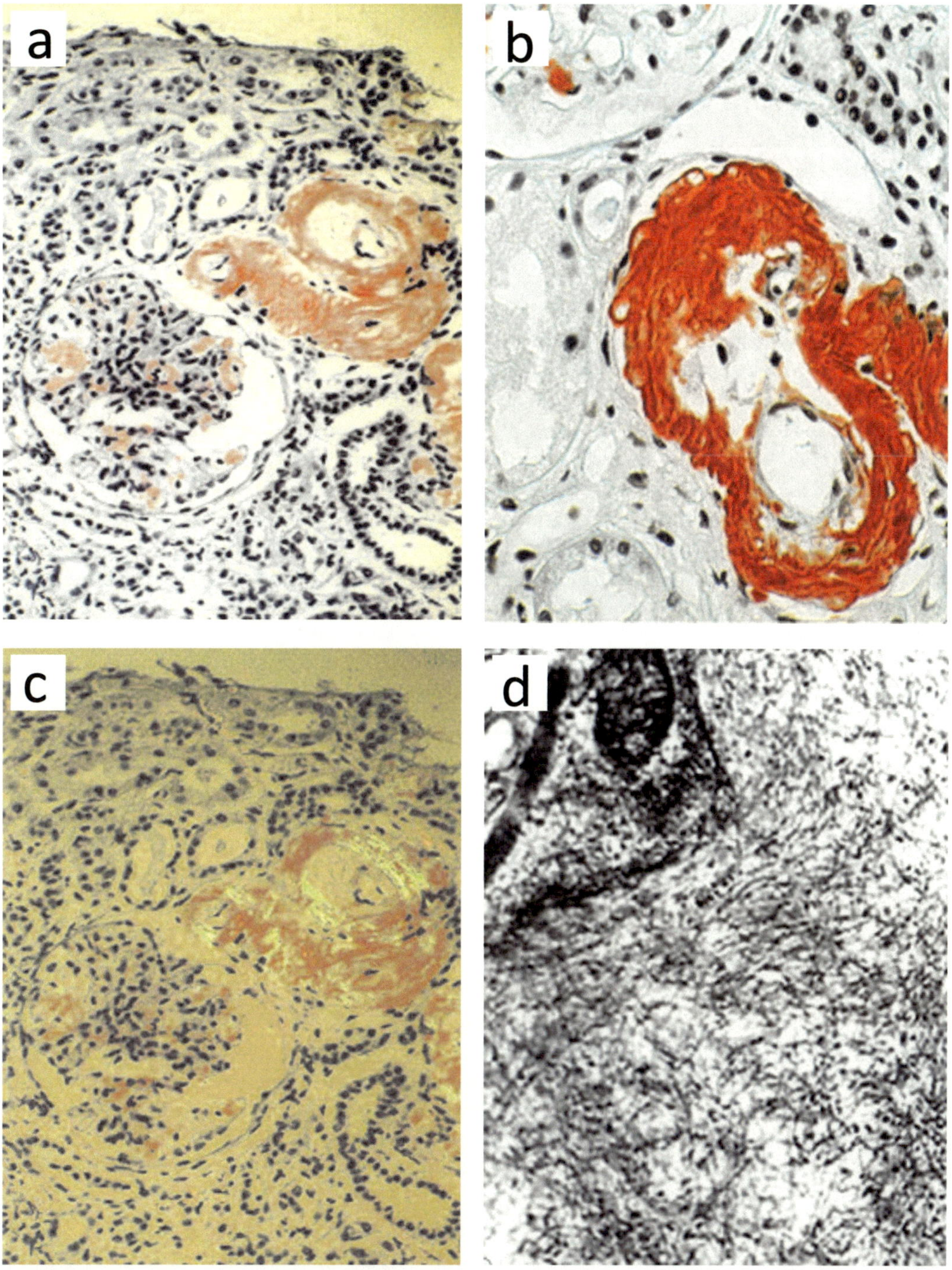

Amyloid substance is reactive with Congo red stain (a) and Dylon stain (b), and shows apple-green fluorescence under a polarizing microscope (c). Electron microscopy shows thin amyloid fibrils with a diameter of about 10 nm in AA and AL amyloidosis.

Fig. 2. Histological diagnosis of renal amyloidosis

it is obtained from blood donors, and it is possible to perform limited facilities. Additionally, it is less helpful for detecting cardiac amyloid. The fourth step is to initiate treatment. If AA amyloid is revealed in any organ, the treatment should be focused on systemic amyloidosis, while giving due attention to any underlying chronic inflammatory diseases. If AA amyloidosis is related to tuberculosis or FMF, treatment of these underlying diseases should also be started. It is important to introduce specific therapies for individual diseases in such cases.

5. Clinical features

The clinical features of amyloidosis are compatible with the infiltration of amyloid deposits. AA amyloidosis is a serious disease with a significant mortality due to end-stage renal disease, heart failure, bowel perforation, or GI bleeding [70,79]. Common clinical features of AA amyloidosis are proteinuria, loss of renal function, and gastrointestinal disorders. A clinical diagnosis of amyloidosis is usually suspected if proteinuria, renal insufficiency, or intractable diarrhea is present. Attention should also be paid to long-lasting and high inflammatory disease activity. Although AA amyloid can sometimes be detected in patients with arthritis in the absence of other clinical features, the clinical importance of such "silent" deposits remains to be determined. Renal involvement is a well-known complication of amylodiosis with RA. It is usually manifested as proteinuria or nephrotic syndrome with a variable degree of renal impairment that may progress to end-stage renal disease (ESRD). If proteinuria worsens to about 0.5 g/day, amyloidosis should be suspected even if other reasons are plausible. In RA, several underlying renal disorders accompanying renal amyloidosis have been observed [80], including MesPGN, MN, TBMD, and interstitial nephritis [80]. Crescentic glomerulonephritis is a rare underlying disease in RA patients, and can result in rupture of the fragile glomerular basement membrane due to amyloid deposition [81]. Usually, MesPGN and interstitial nephritis are associated with mild to moderate proteinuria, and MN with severe proteinuria. TBMD shows no proteinuria, and usually hematuria alone is evident. Histological investigation frequently demonstrates renal amyloidosis concomitant with these underlying diseases [80]. In renal tissue, primary amyloid deposition may be limited to the blood vessels or tubules. Such patients present with renal failure but little or no proteinuria [82]. These deposits lead to narrowing of the vascular lumina [83]. Glomerular deposits are more common, and are associated with a poor renal outcome in patients with AA and RA. One report has described that 27 patients with renal amyloidosis due to RA had glomerular deposits, and that 85 percent of them showed progression to ESRD during a five-year observation period. However, patients with vascular and tubular amyloid deposits showed no deterioration of renal function [84]. Such patients with vascular and tubular amyloid deposits usually present with slowly progressive chronic kidney disease with little or no proteinuria, and their prognosis appears to be more favorable [84]. The kidneys are usually enlarged slightly when nephrotic, but show a decrease in size as ESRD ensues.

GI symptoms, such as alternating periods of constipation and diarrhea or bleeding, may frequently suggest early localization of amyloid deposits and warrant further investigation. Abdominal distention and appetite loss are also frequently observed. Diminished peristalsis and malabsorption are common results of amyloid deposition, and can lead to nausea, vomiting, diarrhea, or hypoalbuminemia [85]. Endoscopy may demonstrate erosion, ulceration, mucosal weakness, or micro-polyposis, but sometimes no abnormality is evident in patients with mild amyloid deposition [61,86]. Fatal pancreatitis can sometimes occur at the end-stage of renal disease, and this is due to vascular obstruction in the pancreas by amyloid deposits [87]. Liver involvement can be manifested as weight loss, fatigue, and abdominal pain. About one-fourth of patients with amyloidosis have hepatic disease. Clinical signs may include only mild hepatomegaly with elevation of the serum alkaline phosphatase level [88]. However, most patients show concurrent extrahepatic manifestations.

In the cardiovascular system, amyloid deposition is limited to the heart. In cases of unexplained heart failure, only small amounts of amyloid deposition are observed around the vascular walls. In contrast, in AL amyloidosis, massive cardiac involvement is invariably evident. Unlike the situation in AL amyloidosis, cardiac involvement in reactive AA amyloidosis is not so common, affecting only about 10% of patients, and clinically overt heart failure is usually present in the terminal phase of the disease course, in addition to ESRD [89]. Restrictive cardiomyopathy or ischemic heart disease is rarely the cause of death [90]. Hypertension is frequent, and hypotension is rare in such patients, except in those with end-stage renal failure. Hypothyroidism due to amyloid deposition is sometimes observed [91]. In AA amyloidosis, involvement of the musculoskeletal system is rare. Usually, most of the symptoms are due to RA itself, and amyloid deposits do not elicit musculoskeletal symptoms. Central nervous system involvement is also unusual. Infiltration of subcutaneous fat is generally asymptomatic, but provides a convenient site for biopsy.

6. Management and treatment

Clinicians should remain vigilant for early signs of amyloidosis. For this purpose, patients with chronic rheumatic disorders, including those with elevated levels of inflammatory markers despite adequate symptom control by specific therapy, should undergo periodic urinalysis or assessments of 24-hour urinary protein excretion. If proteinuria exceeds 1(+) or increases to 0.5 g/day, screening for amyloidosis should be performed, including abdominal fat aspiration, or GI or rectal biopsy, to search for amyloid deposits [42]. Occasionally, GI symptoms, such as alternating periods of constipation and diarrhea or bleeding, may suggest early localization of amyloid deposits and warrant further investigation. If possible, GI endoscopy is recommended, because of its diagnostic yield. If a positive biopsy result is obtained after Congo red staining, accurate immunohistochemical characterization of amyloid as the AA type is mandatory. Once amyloidosis has developed, the SAA concentration over the course of the disease represents the main factor affecting renal progression and survival [36,92]. A previous study has revealed a relationship between turnover and regression of amyloid deposits and the corresponding clinical benefit, in terms of both organ function and survival [36].

AA amyloidosis occurs in patients who have persistently high plasma SAA concentrations, as part of the acute-phase response to a wide range of diseases. The natural history of AA amyloidosis is typically progressive, leading to organ failure and death, in patients whose underlying inflammatory disease remains active. By contrast, patients in whom the serum SAA concentration falls to within the reference range as a result of anti-inflammatory therapy show regression of amyloid deposits, stabilisation or recovery of amyloidotic organ function, and excellent long-term survival [93]. The therapeutic approach to AA involves treatment of the RA inflammatory process. It is important to control the level of SAA protein, which is the precursor of AA amyloid. It appears that reduction of the SAA level to less than 10 mg/L allows resorption of the deposits and prevents further accumulation [92]. Frequent monitoring of SAA, when available, is therefore recommended in patients with AA amyloidosis as a guide to treatment strategy and follow-up. Alternatively, quantification of CRP may provide a valid marker for monitoring the effective suppression of underlying inflammation in these patients. The therapeutic strategy is shown in Table 2. It may be assumed that tight control of RA with any other DMARDs such as methotrexate (MTX), cyclophosphamide, azathioprine, tacrolimus, mycophenolate mofetil, and a combination of DMARDs would have a similar impact. A small retrospective study has indicated that cyclophosphamide may confer a significant survival benefit in patients with RA and renal AA amyloidosis [94]. In that study, six of 15 patients received monthly pulse cyclophosphamide following confirmation of renal involvement. These patients treated with cyclophosphamide survived longer than those administered non-alkylating drugs [94]. Trends toward decreased proteinuria and maintenance of renal function have also been noted with cyclophosphamide. Similar results have been confirmed in a cohort study reported from Japan [95]. Prospective studies are required to properly assess the role and toxicity of this agent in this setting. Recent studies have indicated the therapeutic benefit of anti-TNF or anti-IL-6 agents for AA amyloidosis secondary to inflammatory arthritides, including RA [93,96,97,98,99,100]. These agents strongly inhibit the production of SAA. If possible, for the treatment of reabsorption of amyloid deposits, and, possibly, recovery of target organ function, treatment with biologics has been recommended. Tocilizumab has an excellent inhibitory effect on disease activity and joint destruction, and is therapeutically beneficial for the symptoms of AA amyloidosis, especially intractable diarrhea [101]. Although there are no data for the effect of abatacept on AA amyloidosis, it may be effective in theory. AA amyloid deposits exist in a state of dynamic turnover, and the outcome is favorable when the SAA concentration is maintained at below 10 mg/L. The potential for amyloid to regress and for the function of amyloidotic organs to recover support the use of therapeutic strategies to decrease the supply of amyloid fibril precursor proteins in amyloidosis generally [36]. The use of biologics is not part of the conventional treatment approach, and they are chosen according to the conditions in individual patients, such as renal and pulmonary function. If there is any risk of infection, short-acting biologics are desirable. Especially, in the case of tocilizmab, infection may be difficult to find, and clinicians need to be vigilant. Treatment with biologic agents is prohibited in certain circumstances, such as severe infections or demyelinating diseases. The treatment of patients with coexisting RA and hepatitis B poses a difficult therapeutic challenge because of the risk that treatment of the RA could aggravate hepatic disease and increase viremia. In general, the use of biologics such as anti-TNF and anti-IL-6 is contraindicated in patients who are HBV carriers or have chronic hepatitis B. However, in clinical practice, it is necessary to use anti-TNF in these patients. The existing data suggest that treatment of such patients with etanercept and tocilizmab co-administered with lamivudine or entecavir is safe [102,103]. If treatments for the organ damage, such as immunosuppressive agents or anti-cytokine therapy, are unavailable, medium-dose steroid (prednisolone 10~40 mg daily) is effective. However, it is important to establish a diagnosis in the early stage without organ damage, and robust treatment for RA is the most reasonable approach. A recent report has indicated that eprodisate is a useful antifibril compound for treatment of AA amyloidosis, significantly delaying progression to HD or ESRD [104].

Control SAA synthesis
(1) Tight control of disease activity of RA
a) DMARDs: MTX as the anchor drug
b) Immunosupressant: cyclophosphamide, azathiopurine, tacrolimus, MMF
c) Biologics: anti-TNF, anti-IL-6, abatacept
d) Antifibril drug: eprosidate
Supportive treatment
(1) Cardiac
a) Congestive heart failure*: Salt restriction, Diuretics
b) Arrhythmia: Pacemaker, Automatic implantable cardiac defibrillator, Antiarrythmics
(2) Renal
a) Nephrotic syndrome: Salt restriction, Maintain dietary protein, ACE inhibiter, ARB
b) Renal failure: Dialysis (HD,CAPD) : Programmed initiation**
(3) Gastrointestinal
a) Diarrhea: Steroid, codeine phosphate, lactate bacteria, octreotide, parenteral nutrition, anti-IL-6
(4) Others
a) DMSO: resoluble amyloid deposits (very limited)
b) HB carrier : Etanercept with anti-viral agents is relatively safe.

SAA serum amyloid A protein, RA rheumatoid arthritis, DMARDs disease-modifying antirheumatic Drugs, MTX methotrexate, MMF mycophenolate mofetil, TNF tumor necrosis factor, IL-6 interleukin-6, ACE angiotensin converting enzyme, ARB angiotensin receptor blocker, HD hemodialysis, CAPD continuous ambulatory peritoneal dialysis, DMSO dimethyl sulfoxide
*If co-existence of renal failure, CHDF (Continuous hemodiafiltration) is effective.
** To avid the trouble for the HD initiation, programmed initiation is recommended

Table 2. Treatment for AA amyloidosis

When considering supplementary treatment, cardiac amyloidosis is major therapeutic problem. Loop diuretics are the main therapeutic agents for the managements of volume overload. However, many patients with cardiac amyloidosis mostly have concomitant renal amyloidosis, making it difficult to maintain a balance between edema and intravascular contraction. Antihypertensive treatment is also important. A recent report has indicated that etanercept was effective in a patient with cardiac amyloidosis associated with RA [100]. Heart failure is known to be a contraindication for the heart failure [105], but the condition under the control of heart failure, biologics may be effective. With regard to renal impairment in patients with RA and amyloidosis, the serum creatinine (Cr) level is relatively low because of reduced muscle volume. Gender, long-lasting inflammation and RA, together with a low level of serum protein, may be associated with a decrease of muscle volume, and these in turn affect the level of serum Cr. This may partly explain why the serum Cr level is not elevated in comparison with creatinine clearance (Ccr) in patients with RA-associated amyloidosis [106]. Measurement of the serum Cr level is convenient in an outpatient setting, and is considered useful for accurate estimation of renal function even in these states. Measurement of cystatin C and calculation of estimated glomerular filtration rate (eGFR) are also useful [107]. Care must be taken not to underestimate the level of Cr. If renal dysfunction has progressed to some extent, almost all cases will follow a final common pathway to renal failure. Clinicians should always be mindful of the serum Cr level, and initiate treatment of renal amyloidosis as early as possible [97]. For the treatment of renal amyloidosis, it is important to estimate renal function accurately. Because the muscle volume in RA patients is relatively low, the serum Cr concentration does not reflect renal function. Even if the serum Cr level is normal, such patients may still have renal damage. If patients are in a nephrotic state, angiotensin converting enzyme (ACE) inhibitor and/or angiotensin II receptor antagonist (ARB) are effective for reducing the level of urinary protein. For patients with renal failure, dialysis is needed. The prognosis of those who require dialysis is not good, although some data suggest a survival benefit among patients with AA amyloidosis [70]. The poor prognosis of these patients is due mainly to a large number of sudden deaths immediately after introducing HD therapy [108,109]. Additionally, unplanned initiation of HD is significantly associated with poor survival. Therefore, properly planned initiation of HD is highly recommended. To circumvent the problem of HD initiation while ensuring its safety, the procedure for planned introduction is shown in Figure 3. Programmed initiation of HD will improve the prognosis of patients with ESRD [110]. Continuous ambulatory peritoneal dialysis (CAPD) can also be considered for patients with ESRD, as it has an advantage in preserving the functionality of the kidneys and avoiding hypotension associated with HD. However, in RA patients, disability of the hands due to chronic inflammation, and also the risk of peritonitis, should be considered [111]. Renal transplantation has been performed successfully for a number of patients with renal failure and AA amyloidosis, but only on a very limited basis [112]. In the near future, renal transplantation may become a recommended therapy for such patients. For treatment of GI symptoms, mostly intractable diarrhea, medium- to high-dose steroid (prednisolone 10~40 mg daily) is effective. Parenteral nutrition is also effective for this condition. Anti-IL-6 therapy is reportedly highly effective for intractable diarrhea [101]. However, immunosuppressive therapies, including biologics, may be associated with serious infection in amyloidosis patients. Advanced age is an important risk factor for infection in patients with RA. Some of the increased risk may be related to steroid usage. Additionally, such patients generally show low protein levels or hypoalbuminemia. These factors may lead to serious infection and/or opportunistic infection. It is possible that infection may exacerbate elevation of the SAA level and lead to additional organ damage. Preventive therapy against infection should always be borne in mind. Dimethyl sulfoxide (DMSO) has been proposed as a therapeutic agent that may solubilize AA deposits, and a number of patients have been treated with DMSO in an uncontrolled trial. There appeared to be salutary effects in some patients, but the accompanying body odor made the treatment unacceptable [113]. Recently, treatment with DMSO has been very limited. Earlier diagnosis of amyloidosis leads to better treatment and an improved chance of recovery.

7. Outcome

Survival after the diagnosis of AA amyloidosis secondary to RA seems to be 4–5 years [108,114]. Recently, however, a median survival period of more than 10 years after diagnosis has been reported [115]. Survival seems to depend on the timing of diagnosis, and this may partly explain the great individual variation in observed survival time, leading to the notion that an active diagnostic attitude for AA amyloidosis should be adopted in patients with RA. Treatment strategy is also important. Infection and renal failure are generally common causes of death in RA patients with AA amyloidosis [116,117]. A higher risk of severe infection is a substantial problem in the management of such patients. Potent immunosuppressive treatment may sometimes result in infection, and in such cases, prophylactic treatment with an antituberculosis agent is recommended. Increased production of SAA is a strong risk factor for ESRD and death, but this may be ameliorated by anti-inflammatory treatment. A relationship between SAA concentration, renal function and whole-body amyloid burden has been revealed. Outcome has been shown to be favorable in patients with AA amyloidosis when the SAA concentration is maintained below 10 mg/L [115]. Factors associated with poor prognosis are well known to include age at onset of RA and amyloidosis, female gender, a reduced serum albumin concentration, end-stage renal failure, the level of disease activity including serum levels of CRP and IgG, and the SAA concentration during follow-up [117]. Steroid dosage, and markers of renal function that are correlated with renal disease, such as BUN, Cr, and Ccr, at the time of detection of amyloidosis are important factors predictive of survival [108].

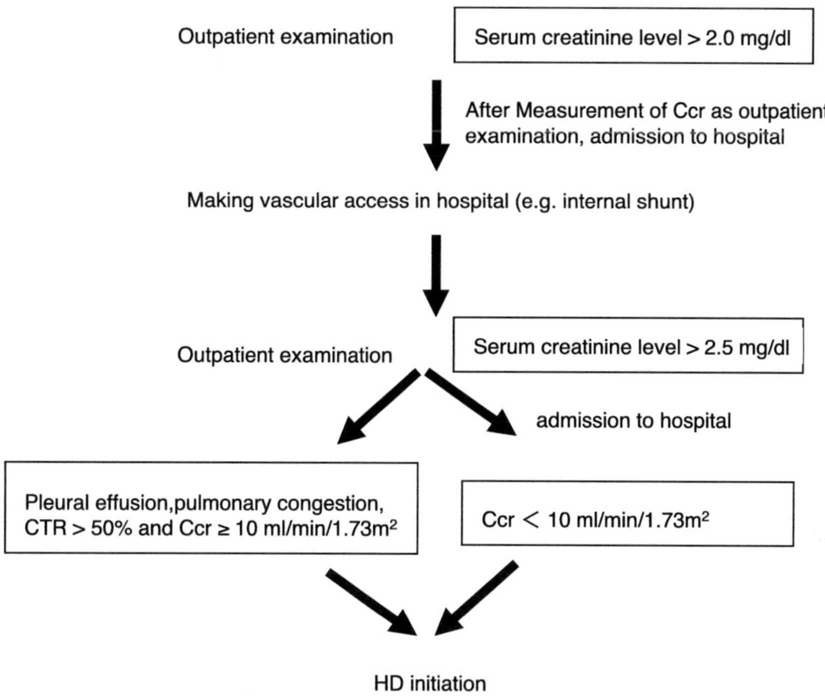

Schematic representation of the program used for our patients with end-stage renal disease due to reactive amyloidosis associated with rheumatoid arthritis. Ccr: creatinine clearance, CTR: cardiothoracic ratio

Fig. 3. Program of hemodialysis initiation

The results of dialysis for AA amyloidosis are extremely poor, and trouble with the initiation of HD in fact worsens prognosis, due to a rapid decline of renal function in the year preceding dialysis. Reported median survival after initiation of HD is more than 1 year [118], or more than 5 years [119]. These reports indicate that strict treatment and care will improve the clinical outcome. Amyloidotic cardiac involvement has been shown to be a poor prognostic factor [120,121]. Heart failure is one of the severe complications in these patients. Patients with heart failure usually have concomitant multiple organ failure, as well as renal failure, in the later phase of the RA disease course. To improve the outcome of these patients, frequent examinations for infection and acute inflammatory reactants such as CRP and SAA are necessary.

8. Conclusion

The best approach to treatment of amyloidosis is to prevent progression by controlling the serum level of SAA. In AA amyloidosis, proteinurea, renal dysfunction and GI symptoms are diagnostically informative. It is important not to overlook these symptoms, and to confirm the presence of amyloidosis by organ biopsy. Treatment with biologic agents plays a key role, especially for decreasing the production of SAA, along with prophylactic administration of anti-tuberculosis and anti-fungal agents. Monitoring of adverse events such as infection is an important part of the standard strategy associated with biologics treatment and checks for chronic inflammatory disorders should be conducted routinely. Physicians should make consideration to use biologics out of difficulties such as hepatitis B. These efforts should help to improve the outcome of patients with AA amyloidosis, achieve stabilization or regression of amyloid deposits, and prolong survival.

9. Acknowledgement

This work was supported in part by a Grant-in-Aid for scientific research from the Japanese Ministry of Health, Labour, and Welfare. The authors thank Professor Shinichi Nishi, M.D., Kobe University, for the photographs of renal tissue.

10. References

[1] Mueller OS. Amyloidosis. Current rheumatology diagnosis & treatment. 2nd ed. USA: Mc Graw Hill; 2007.
[2] Kyle RA. Amyloidosis: a convoluted story. Br. J Haematol. 2001; 114:529-538.
[3] Sipe JD, Benson MD, Buxbaum JN, et al. Amyloid fibril protein nomenclature: 2010 recommendations from the nomenclature committee of the International Society of Amyloidosis. Amyloid. 2010; 17: 101-104.
[4] Missen GA, Taylor JD. Amyloidosis in rheumatoid arthritis. J pathol Bact. 1956;71:179-192.
[5] Scheinberg MA, Hubscher O, Morteo OG, et al. Serum amyloid protein levels in south american children with rheumatoid arthritis: a co-operative study. Ann Rheum Dis. 1980; 39: 228–230.
[6] van Eijk IC, de Vries MK, Levels JH, et al. Improvement of lipid profile is accompanied by atheroprotective alterations in high-density lipoprotein composition upon tumor necrosis factor blockade: a prospective cohort study in ankylosing spondylitis. Arthritis Rheum. 2009;60:1324-1330.
[7] Greenstein AJ, Sachar DB, Panday AK. Amyloidosis and inflammatory bowel disease. A 50-year experience with 25 patients. Medicine (Baltimore). 1992;71:261-270.
[8] Ensari C, Ensari A, Tümer, et al. Clinicopathological and epidemiological analysis of amyloidosis in Turkish patients. Nephrol Dial Transplant. 2005;20:1721-1725.
[9] Pras M, Franklin EC, Shibolet S, et al. Amyloidosis associated with renal cell carcinoma of the AA type. Am J Med. 1982; 73:426-428.
[10] Piskin O, Alacacioglu I, Ozkal S, et al. A patient with diffuse large B-cell non-Hodgkin's lymphoma and AA type amyloidosis. J BUON. 2008; 13:113-116.
[11] Ogita, M, Hoshino, J, Sogawa, Y, et al. Multicentric Castleman disease with secondary AA renal amyloidosis, nephrotic syndrome and chronic renal failure, remission

after high-dose melphalan and autologous stem cell transplantation. Clin Nephrol. 2007; 68:171-176.
[12] Skinner, M, Pinnette, A, Travis, WD, et al. Isolation and sequence analysis of amyloid protein AA from a patient with cystic fibrosis. J Lab Clin Med. 1988; 112:413-417.
[13] Simms RW, Prout MN, Cohen AS. The epidemiology of AL and AA amyloidosis. Baillieres Clin Rheumatol 1994; 8: 627–634.
[14] Hazenberg BP, Van Rijswijk MH. Where has secondary amyloid gone? Ann Rheum Dis. 2000; 59: 577–579.
[15] Lender M, Wolf E. Incidence of amyloidosis in rheumatoid arthritis. Scand J Rheumatol. 1972;1:109-112.
[16] Koivuniemi R, Paimela L, Suomalinen R, et al. Amyloidosis is frequently undetected in patients with rheumatoid arthritis. Amyloid. 2008;15:262–268.
[17] Toyoshima H, Kusaba T, Yamaguchi M. Cause of death in autopsied RA patients. Rheumachi. 1993;33:209-214.
[18] Kobayashi H, Tada S, Fuchigami T, et al. Secondary amyloidosis in patients with rheumatoid arthritis: diagnostic and prognostic value of gastroduodenal biopsy. Br J Rheumatol. 1996;35:44–49.
[19] Kuroda T, Tanabe N, Sakatsume M, et al. Comparison of gastroduodenal, renal and abdominal fat biopsies for diagnosing amyloidosis in rheumatoid arthritis. Clin Rheumatol. 2002;21:123–128.
[20] Wakhlu A, Krisnani N, Hissatia P, et al. Prevalence of secondary amyloidosis in Asian north Indian patients with rheumatoid arthritis. J Rheumatol. 2003;30:948–951.
[21] Okuda Y, Takasugi K. Diagnostic and prognostic study of secondary amyloidosis complication rheumatoid arthritis. Amyloid and Amyloidosis. Parthenon Publishing Group. New York. pp426-428,1998.
[22] Bolloti V, Mangione P, Merline G. Immunoglobulin light chain amyloidosis-the archtype of structural and pathologic variability. J Struct Biol. 2000;130:280-289.
[23] Lansbury PT. Evolition of amyloid：What normal protein foldint may tell us about fibrinogenesis and disease. Proc Natl Acad Sci USA. 1999;96:3342-3344.
[24] Westermark GT, Westermark P. Serum amyloid A and protein AA: molecular mechanisms of a transmissible amyloidosis. FEBS Letter. 2009;583:2685-2690
[25] Yoshida T, Zhang P, Fu X, et al. Slaughtered aged cattle might be one dietary source exhibiting amyloid enhancing factor activity. Amyloid. 2009;16:25-31.
[26] Röcken C, Menard R, Bühling F, et al. Proteolysis of serum amyloid A and AA amyloid proteins by cysteine proteases: cathepsin B generates AA amyloid proteins and cathepsin L may prevent their formation. Ann Rheum Dis. 2005;64:808-815.
[27] Cunnane G. Amyloid precursors and amyloidosis in inflammatory arthritis. Curr Opin Rheumatol. 2001;13:67–73.
[28] Malle E, Steinmetz A, Raynes JG. Serum amyloid A (SAA): an acute phase protein and apolipoprotein. Atherosclerosis. 1993;102:131–146.
[29] Uhlar CM, Whitehead AS. Serum amyloid A, the major vertebrate acute-phase reactant. Eur J Biochem. 1999;265:501–523.
[30] Gallo G, Wisniewski T, Choi-Miura NH, et al. Potential role of apolipoprotein-E in fibrillogenesis. Am J Pathol. 1994;145:526–530.
[31] Husby G, Marhaug G, Dowton B, et al. Serum amyloid A (SAA): biochemistry, genetics and the pathogenesis of AA amyloidosis. Amyloid. 1994;1:119–137.
[32] Kelly JW. Alternative conformations of amyloidogenic proteins govern their behavior. Curr Opin Struct Biol. 1996; 6:11-17.

[33] Dobson CM. Protein folding and disease: a view from the first Horizon Symposium. Nat Rev Drug Discov. 2003, 2:154-160.

[34] Vallon R, Freuler F, Desta-Tsedu N, et al. Serum amyloid A (apoSAA) expression is up-regulated in rheumatoid arthritis and induces transcription of matrix metalloproteinases. J Immunol. 2001;166:2801-2807.

[35] Ray A, Schatten H, Ray BK. Activation of Sp1 and its functional co-operation with serum amyloid A-activating sequence binding factor in synoviocyte cells trigger synergistic action of interleukin-1 and interleukin-6 in serum amyloid A gene expression. J Biol Chem. 1999;274:4300-4308.

[36] Lachmann HJ, Goodman HJ, Gilbertson JA,et al. Natural history and outcome in systemic AA amyloidosis. N Engl J Med. 2007;356:2361-2371.

[37] O'Hara, R, Murphy, EP, Whitehead, AS, et al. Local expression of the serum amyloid A and formyl peptide receptor-like 1 genes in synovial tissue is associated with matrix metalloproteinase production in patients with inflammatory arthritis. Arthritis Rheum. 2004; 50:1788-1799.

[38] Thorn, CF, Lu, ZY, Whitehead, AS. Regulation of the human acute phase serum amyloid A genes by tumour necrosis factor-alpha, interleukin-6 and glucocorticoids in hepatic and epithelial cell lines. Scand J Immunol. 2004; 59:152-158.

[39] Ray, A, Shakya, A, Kumar, D, et al. Inflammation-responsive transcription factor SAF-1 activity is linked to the development of amyloid A amyloidosis. J Immunol. 2006; 177:2601-2609.

[40] Thorn CF, Whitehead AS. Differential glucocorticoid enhancement of the cytokine-driven transcriptional activation of the human acute phase serum amyloid A genes, SAA1 and SAA2. J Immunol. 2002;169:399-406.

[41] Nakamura T, Higashi S, Tomoda K, et al. Significance of SAA1.3 allele genotype in Japanese patients with amyloidosis secondary to rheumatoid arthritis. Rheumatology (Oxford). 2006;45:43-49.

[42] Obici, L, Raimondi, S, Lavatelli, F, et al. Susceptibility to AA amyloidosis in rheumatic diseases: a critical overview. Arthritis Rheum. 2009; 61:1435-1440.

[43] Baba S, Takahashi T, Kasama T, et al. Identification of two novel amyloid A protein subsets coexisting in an individual atient of AA-amyloidosis. Biochim Biophys Acta. 1992; 180:195–200.

[44] Baba S, Takahashi T, Kasama T, et al. A novel olymorphism of human serum amyloid A protein, SAA1 gamma, is characterized by alanines at both residues 52 and 57. Arch Biochem Biophys. 1993;303:361–366.

[45] Xu Y, Yamada T, Satoh T, et al. Measurement of serum amyloid A1 (SAA1), a major isotype of acute phase SAA. Clin hem Lab Med. 2006;44:59–63.

[46] Moriguchi M, Terai C, Koseki Y, et al. Influence of genotypes at SAA1 and SAA2 loci on the development and the length of latent period of secondary AAamyloidosis in patients with rheumatoid arthritis. Hum Genet. 1999;105:360–366.

[47] Utku U, Dilek M, Akpolat I, et al. SAA1 a/a alleles in Behcet's disease related amyloidosis. Clin Rheumatol. 2007;26:927–929.

[48] Yamada T, Okuda Y, Takasugi K, et al. An allele of serum amyloid A1 associated withamyloidosis in both Japanese and Caucasians. Amyloid. 2003;10:7–11.

[49] Nakamura T. Amyloid A amyloidosis secondary to rheumatoid arthritis: an uncommon yet important complication. Curr Rheumatol Rev. 2007;3:231–241.

[50] Baba S, Masago SA, Takahashi T, et al. A novel allelic variant of serum amyloid A, SAA1c: genomic evidence, evolution, frequency, and implication as a risk factor for reactive systemic AA-amyloidosis. Hum Mol Genet. 1995;4:1083–1087.
[51] Moriguchi M, Kaneko H, Terai C, et al. Relative transcriptional activities of SAA1 promoters polymorphic at position -13T(T/C): potential association between increased transcription and amyloidosis. Amyloid. 2005;12:26–32.
[52] Ajiro J, Narita I, Sato S, et al. SAA1 gene polymorphisms and the risk of AA amyloidosis on Japanese patients with rheumatoid arthritis. Mod Rheumatol. 2006;16:294–299.
[53] Hasegawa H, Nishi S, Ito S, et al. High prevalence of serum apolipoprotein E4 isoprotein in rheumatoid arthritis patients with amyloidosis. Arthritis Rheum. 1996;39:1728–1732.
[54] Coker AR, Purvis A, Baker D, et al. Molecular chaperone properties of serum amyloid P component. FEBS Letter. 2000;473:199–202.
[55] Elghetany MT, Saleem A, Barr K. The Congo red stain revisited.Ann Clin Lab Sci. 1989;19:190–195.
[56] Puchtler H, Waldrop FS, Meloan SN. A review of light, polarization and fluorescence microscopic methods for amyloid. Appl Pathol. 1985;3:5–17.
[57] Shirahama T, Cohen AS. High-resolution electron microscopic analysis of the amyloid fibril. J Cell Biol. 1967;33:679–708.
[58] Sipe JD, McAdam KP, Torain BF, et al. Conformational flexibility of the serum amyloid precursor SAA. Br J Exp Pathol. 1976;57:582-592.
[59] Gomez-Casanovas E, Sanmarti R, Sole M, et al. The clinical significance of amyloid fat deposit in rheumatoid arthritis. A systemic long-term follow up study using abdominal fat aspiration. Arthritis Rheum. 2001;44:66–72.
[60] Hachulla E, Janin A, Flipo RM, et al. Labial salivary gland biopsy is a reliable test for the diagnosis of primary and secondary amyloidosis. A prospective clinical and immunohistologic study in 59 patients. Arthritis Rheum. 1993;36:691-697.
[61] Tada S, Iida M, Iwashita A, et al. Endoscopic and biopsy findings of the upper digestive tract in patients with amyloidosis. Gastrointest Endosc. 1990;36:10-14.
[62] Falk RH, Comenzo RL, Skinner M. The systemic amyloidoses. N Engl J Med. 1997;337:898-909.
[63] Rocken C, Shakespeare A. Pathology, diagnosis and pathogenesis of AA amyloidosis. Virchows Arch. 2002;440:111-122.
[64] Murakami T, Yi S. Amyloidosis and hepatic amyloidosis. Nippon Rinsho. 1993;51:453-457.
[65] Libbey CA, Skinner M, Cohen AS. Use of abdominal fat tissue aspirate in the diagnosis Arch Intern Med 1983;143:1549-1552.
[66] Dubrey SW, Cha K, Simms RW, et al. Electrocardiography and Doppler echocardiography in secondary (AA) amyloidosis. Am J Cardiol. 1996;77:313-315.
[67] Mcalpine JC, Bancroft JD. A histological study of hyaline deposits in laryngeal, aural, and nasal polyps and their differentiation from amyloid. J Clin Pathol. 1964;17:213–219.
[68] Takahashi T, Miura H, Matsu-ura Y, Iwana S, Maruyama R, Harada T. Urine cytology of localized primary amyloidosis of the ureter: a case report. Acta Cytol. 2005;49:319–322.
[69] Iijima S. Primary systemic amyloidosis: a unique case complaining of diffuse eyelid swelling and conjunctival involvement. J Dermatol. 1992;19:113–118.

[70] Getz MA, Kyle RA. Secondary systemic amyloidosis. Response and survival in 64 patients. Medicine. 1991;70:246-254.
[71] Klem PJ, Sorsa S, Happonen RP. Fine-needle aspiration biopsy from subcutaneous fat: an easy way to diagnose secondary amyloidosis. Scand J Rheumatol. 1987;16:429-431.
[72] Bogov B, Lubomirova M, and Kiperova B. Biopsy of subcutaneus fatty tissue for diagnosis of systemic amyloidosis. Hippokratia. 2008;12:236–239.
[73] Kuroda T, Tanabe N, Kobayashi D, et al. Association between clinical parameters and amyloid-positive area in gastroduodenal biopsy in reactive amyloidosis associated with rheumatoid arthritis. Rheum Int. (in press)
[74] Stiles KP, Yuan CM, Chung EM, et al. Renal biopsy in high-risk patients with medical diseases of the kidney. Am J Kidney Dis. 2000;36:419–433.
[75] Stiller D, Katenkamp D, Thoss K. Staining mechanism of thioflavin T with special reference to the localization of amyloid. Acta Histochem. 1972;42:234–245.
[76] Nebut M, Hartmann L. Contribution of thioflavin T in the study of the early histologic lesions of experimental amyloidosis. Ann Biol Clin. 1966;24:1063–1079.
[77] Rogers DR. Screening for amyloid with the thioflavin-T fluorescent method. Am J Clin Pathol. 1965;44:59–61.
[78] Hazenberg BP, van Rijswijk MH, Piers DA, et al. Diagnostic performance of 123I-labeled serum amyloid P component scintigraphy in patients with amyloidosis. Am J Med. 2006;119:355.e15-24.
[79] Kuroda T, Tanabe N, Harada T, et al. Long-term mortality outcome in patients with reactive amyloidosis associated with rheumatoid arthritis. Clin Rheumatol. 2006;25:498-505.
[80] Nakano M, Ueno M, Nishi S, et al. Analysis of renal pathology and drug history in 158Japanese patients with rheumatoid arthritis. Clin Nephrol. 1998;50:154–160.
[81] Nagata M, Shimokama T, Harada A, et al. Glomerular crescents in renal amyloidosis: an epiphenomenon or distinct pathology? Pathol Int. 2001;51:179-186.
[82] Nishi S, Alchi B, Imai N, et al. New advances in renal amyloidosis. Clin Exp Nephrol. 2008;12:93–101.
[83] Falck HM, Törnroth T, Wegelius O. Predominantly vascular amyloid deposition in the kidney in patients with minimal or no proteinuria. Clin Nephrol. 1983; 19:137-142.
[84] Uda H, Yokota A, Kobayashi K, et al. Two distinct clinical courses of renal involvement in rheumatoid patients with AA amyloidosis. J Rheumatol. 2006; 33:1482-1487.
[85] Ebert EC, Nagar M. Gastrointestinal manifestations of amyloidosis. Am J Gastroenterol. 2008;103:776-787.
[86] Tada S, Iida M, Yao T et al. Endoscopic features in amyloidosis of the small intestine: clinical and morphologic differences between chemical types of amyloid protein. Gastrointest Endosc. 1994;40:45-50.
[87] Kuroda T, Sato H, Hasegawa H,et al. Fatal acute pancreatitis associated with reactive AA amyloidosis in rheumatoid arthritis with end-stage renal disease: a report of three cases. Intern Med. 2011;50:739-744.
[88] Ellen C. Ebert C, Klaus D. Hagspiel Gastrointestinal and Hepatic Manifestations of Rheumatoid Arthritis Dig Dis Sci. 2011;56:295–302.
[89] Hazenberg BP, van Rijswijk MH. Clinical and therapeutic aspects of AA amyloidosis. Bailliere's Clin Rheumatol. 1994; 8: 661-690.
[90] Lachmann HJ, Goodman HJB, Gallimore J *et al.* Characteristic and clinical outcome on 340 patients with systemic AA amyloidosis. In Grateau G, Kyle RA, Skinner M

(eds) Amyloid and Amyloidosis:10th International Symposium on Amyloidosis. Tours, France, 2004,173–175

[91] Kanoh T, Shimada H, Uchino H, et al. Amyloid goiter with hypothyroidism. Arch Pathol Lab Med. 1989;113:542-544.

[92] Gillmore JD, Lovat LB, Persey MR, et al. Amyloid load and clinical outcome in AA amyloidosis in relation to circulating concentration of serum amyloid A protein. Lancet. 2001;358:24-29.

[93] Gottenberg JE, Merle-Vincent F, Bentaberry F, et al. Anti-tumor necrosis factor alpha therapy in fifteen patients with AA amyloidosis secondary to inflammatory arthritides: a followup report of tolerability and efficacy. Arthritis Rheum. 2003;48:2019-2024.

[94] Chevrel G, Jenvrin C, McGregor B, et al. Renal type AA amyloidosis associated with rheumatoid arthritis: a cohort study showing improved survival on treatment with pulse cyclophosphamide. Rheumatology (Oxford). 2001; 40:821-825.

[95] Nakamura T, Yamamura Y, Tomoda K, et al. Efficacy of cyclophosphamide combined with prednisolone in patients with AA amyloidosis secondary to rheumatoid arthritis. Clin Rheumatol 2003; 22:371-375.

[96] Okuda Y, Takasugi K. Successful use of a humanized anti-interleukin-6 antibody, tocilizumab, to treat amyloid A amyloidosis complicating juvenile idiopathic arthritis. Arthritis Rheum. 2006;54:2997–3000.

[97] Kuroda T, Otaki Y, Sato H, et al. Improvement of renal function and gastrointestinal amyloidosis treated with Infliximab in a patient with AA amyloidosis associated with rheumatoid arthritis. Rheum Int. 2008;28:1155-1159.

[98] Kuroda T, Wada Y, Kobayashi D, et al. Effective anti-TNF-a therapy can induce rapid resolution and sustained decrease of gastroduodenal mucosal amyloid deposits in reactive amyloidosis associated with rheumatoid arthritis. J Rheumatol. 2009;36:2409-2415.

[99] Nakamura T, Higashi S, Tomoda K, et al. Etanercept can induce resolution of renal deterioration in patients with amyloid A amyloidosis secondary to rheumatoid arthritis.Clin Rheumatol. 2010 ;29:1395-1401.

[100] Wada Y, Kobayashi D, Murakami S, et al. Cardiac AA amyloidosis in a patient with rheumatoid arthritis and systemic sclerosis - the therapeutic potential of biologic reagents. Letter. Scand J Rheumatol. (in press)

[101] Sato H, Sakai T, Sugaya T, et al. Tocilizumab dramatically ameliorated life-threatening diarrhea due to secondary amyloidosis associated with rheumatoid arthritis. Clin Rheumatol. 2009;28:1113-1116.

[102] Kuroda T, Kobayashi D, Sato H, et al. Effect of etanercept and entecavil in a patient with rheumatoid arthritis who is a hepatitis B carrier: A review of the literature. Rheum Int. (in press)

[103] Kishida D, Okuda Y, Onishi M, et al. Successful tocilizumab treatment in a patient with adult-onset Still's disease complicated by chronic active hepatitis B and amyloid A amyloidosis. Mod Rheumatol. 2011;21:215-218.

[104] Dember LM, Hawkins PN, Hanzenberg BPC, et al. Eprodisate for the treatment of renal disease in AA amyloidosis. N Engl J Med. 2007;356:2349–2360.

[105] Mann DL, McMurray JJ, Packer M, et al. Targeted anticytokine therapy in patients with chronic heart failure: results of the Randomized Etanercept Worldwide Evaluation (RENEWAL). Circulation. 2004;109:1594-1602.

[106] Moriguchi M, Terai C, Koseki Y, et al. Renal function estimated from serum creatinine is overestimated in patients with rheumatoid arthritis because of their muscle atrophy. Mod Rheumatol. 2000;10:230–234.
[107] Sato H, Kuroda T, Tanabe N, et al. Cystatin C is a sensitive marker for detecting a reduced glomerular filtration rate when assessing chronic kidney disease in patients with rheumatoid arthritis and secondary amyloidosis. Scand J Rheumatol. 2010;39:33-37.
[108] Kuroda T, Tanabe N, Sato H, et al. Outcome of patients with reactive amyloidosis associated with rheumatoid arthritis in dialysis treatment. Rheumatol Int 2006;26:1147–1153.
[109] Hezemans RL, Krediet RT, Arisz L. Dialysis treatment in patients with rheumatoid arthritis. Neth J Med.1995;47:6-11.
[110] Kuroda T, Tanabe N, Kobayashi D, et al. Programmed initiation of hemodialysis for systemic amyloidosis patients associated with rheumatoid arthritis. Ruheumatol Int. (in press)
[111] Martinez-Vea A, García C, Carreras M, et al. End-stage renal disease in systemic amyloidosis: clinical course and outcome on dialysis. Am J Nephrol. 1990;10:283-289.
[112] Heering P, Hetzel R, Grabensee B, et al. Renal transplantation in secondary systemic amyloidosis. Clin Transplant. 1998;12:159-164.
[113] van Rijswijk MH, Ruinen L, Donker AJ,et al. Dimethyl sulfoxide in the treatment of AA amyloidosis. Ann N Y Acad Sci. 1983;411:67-83.
[114] van Gameren II, Hazenberg BP, Bijzet J, et al. Amyloid load in fat tissue reflects disease severity and predicts survival in amyloidosis. Artritis Care Res (Hoboken). 2010;62:296-301.
[115] Lachmann HJ, Goodman HJ, Gilbertson JA, Natural history and outcome in systemic AA amyloidosis. N Engl J Med. 2007;356:2361-2371.
[116] Suzuki A, Ohosone Y, Obana M, et al. Cause of death in 81 autopsied patients with rheumatoid arthritis. J Rheumatol. 1994;21:33–36.
[117] Joss N, McLaughlin K, Simpson K, et al. Presentation, survival and prognostic markers in AA amyloidosis. Q J Med. 2000;93:535–542.
[118] Bergesio F, Ciciani AM, Manganaro M, et al. Renal involvement in systemic amyloidosis: an Italian collaborative study on survival and renal outcome. Nephrol Dial Transplant. 2008;23:941-951.
[119] Bollée G, Guery B, Joly D, et al. Presentation and outcome of patients with systemic amyloidosis undergoing dialysis. Clin J Am Soc Nephrol. 2008;3:375-381.
[120] Shah KB, Inoue Y, Mehra MR. Amyloidosis and the heart. Arch Intern Med 2006; 166: 1805-1813.
[121] Falk RH. Diagnosis and management of the cardiac amyloidoses. Circulation. 2005; 112: 2047-2060.

4

Apolipoprotein A-I Associated Amyloidoses: The Intriguing Case of a Natively Unfolded Protein Fragment

Daria Maria Monti[1,2], Renata Piccoli[1,2] and Angela Arciello[1,2]
[1]*Department of Structural and Functional Biology, University of Naples Federico II, School of Biotechnological Sciences, Naples*
[2]*Istituto Nazionale di Biostrutture e Biosistemi (INBB), Italy*

1. Introduction

Nowadays, a main challenge for scientists is that of drawing a comprehensive picture, in which common traits shared by the amyloidogenic proteins identified so far, structurally and functionally different from one another, are depicted. From a structural point of view, a clear relationship between protein sequences and aggregation does not exist, although proteins able to aggregate in general are characterized by a low sequence complexity (Wootton & Federhen, 1996) and/or high net charge coupled with low mean hydrophobicity (Gast et al., 1995), as well as by the abundance of residues favouring the β-sheet secondary structure (Steward et al., 2002). From a functional point of view, amyloidogenic proteins are associated to a variety of cellular functions and activities, and in some cases their biological function is unknown. As for the localization of the disease, amyloidoses may be localized in the nervous system, as those implicated in neurodegenerative diseases, or may be systemic when target tissues for amyloid deposition are in peripheral organs.

Two main classes of fibrillogenic proteins have been identified: those with a compact folding in their native state and those that are partially unfolded. Studies on pre-amyloid order-disorder transitions are central to understand both the assembly mechanisms and the disease molecular bases. In the case of amyloidogenic proteins that are natively folded, destabilizing mutations and/or changes in solution conditions are key factors responsible for the induction of fibrillogenesis, as in the case of β_2-microglobulin ($A\beta_2M$) or the prion protein APrP (Chiti & Dobson, 2006). On the other hand, several amyloidogenic proteins or polypeptides are intrinsically disordered. Such proteins include the *β*-Amyloid peptide (Aβ), islet amyloid polypeptide (AIAPP) and α-synuclein (Abedini & Raleigh, 2009). These "natively unfolded" (Weinreb et al., 1996) proteins emerged as proteins lacking of almost any secondary structure and were shown to be extremely flexible and disordered under physiological conditions (Uversky, 2002). The main feature of these proteins is the intrinsic structural plasticity, as a disorder to order transition may occur upon functioning (Abedini & Raleigh, 2009).

In some cases, natively folded proteins generate unfolded fragments associated to the amyloid pathology. This may occur when a specific mutation diverts the fate of a globular protein converting it to the precursor of fragments responsible for fibril formation. Is this the case of Apolipoprotein A-I (ApoA-I) and its amyloidogenic N-terminal fragment.

1.1 Apolipoprotein A-I

ApoA-I is synthesized by the liver and the intestine as a *pre-pro*-protein. After the cleavage of the *pre-* and *pro-* peptides, the mature protein (28 kDa) is secreted in the plasma, where it is either associated to lipids, or in a lipid-free state (5-10%) (Brouillette et al., 2001). ApoA-I plays a critical role in lipid metabolism (Fielding & Fielding, 1995), both in delivering cholesterol to steroidogenic tissues and in transporting it from the periphery to the liver for catabolism, in the so called reverse cholesterol transport. Therefore, ApoA-I plays an anti-atherogenic role *in vivo*, with a protecting effect against cardiovascular diseases (Pastore et al., 2004).

During HDL biogenesis, the primary acceptor of cholesterol and phospholipids from macrophages is lipid-free or lipid-poor ApoA-I, containing up to four phospholipid molecules (Duong et al., 2008). In this state, ApoA-I is the preferred substrate of the plasma membrane transporter ATP-binding cassette A1 (ABCA1) (Adorni et al., 2007; Mulya et al., 2007; Sacks et al., 2009). The conversion of unesterified cholesterol into cholesteryl ester by the enzyme lecithin:cholesterol acyltransferase (LCAT) is responsible for the conversion of the nascent, discoidal HDL into mature spherical HDL, with ApoA-I representing roughly 70% of HDL protein mass. Circulating HDL are remodelled by the action of proteins and enzymes, such as cholesteryl ester transfer protein (Rye et al., 1997), LCAT (Liang et al., 1995; Liang et al., 1996), phospholipid transfer protein (Lusa et al., 1996; Ryan et al., 1992) and hepatic lipase (Clay et al., 1992). Plasma HDL remodelling can result in the destabilization of HDL and the release of lipid-free/lipid-poor ApoA-I. Furthermore, the selective uptake of lipids from HDL through scavenger receptor B type 1 (SRB1) can yield lipid-poor ApoA-I (Acton et al., 1996). It has been demonstrated that the production of lipid-free/lipid-poor ApoA-I from mature HDL and relipidation by ABCA1 is a dynamic process in the arterial wall, which is critical in protecting macrophages from cholesteryl ester accumulation (Cavigiolio et al., 2010). Nevertheless, the molecular mechanism of the atheroprotective action of ApoA-I, as well as HDL biogenesis, is not fully understood.

HDL catabolism requires disassembly of protein and lipid components. While HDL lipid clearance is well described (Obici et al., 2006), less is known about the catabolism of the HDL protein moiety. Numerous tissue uptake studies support the view that kidneys are the principal site of ApoA-I degradation (Glass et al., 1983).

The conformational transition from the lipid-free to the lipid-bound state of ApoA-I (Cavigiolio et al., 2010) is made possible by the conformational plasticity of the protein (Obici et al., 2006). In fact, different are the structures proposed for ApoA-I as a lipid-bound or a lipid-free protein (Borhani et al., 1997; Silva et al., 2005; Ajees et al., 2006). In the absence of lipids, ApoA-I can assume a compact four-helix bundle (Silva et al., 2005), while, upon lipidation, the amphipathic α-helices substitute protein-protein contacts for protein-lipid interactions. This induces the opening of the helical bundle into an extended belt-like α-helix, which wraps around the perimeter of the nascent HDL particle (Borhani et al., 1997). Therefore, conformational plasticity of full-length ApoA-I is a functionally relevant feature, strictly related to the complex mechanism of its biological action.

1.2 The genetic basis of ApoA-I-associated amyloidosis

A variety of mutations in ApoA-I gene have been associated with familial hypercholesterolemia (Sorci-Thomas & Thomas, 2002), a prototypic "loss of function" genetic disease, whereas other mutations have been associated with familial systemic amyloidosis, a "gain of function" genetic disease (Obici et al., 2006), in that new pathological properties are associated to the protein.
Sixteen variants of ApoA-I are responsible for systemic amyloidoses, which are characterized by amyloid deposition in peripheral organs, such as heart, liver or kidneys (Obici et al., 1999; Obici et al., 2006; Eriksson et al., 2009). Although patients are invariably heterozygous for the mutated gene, only the variant isoform was detected in amyloid deposits.
In Figure 1, the map of the sixteen ApoA-I mutations associated to amyloidosis is represented.

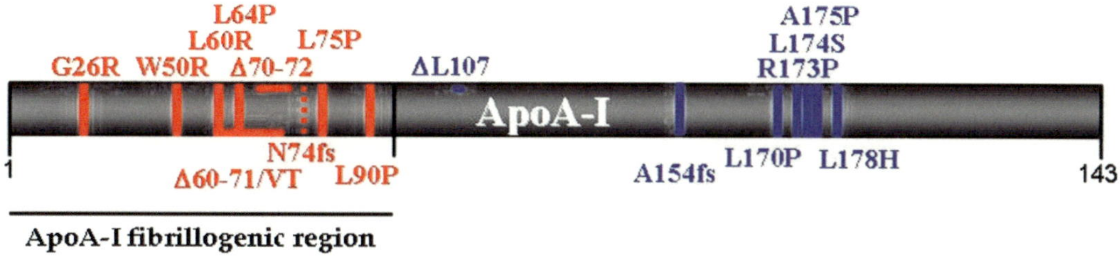

Fig. 1. ApoA-I mutations associated to systemic amyloidoses. In red, the mutations located within the N-terminal fibrillogenic region ("inside mutations"). In blue, the "outside mutations". Δ, deletion mutation; fs, frameshift mutation.

For all these variants, amyloid fibrils isolated *ex vivo* were found to be mainly constituted by N-terminal fragments of AApoA-I, 90-100 residue long. Thus, ApoA-I variants represent the precursors of N-terminal fragments of the protein responsible for fibril formation.
The amyloidogenic mutations described so far in patients can be divided in two groups (see Figure 1): those located within the N-terminal portion of the protein that is eventually found in fibrils (''inside mutations''), and those located externally to this region (''outside mutations'') (Obici et al., 2006). Wherever an amyloidogenic mutation is located, internally or externally to the N-terminal region, a protein fragment corresponding to the N-terminal end of the protein is released, leading to the formation of fibrillar deposits. However, nothing is known about the mechanism leading *in vivo* to the release of the fibrillogenic polypeptide from a full-length amyloidogenic variant of ApoA-I, nor in which context it occurs.
The fragment corresponding to sequence 1-93 was found to be the most abundant species among all the specimens investigated so far (Obici et al., 1999). Therefore, our studies focused on this N-terminal AApoA-I peptide, denoted here as [1-93]ApoA-I, to shed light on structural and functional features relevant to the understanding of the molecular basis of the pathology. The amino acid sequence of polypeptide [1-93]ApoA-I is shown in Figure 2A.

To predict the aggregation propensity of the fibrillogenic polypeptide [1-93]ApoA-I, we performed *in silico* analyses using various algorithms. First, by the Prot Param algorithm (Guruprasad et al., 1990), the instability index of [1–93]ApoA-I was calculated and found to be 46.7, a value that classifies the polypeptide as "unstable". The propensity of [1–93]ApoA-I to generate fibrils was analysed using the TANGO algorithm (Fernandez-Escamilla et al., 2004) (Figure 2B). The aggregation score, describing the overall protein propensity to aggregate (25°C, 0.01 M ionic strength), was found to be 372 and 428, at pH 7.0 and 4.0, respectively. This is indicative of high propensity of [1–93]ApoA-I to generate β-cross aggregated structures at both pH values, with a higher propensity at pH 4.0, as expected.

Moreover, at both pH values the region 13-25 shows the highest propensity to generate β-cross aggregates, as shown in Figure 2B. The high aggregation potential of region 13-25 was confirmed by other algorithms (Maurer-Stroh et al., 2010; Chou & Fasman, 1978). The data are also consistent with theoretical predictions obtained by the Zyggregator method (Tartaglia et al., 2008), indicating that residues 15-20 represent the most aggregation-prone region at pH 4.0 (Raimondi et al., 2011).

A

1- D E P P Q S P W D R V K D L A T V Y Y V D V L K D S G R D Y V S Q F E G -35

36- S A L G K Q L N L K L L D N W D S V T S T F S K L R E Q L G P V T Q E -70

71- F W D N L E K E T E G L R Q E M S K D L E E V -93

B

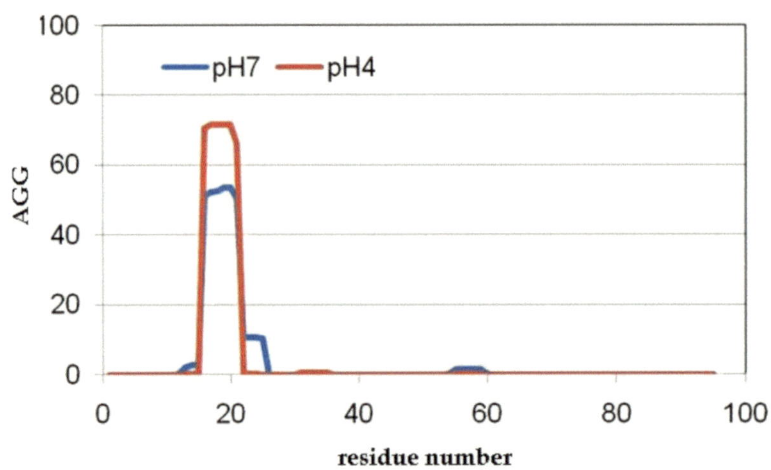

Fig. 2. AApoA-I fibrillogenic polypeptide. A, Amino acid sequence of [1-93]ApoA-I. Underlined are the sequence positions where the mutations identified in patients occur. B, Aggregation propensity (AGG) of [1-93]ApoA-I predicted by the TANGO algorithm at pH 7.0 and pH 4.0.

2. Structural and functional features of AApoA-I fibrillogenic polypeptide

2.1 A recombinant version of AApoA-I fibrillogenic polypeptide: An essential tool for structural and functional studies

The 93-residue fibrillogenic domain of AApoA-I, extracted from amyloid deposits of a patient who underwent a heart transplant for end-stage heart failure, was found to be a natively unfolded protein in water at neutral pH (Andreola et al., 2003). Acidic conditions (pH 4.0) were able to switch on a complex fibrillogenic pathway, consisting of extensive structural rearrangements of the polypeptide, that shifts from a random coil structure to an unstable helical conformation, and then aggregates into a β-sheet based polymeric structure (Andreola et al., 2003). Nevertheless, detailed structural and functional studies on the polypeptide extracted from *ex vivo* fibrils were made impossible due to the paucity of the available material.

Despite the intrinsic instability of the fibrillogenic polypeptide of AApoA-I due to its natively unfolded structure, we succeeded in the production of a recombinant version of the polypeptide, opening the way to structural and functional studies (Di Gaetano et al., 2006). The 1–93 fragment of AApoA-I was expressed in bacterial cells following an experimental strategy aimed at reducing the intracellular degradation of the polypeptide during its production. It was expressed in prokaryotic cells as a chimeric protein obtained by fusing the 93 residues polypeptide to glutathione S-transferase (GST). The [1–93]ApoA-I moiety was then released from the chimeric protein by targeted proteolysis, making use of a unique cleavage site positioned between the GST and the [1–93]ApoA-I sequences (Di Gaetano et al., 2006).

Conformational analyses of the recombinant polypeptide in solution by far-UV CD spectroscopy indicated that in physiological-like conditions the protein is largely unfolded. A pH switch from 7.0 to 4.0 induces a predominant α-helical structure, through the conversion of the protein from a random coil to a helical/molten globule state. This transition, complete within 2 seconds and fully reversible when the pH is returned to 7.0, is followed by the appearance of a significant β-sheet component. The helical conformers are thought to be key intermediates in the multistep fibrillogenic process. These observations are in good agreement with the behaviour of the natural polypeptide isolated from *ex vivo* fibrils (Obici et al., 1999).

The helical/molten globule intermediate displays a strong propensity to oligomerize, as demonstrated by atomic force microscopy (AFM) analyses. [1-93]ApoA-I, in fact, generates typical amyloid fibrils upon incubation at pH 4.0 for lengths of time comparable to those described for the natural polypeptide (Di Gaetano et al., 2006). Recently, we found that amyloid fibrils can also be obtained at neutral pH. Upon incubation of the polypeptide for 2 weeks at 37°C in buffer at pH 6.4, in the presence of 20% (v/v) trifluoroethanol (TFE), typical amyloid fibrils were obtained. In Figure 3, fibrils images obtained by AFM, following the procedure previously described (Arciello et al., 2011), are shown.

As the main features of the natural polypeptide were found to be preserved in the recombinant version of the fibrillogenic polypeptide, a valuable tool was available to generate the recombinant forms of all the variants of the polypeptide identified so far in patients affected by AApoA-I associated amyloidoses. This made possible the analysis of the structural and functional properties of the fibrillogenic polypeptides and their relationships, relevant for the comprehension of the disease.

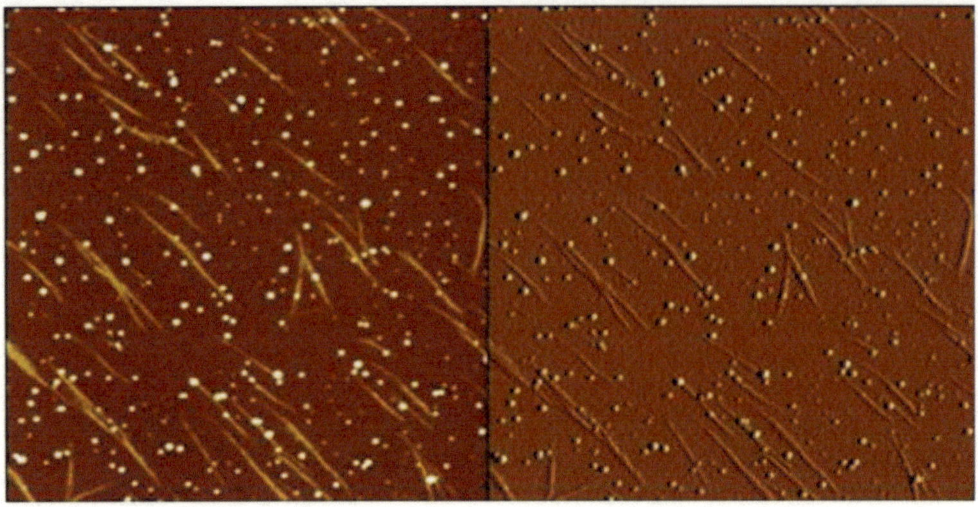

Fig. 3. AFM analysis of [1-93]ApoA-I fibrils.Tapping mode AFM image (left, height data; right, amplitude data) of [1-93]ApoA-I fibrils, obtained after 2 weeks incubation of [1-93]ApoA-I (0.3 mg/ml) at 37°C in 20% (v/v) TFE in 12 mM sodium phosphate buffer, pH 6.4. Amyloid fibrils are detected together with spheroidal aggregates. Scan size 4.0 µm, Z range 10 nm.

So far, in patients affected by AApoA-I associated amyloidoses, nine "inside mutations" have been identified, each identifying a variant of [1-93]ApoA-I polypeptide. Six variants (G26R, W50R, L60R, L64P, L75P and L90P) present a single residue substitution. Two variants contain sequence deletions, at positions 70-72 (variant Δ70-72) or at positions 60-71 (variant Δ60-71/VT); in the latter case the deleted residues are replaced by a Val-Thr sequence. The ninth variant, recently reported (Eriksson et al., 2009), is associated to a frameshift mutation (Asn74fs). It has to be noticed that the replacement of a hydrophobic residue either with a positively charged residue (arginine), or with an α-helical interrupting residue (proline) often occurs.

2.2 Intrinsic factors influencing amyloid formation: mutations induce AApoA-I susceptibility to proteolysis

We expressed and purified recombinant forms of all the isoforms of [1-93]ApoA-I, with the exception of the truncation mutation Asn74fs. The polypeptide variants were analysed in comparison to the wild-type polypeptide to investigate the effects of each individual mutation on the aggregation propensity of the polypeptide. We investigated the induction of structural transitions by acidic conditions (pH 4.0), along with structural properties of the aggregated material, and found that all the variants adopt a highly disordered structure at neutral pH, whereas acidification of the solution induces conformational changes and the subsequent aggregation into the cross-β structure aggregates. Nevertheless, differing results were obtained when the aggregation rate of the variants was analysed: two mutations (Δ70-72 and L90P) almost abrogate the lag phase of the aggregation process; three mutations (Δ60-71, L75P and W50R) significantly accelerate the aggregation rate by two-three fold, while the remaining three variants (L64P, L60R and G26R) are not significantly different from the wild-type polypeptide.

Our results indicate that an amyloidogenic mutation may, or may not, increase the aggregation propensity of the polypeptide. Thus, the paradigm amyloidogenic mutation-increased aggregation propensity has not to be taken as a general rule. Instead, a different scenario was provided by *in silico* analyses. Sequence-based predictions of aggregation propensities and stabilities of the pathogenic variants of full-length ApoA-I revealed in almost all the variants an increase of conformational fluctuations and chain flexibility in the proximity of the region of the protein spanning approximately residues 88-110, with the consequent exposure of a putative cleavage site to a proteolytic attack that releases the fibrillogenic moiety (Raimondi et al., 2011). Therefore, all the amyloidogenic structural modifications occurring at the N-terminal region of AApoA-I have a common feature, that of dramatically affecting the stability of the whole protein, favouring the cleavage that generates the N-terminal fibrillogenic fragment. In addition, some of the mutations increase the aggregation rate of the fibrillogenic polypeptide.

2.3 Extrinsic factors that influence amyloid formation: Effects of a lipid environment

2.3.1 General aspects of membrane interaction and protein aggregation

The elucidation of the structural properties of the fibrillogenic polypeptide is a central issue in the comprehension of the pathology. To this regard, the identification of structural or environmental factors, able to activate the pathological pathway leading to amyloid fibrils, is of enormous importance to pursue strategies aimed at inhibiting this process.

Extracellular amyloid deposition *in vivo* takes place in a heterogeneous environment, in which components of the cell membrane and/or the extracellular matrix may have a central role. From a general point of view, the interaction of proteins with biological superstructures, like membranes, may dramatically affect their structural organization. The general concept that biological surfaces may influence and direct molecular assemblies is gaining increasing attention. It is known that the interaction of natively folded proteins with groups exposed on a membrane surface often modifies their conformational states (Fantini & Yahi, 2010; Shanmugam & Jayakumar, 2004; Kakio et al., 2004). On the other hand, unfolded polypeptide chains can gain ordered structures at the membrane surface or inside the bilayer (Fantini & Yahi, 2010). Conversely, proteins can alter membrane fluidity, and/or permeate the membrane bilayer and can even extract lipids from it (Hou et al., 2005).

A dramatically different behaviour may be expected for a protein in a bulk solution with respect to that in a physiological environment. It is known that the hydrophobic interior of the plasma membrane can induce structural changes in soluble intrinsically disordered proteins and peptides by favouring secondary structures often leading to aggregate nucleation (Kazlauskaiteet al., 2003; Fernandez-Escamilla et al., 2004; Shanmugam & Jayakumar, 2004; Kakio et al., 2004). The well known stability of protein α-helical structures within a membrane lipid bilayer is in line with the concept that the early formation of multimeric species is often promoted by the association of polypeptide molecules through helix-helix interaction. From this point of view, a general mechanism of membrane-catalyzed amyloid formation can be envisaged.

To this regard, factors able to induce α-helical conformers may accelerate amyloid formation. Conversely, factors able to bind to, and stabilize, helical regions by entrapping the helical intermediates in a minimum energy (kinetic trap), may have an opposite effect, i.e. that of slowing down the fibrillogenic process. Therefore, targeting helix-helix interactions can be a valuable strategy to inhibit amyloid formation.

2.3.2 Effects of cholesterol on [1-93]ApoA-I aggregation

It is known that the *in vivo* role of ApoA-I is mediated by its interactions with lipids, that are fundamental in the maintenance of the protein native structure. It is known that the N-terminal region of ApoA-I contributes to lipid binding in the native protein (Frank & Marcel, 2000; Tanaka et al., 2006). To this regard, recently we analysed the effects of lipids on the propensity of [1-93]ApoA-I to undergo fibrillogenesis and found that a lipid environment affects [1-93]ApoA-I aggregation pathway by inducing and stabilizing helical intermediates (Monti et al., 2010). In particular, by far-UV CD spectroscopy, we observed that the presence of a lipid-mimicking detergent, namely Triton X-100, greatly affects the conformational state of [1-93]ApoA-I. We found that at pH 8.0 [1-93]ApoA-I, which is predominantly in a random coil state, adopts a helical conformation in the presence of Triton X-100. This α-helical state remains unchanged upon acidification to pH 4.0. Interestingly, we observed that in the presence of Triton X-100 the polypeptide does not aggregate over time, rather a shift towards a random coil conformation occurs. Therefore, Triton X-100 induces and stabilizes helical conformers of [1-93]ApoA-I, thus hampering aggregation. We also demonstrated that the fibrillogenic pathway of [1-93]ApoA-I can be activated even under pathophysiological conditions, as we found that [1-93]ApoA-I at pH 6.4 is predominantly in an α-helical state and aggregates over time. Again, in the presence of Triton X-100 aggregation of [1-93]ApoA-I at neutral pH was found to be strongly impaired.

Furthermore, we investigated the effects of cholesterol, a natural ApoA-I ligand, on [1-93]ApoA-I aggregation and found that cholesterol acts as an inducer of helical conformers and an inhibitor of protein aggregation in a concentration-dependent and time-dependent manner (Monti et al., 2010). When the percentage of helical species was calculated in the presence of increasing concentrations of cholesterol both at pH 8.0 and 6.4, a positive correlation was observed. In Figure 4A and B, the results of typical experiments are shown. At pH 6.4, i.e. in conditions favouring aggregation, in the absence of cholesterol a significant decrease of helical species is observed after 7 days incubation, consistent with protein aggregation (Figure 4B). In the presence of cholesterol, at concentrations close to the physiological value (1.6 mM in HDL), the aggregation process is significantly slowed down, as shown in Figure 4B.

An inverse correlation exists between the α-helical content and the aggregation rate of the polypeptide, so that the fibrillogenic process is strongly affected by a hydrophobic environment that favours the formation of α-helices.

The behaviour of [1-93]ApoA-I is in line with that of other amyloidogenic proteins, whose conformations were reported to be strongly affected by the interaction with cholesterol. It is known that cholesterol and sphingolipids are the most abundant molecules of lipid rafts. Amyloid protein precursor (AβPP) and secretases preferentially localize into ganglioside and cholesterol-rich membrane microdomains (lipid rafts) (Lee et al., 1998; Ehahalt et al., 2003; Kakio et al., 2003). Accordingly, it has been proposed that aggregation of soluble Aβ peptides and APrP is a raft-associated process (Ehahalt et al., 2003) and that an alteration of cholesterol homeostasis is a shared primary cause of several neurodegenerative diseases (Vedhachalam et al., 2007).

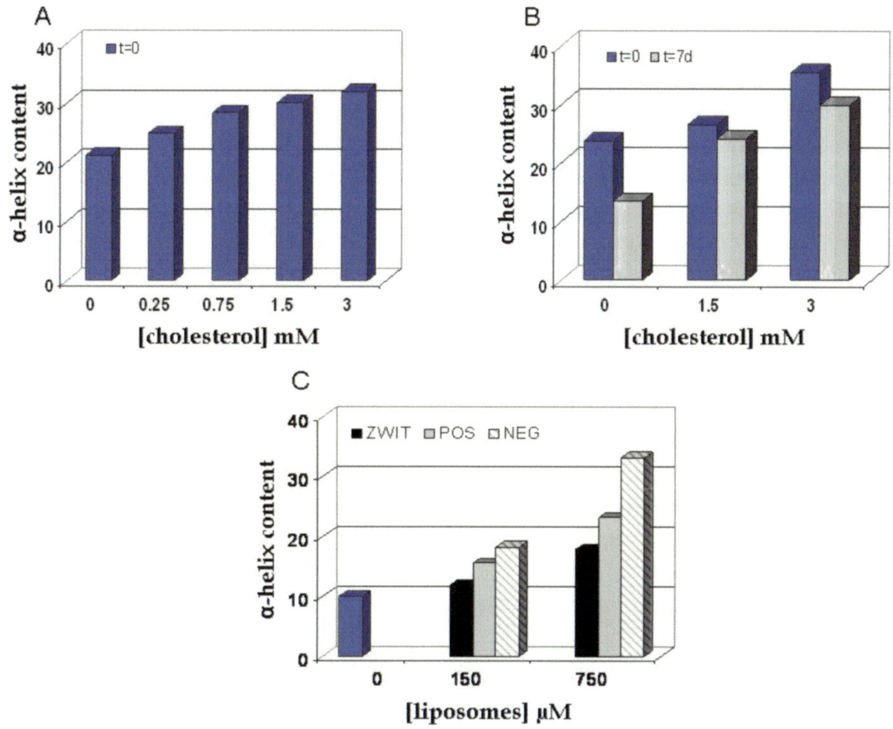

Fig. 4. Analysis of the effects of cholesterol and artificial membranes on [1-93]ApoA-I conformational state by far-UV CD spectroscopy. A, [1-93]ApoA-I (0.3 mg/ml) α-helical content in the presence of increasing concentrations of cholesterol in 3 mM glycine, 3 mM sodium acetate, and 3 mM sodium phosphate at pH 8.0. B, cholesterol concentration-dependence and time-dependence of [1-93]ApoA-I (0.3 mg/ml) α-helical content in 3 mM glycine, 3 mM sodium acetate, and 3 mM sodium phosphate at pH 6.4. C, [1-93]ApoA-I (0.3 mg/ml) α-helical content in the presence of zwitterionic (ZWIT), positively charged (POS) and negatively charged (NEG) liposomes in buffer at pH 6.4. The lipid-to-protein molar concentration ratio was 10:1 (150 μM liposome concentration) or 50:1 (750 μM liposome concentration). Helical content was estimated using CDPro program pack (Sreerama & Woody, 2000).

Consistent with these data are those obtained with the prion protein. In fact, PrP^c to $APrP^{sc}$ pathological conversion seems to occur on the cell surface or during/after internalization of PrP^c, and cellular cholesterol depletion, which impairs association of PrP^c with rafts, inhibits the formation of the scrapie form in neuroblastoma cells (Taraboulos et al., 1995). However, it was also reported that the impairment of raft-association by cholesterol depletion during the early stage of PrP biosynthesis leads to protein misfolding in the ER (Sarnataro et al., 2004), suggesting a role for cholesterol as a lipochaperone. It has also been demonstrated that binding of PrP to raft-like artificial membranes induces the formation of an α-helical structure (Sanghera & Pinheiro, 2002).
Furthermore, α-synuclein, a fibrillogenic protein responsible for Parkinson's disease (PD), has been suggested to be associated with caveolae or caveolae-like domains (lipid raft domains containing caveolin), since it was found to regulate several signalling proteins

localized in these regions (Lusa et al., 1996; Ryan et al., 1992; Clay et al., 1992). Specific association of α-synuclein with lipid rafts suggests an important role for these membrane domains in the normal function of α-synuclein and raises the possibility that a perturbation of raft association could induce changes in α-synuclein conformation that contribute to PD pathogenesis (Martinez et al., 2007).

Moreover, an inverse correlation was envisaged between neurodegeneration and content in cholesterol (Lee et al., 1998; Martins et al., 2008), since reduced levels of cholesterol are present in the brains of Alzheimer disease (AD) patients (Mason et al., 1992). On the contrary, an increased membrane rigidity due to the presence of cholesterol has a protective action against aggregate cytotoxicity and membrane perturbation (Cecchi et al., 2005; Zampagni et al., 2010).

In conclusion, cholesterol can modulate conformational changes of specific proteins or peptides and influence their aggregation propensity. From a general point of view, the interaction of amyloidogenic proteins with lipid rafts may play a key role in the pathogenesis of amyloid diseases.

2.3.3 Effects of liposomes on [1-93]ApoA-I aggregation

Although the mechanisms underlying amyloid diseases remain largely unknown, common features shared by some amyloidogenic proteins and peptides are emerging. One of these features is the key role of biological membranes in inducing helical structures in natively unstructured polypeptides.

Mechanistic studies with well defined model membranes have shown that natively unfolded polypeptides, upon interaction with surfaces, readily adopt helical structures that represent key intermediates in amyloid formation process (Abedini & Raleigh, 2009). In particular, anionic surfaces and anionic phospholipid-rich membranes can play key roles either in triggering protein fibrillogenesis by acting as conformational catalysts for amyloid fibrils deposition (Fantini & Yahi, 2010), or as inhibitors of fibrillogenesis (Zhu & Fink, 2003).

We demonstrated that the conformation of the fibrillogenic polypeptide [1-93]ApoA-I is largely affected by membrane-mimicking structures, such as liposomes (Monti et al., 2010). Zwitterionic, negatively charged, and positively charged liposomes were prepared, made of POPC (1-Palmitoyl-2-oleoyl-sn-glycero-3-phosphocholine), POPC/POPS (POPS, 1-Palmitoyl-2-oleoyl-sn-glycero-3-phospho-L-serine) and POPC/DOTAP (DOTAP, 1,2,-Dioleoyl-3-trimethylammonium-propane), respectively. The POPC/POPS and POPC/DOTAP molar ratio was 85:15. We performed conformational analyses of [1-93]ApoA-I at pH 8.0 at 37°C in the presence of increasing concentrations of each liposome type and found a significant concentration-dependent increase of [1-93]ApoA-I helical content, particularly evident in the case of negatively charged liposomes (Figure 4C).

It has to be noticed that [1-93]ApoA-I is very rich in charged residues. Thus, interaction with charged lipids, either positive or negative, might mask intramolecular repulsion effects and favour the conformational transition towards a helical state. Furthermore, our data indicate a negative effect of liposomes on polypeptide aggregation, suggesting that membrane composition influences the fate of AApoA-I fibrillogenic polypeptide.

To this regard, the identification of molecules able to have an effect on the critical balance between folded and partially unfolded states of the fibrillogenic polypeptide would allow the development of therapies targeted to amyloidoses. To this purpose, biomimetic membranes appear of interest as effectors/modulators of the fibrillogenic process.

Our data are in line with previous observations regarding α-synuclein. Evidence was provided that α-synuclein preferentially interacts with small unilamellar vesicles (SUVs) containing acidic phospholipids, which induce and stabilize helical conformers (Wang et al., 2000). On the other hand, no interaction of α-synuclein with zwitterionic vesicles was detected (Wang et al., 2000). It has also been reported that helical conformation of α-synuclein is a prerequisite for its binding to lipids. Thus, interaction of α-synuclein with lipid vesicles might lead to preferential binding to membranes and induction of helix with a concomitant inhibition of fibrillogenesis (Zhu & Fink, 2003). It has also been demonstrated that, upon PrP binding to raft-like artificial membranes, the formation of α-helical structures is induced (Sanghera & Pinheiro, 2002), similarly to the fibrillogenic polypeptide [1-93]ApoA-I.
In conclusion, our observations, in line with those collected for other fibrillogenic proteins, indicate that protein-lipid interactions induce and stabilize helical conformers, interfering with aggregation.

2.4 Membrane interaction, internalization and intracellular pathway of AApoA-I fibrillogenic polypeptide

Of primary importance in the comprehension of amyloid diseases is the elucidation of the cascade of biochemical events triggered by the exposure of cells to fibrillogenic proteins or polypeptides. Upon its release, [1-93]ApoA-I is expected to accumulate in the extracellular space. The possibility that the fibrillogenic polypeptide of AApoA-I interacts with membranes of target cells and enters the cell compartment, mimicking ApoA-I full-length protein, has to be taken into account. Recently we analysed the intracellular pathway of [1-93]ApoA-I in comparison to full-length ApoA-I using cardiac cells. Since in the case of AApoA-I associated amyloidoses the heart is a natural target for aggregate deposition *in vivo*, cardiomyoblasts were chosen as an experimental system.
We provided evidence that the polypeptide partially co-localizes with ABCA1 on rat cardiomyoblasts cell membranes (Arciello et al., 2011). Similar results were obtained for ApoA-I, in agreement with recent reports showing that the majority of cell-associated ApoA-I does not co-localize with ABCA1, although no internalization was observed in cells ABCA1$^{-/-}$ (Zha et al., 2001). To explain this observation, a model was recently proposed (Denis et al., 2008; Vedhachalam et al., 2007) in which the interaction of a small fraction of lipid-free ApoA-I to ABCA1 is sufficient to activate ABCA1 lipid translocase activity, which in turn promotes the formation of specialized lipid domains, acting as high affinity binding sites for ApoA-I (Vedhachalam et al., 2007). Nevertheless, whether or not ABCA1 has to be considered as an ApoA-I receptor is still ambiguous, as ABCA1 could have a role in inducing modifications of membrane lipid distribution facilitating ApoA-I docking (Vedhachalam et al., 2007).
We demonstrated that the fibrillogenic polypeptide recognizes specific binding sites on cardiac cell membranes and that this binding represents a key step for [1-93]ApoA-I internalization (Arciello et al., 2011). The apparent affinity constant calculated for the binding of the polypeptide to rat cardiomyoblasts ($K_d = 5.90 \times 10^{-7}$ M) was found to be similar to those previously reported for lipid-free full-length ApoA-I binding to different cell types, such as HepG2 cells ($K_d = 0.84 \times 10^{-7}$ M) (Barbaras et al., 1994), or bovine aortic endothelial cells BAECs ($K_d = 0.8 \times 10^{-7}$ M) (Rohrer et al., 2006).
Interestingly, we demonstrated that, following binding, the polypeptide is internalized in cardiomyoblasts.

A comparative analysis of the internalization routes of the polypeptide and the full-length protein revealed that: (i) the polypeptide is internalized mostly by chlatrin-mediated endocytosis and by lipid rafts, whereas a significant involvement of macropinocytosis could be excluded; (ii) ApoA-I is internalized *via* chlatrin-coated pits and macropinocytosis, whereas internalization through lipid rafts was not observed (Arciello et al., 2011).

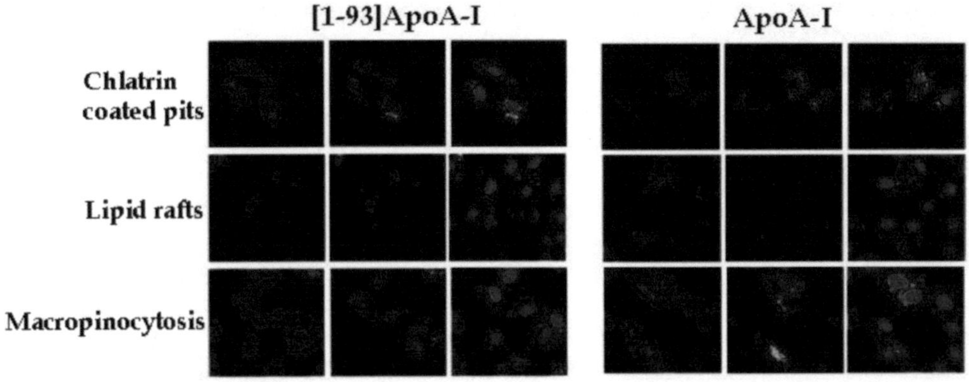

Fig. 5. Analysis of the internalization routes of the fibrillogenic polypeptide [1-93]ApoA-I and full-length ApoA-I by confocal microscopy. To analyse clathrin-mediated endocytosis, cardiomyoblasts (H9c2 cells) were transiently transfected with an expression vector for Rab5 conjugated to the red fluorescent protein. After 24 h, cells were incubated 6 h at 37°C either with FITC-labelled [1-93]ApoA-I (3 µM), or ApoA-I (1 µM). For lipid rafts-mediated internalization, cells were incubated 4 h at 37°C with rhodamine- lebelled proteins (3 µM [1-93]ApoA-I, 1 µM ApoA-I) in the presence of FITC-insulin (0.1 mg/ml). To analyse macropinocytosis, cells were incubated 4 h at 37°C with rhodamine-labelled proteins as above, in the presence of FITC-dextran (5 mg/ml). Nuclei were stained with Hoechst (blue).

Thus, evidence was provided that the pathogenic polypeptide translocates from the extracellular space, where fibrils form and grow, to the intracellular space. ApoA-I and its fribrillogenic polypeptide share the endocytic route to gain access to the intracellular compartment, whereas lipid rafts and macropinocytosis represent specific routes for the fibrillogenic polypeptide and the full-length protein, respectively. Considering that lipid rafts are rich in cholesterol, which is able to induce and stabilize [1-93]ApoA-I helical states, the polypeptide internalization mediated by lipid rafts may have a key role in the pathogenesis of the disease. On the other hand, our data extend the knowledge on ApoA-I mechanism of action as, while it is known that ApoA-I interacts with plasma membrane lipid rafts to control cholesterol export (Gaus et al., 2004), we provided evidence for the first time that these domains are not involved in ApoA-I internalization.

Understanding the fate of internalized [1-93]ApoA-I is fundamental to deeply inspect the molecular bases of the pathology. It has been reported that ApoA-I, once internalized in endosomes, is resecreted to the medium as HDL. Endosomes represent an intracellular reservoir of cholesterol where ApoA-I binds to lipids to be secreted through a retroendocytic pathway involving Rab4 containing endosomes (Mukherjee et al., 1998). We found that ApoA-I and its fibrillogenic polypeptide follow different pathways, as ApoA-I was found to co-localize with Rab4, consistently with the recycling pathway (Mukherjee et al., 1998), whereas no evidence of co-localization with Rab4 was obtained for the polypeptide.

We thus analysed the intracellular fate of the pathogenic polypeptide by fluorescence microscopy. After a prolonged exposure (24 h) of cardiomyoblasts to the fibrillogenic polypeptide, the disappearance of the intracellular fluorescent signal, indicative of a massive degradation of [1-93]ApoA-I, was observed. To define the degradation route, we analysed the involvement of proteasome and lysosomes activities. In the presence of specific inhibitors of protein degradation mediated by either proteasome or lysosomes, a significant persistence of [1-93]ApoA-I associated fluorescent signal was observed. This suggests that the fibrillogenic fragment is targeted to both these stations for degradation (Arciello et al., 2011). Different results were obtained instead in the case of full-length ApoA-I, as the protein does not appear to be significantly degraded once internalized. However, we observed a strong co-localization of ApoA-I with lysosomes, in agreement with recent reports (Cavelier et al., 2006; Denis et al., 2008). Although the question concerning the physiologic role of ApoA-I in lysosomes remains controversial, it might be considered that, even if lysosomes are best known for their role in degradation, they may also fuse with the plasma membrane to release their content in the extracellular medium (Luzio et al., 2007). Some authors demonstrated that ApoA-I reaches lysosomes to be degraded (Pastore et al., 2004; Rye & Barter, 2004), while other studies support the idea that ABCA1-bound ApoA-I traffics through late endosomal vesicles and/or lysosomes. Being these stations an intracellular reservoir of cholesterol, nascent lipoprotein particles may be formed at this level and then secreted in the extracellular space (Oram, 2008; Chen et al., 2001; Chen et al., 2005).

As it is conceivable that the accumulation of the fibrillogenic polypeptide in the extracellular space leads to fibrils deposition, the question was raised: are [1-93]ApoA-I fibrils able to enter cardiac cells? We thus produced fluorescent fibrils *in vitro* by incubating the fluorescein-labelled polypeptide under suitable conditions to induce fibrillogenesis (see Fig. 3). When fibrils were tested on cardiomyoblasts, no evidence of internalization was found.

We also tested the effects of the polypeptide, either in its unaggregated form or in the fibrillar state, on cell viability. In both cases, no effects on cardiomyoblasts viability were detected. These findings are in line with the evidence that: (i) fibrils are not able to enter cardiac cells; (ii) the unaggregated polypeptide, which enters the cells, undergoes rapid intracellular degradation. The latter observation is also in line with our previous experiments of limited proteolysis (Di Gaetano et al., 2006), indicating that the largely unfolded structure of the fibrillogenic polypeptide is responsible for its susceptibility to proteolytic cleavages. This, in turn, is in line with the fact that we succeeded in the production of a recombinant form of the polypeptide in a prokaryotic expression system only upon fusion of [1-93]ApoA-I to a stable bacterial protein to avoid intracellular degradation of the polypeptide (Di Gaetano et al., 2006).

Interestingly, the elucidation of key steps of the intracellular pathway and fate of AApoA-I fibrillogenic polypeptide reveals features common to other amyloidogenic proteins.

In the case of transmissible spongiform encephalopathy, the misfolded form of APrP accumulates in the brain. It is known that, after being exported to the plasma membrane, PrP^c is internalized and recycled back to the surface. However, the compartment where the transition from PrP^c to $APrP^{sc}$ occurs has not yet been clearly identified. It has been suggested that raft-enriched lipids represent the site of scrapie formation (Sarnataro et al., 2004). On the other hand, it is known that $APrP^{sc}$ undergoes proteasomal degradation (Sarnataro et al., 2004), and accumulates in lysosomes, a compartment that might be involved in the transconformational event.

In the case of Parkinson's disease, α-synuclein accumulates inside the cells as fibrillar aggregates named Lewy bodies. However, although α-synuclein is a cytoplasmic protein, a small amount of the protein is secreted by cells and is present in human body fluids. It has been demonstrated that both non-fibrillar oligomeric aggregates and fibrils are able to enter the cells through the endosomal pathway and to be degraded by lysosomes. In contrast to the uptake of protein aggregates, α-synuclein monomers are able to freely diffuse across the plasma membrane and to be resecreted before being degraded by the cellular proteolytic systems. This mechanism might protect neurons from exposure to potentially toxic α-synuclein (Lee et al., 2008). However, it has to be noticed that newly synthesized α-synuclein monomers and dimers, but not protofibrils, can be degraded by the proteasome (Zhang et al., 2008). Once α-synuclein protofibrils are formed, they are able to impair proteasome activity and this phenomenon may eventually result in α-synuclein accumulation in cells (Bennett et al., 1999; Tofaris et al., 2001; McNaught et al., 2002).
Along the internalization and intracellular pathway, common aspects are shared by [1-93]ApoA-I and Aβ. The most abundant forms of Aβ are 40 and 42 residue long (Aβ40/42), whose oligomeric species were found to rapidly bind and internalize in neuronal cells and accumulate in lysosomes. In contrast, aggregated polypeptides were found to associate with cells only weakly (Bateman & Chakrabartty, 2011). Furthermore, soluble Aβ oligomers, but not monomers, inhibit proteasomal activity *in vitro* (Tseng et al., 2008). Thus, an inverse correlation exists between Aβ40/42 aggregation rate and ability to bind to cells and to be internalized (Bateman & Chakrabartty, 2011).
It has to be noticed that cellular mechanisms deputed to protein degradation, i.e. lysosomes, proteasome and autophagy, may be important targets for therapeutic approaches against amyloidoses. It is known that the pathological accumulation of abnormal proteins, improperly folded and able to impair cellular functions, is determined by different causes, such as mutations, protein overproduction or impairment of the protein degradation machineries (Casarejos et al., 2011). Since in several amyloid diseases the impairment of proteasomal activity has been pointed out, a promising therapeutic approach would be that of enhancing the activity of cellular mechanisms for protein clearance.

2.5 A model for [1-93]ApoA-I

Based on the experimental data collected so far, a model representing the possible fates of [1-93]ApoA-I polypeptide in an *in vivo* context is proposed (Figure 6).
From a general point of view, the continuous accumulation of the natively unfolded polypeptide in the cardiac tissue is expected to favour protein aggregation and fibrillogenesis leading to a progressive, massive occupancy of the extracellular space by amyloid deposits, as observed in pathological hearts, from which the natural fibrillogenic polypeptide can be isolated (Obici et al., 1999). During the fibrillogenic process, a dynamic equilibrium between monomeric species and aggregated states has been proposed (Carulla et al., 2005). In the case of [1-93]ApoA-I, internalization in target cells may represent an alternative fate to aggregation, thus subtracting the unaggregated form of [1-93]ApoA-I from the equilibrium. This would direct the polypeptide towards a non pathological route, as, once inside the cells, the fibrillogenic polypeptide is promptly cleared off. Hence, the hypothesis can be raised that internalization and subsequent degradation of the unaggregated polypeptide represent a protective mechanism against fibrillogenesis, able to balance [1-93]ApoA-I progressive aggregation and to slow down the fibrillogenic process.

This phenomenon may be relevant in the slow progression and late onset of AApoA-I-associated amyloidoses.

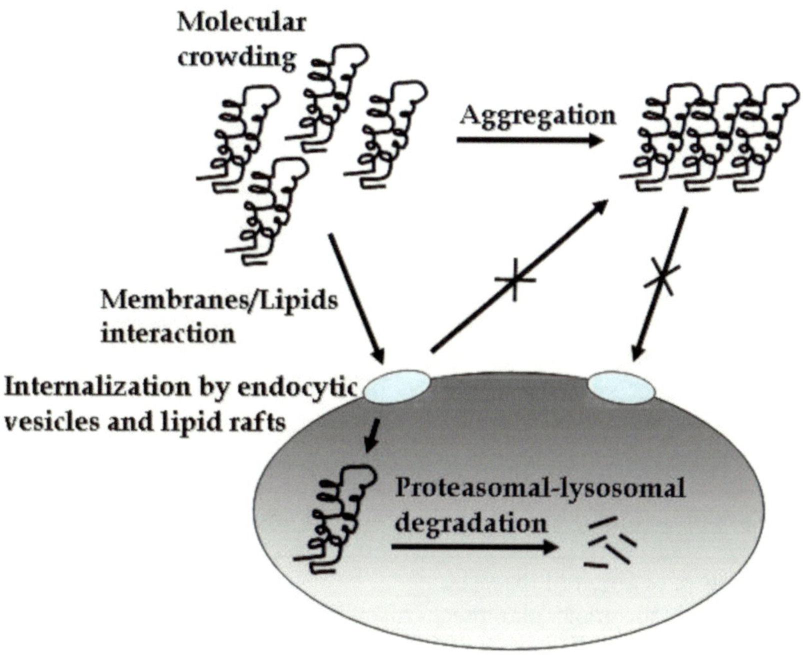

Fig. 6. A schematic representation of the possible fates of AApoA-I fibrillogenic polypeptide. Upon accumulation in the extracellular space of target tissues, the soluble polypeptide is prone to aggregate in fibrillar structures. Viceversa, the interaction with membrane components, presumably lipids, induces conformational changes generating stable helical species with low propensity to aggregation. Upon membrane binding, the polypeptide can gain the intracellular compartment via endocytic vesicles and lipid rafts. Inside the cells, the polypeptide is promptly degraded by the lysosomal and proteasomal machineries. On the contrary, once aggregated in amyloid fibrils, the polypeptide is unable to be internalized.

3. Conclusions

The elucidation of the cascade of biochemical events triggered by the exposure of cells to a fibrillogenic protein is of primary importance in the comprehension of the molecular bases of amyloid diseases. Presently, the molecular mechanism of fibril formation in patients bearing AApoA-I amyloidogenic mutations is largely unknown, as unknown are the molecular bases of the etiology of this pathology.

Our work is aimed at elucidating the molecular bases of the process responsible for fibril deposition in amyloid diseases associated to AApoA-I. ApoA-I plays a key role in lipids metabolism acting as an antiatherogenic factor in humans. Nevertheless, specific mutations convert it into the precursor of a pathogenic polypeptide named [1-93]ApoA-I, whose largely unfolded structure correlates with a high propensity to aggregate in fibrillar deposits. For both the full-length protein and its fibrillogenic fragment, conformational plasticity is an essential feature that makes possible protein adaptation to different environmental conditions.

We shed light on key steps of the possible routes accessible to the pathogenic polypeptide in a physiological-like environment, such as that of cultured cardiomyoblasts, which mimic one of the most frequent target tissues of the pathology, i.e. the heart. We observed that the polypeptide is able to bind lipids undergoing extensive conformational changes. We thus hypothesized that in a cellular environment the interaction of the polypeptide with lipids may play a critical role in slowing down the fibrillogenic process by entrapping the polypeptide in stable helical structures unable to aggregate. Through endocytic vesicles and lipid rafts the polypeptide may be conveyed from the extracellular to the intracellular compartment of target cells. Here, the polypeptide gains access to the protein degradation machinery.

We thus envisaged two distinct mechanisms acting synergistically to prevent the progressive aggregation in fibrillar structures. The interaction of extracellular polypeptide molecules with the cell surface may "freeze" non amyloidogenic conformational states of the polypeptide. On the other side, the activation of the internalization-degradation pathway subtracts polypeptide molecules from the extracellular space, interfering with amyloid deposition.

In this chapter, we underlined some structural and functional features shared by AApoA-I fibrillogenic polypeptide and other natively unfolded amyloidogenic proteins. We believe that pointing out such correlations might greatly contribute to draw a still more comprehensive picture of amyloid diseases.

The comprehension of the molecular mechanisms of the pathology will certainly benefit from future studies aimed at identifying the intracellular partners of the fibrillogenic polypeptide, as well as membrane and extracellular components that may alter the balance between aggregated and unaggregated states of the polypeptide.

4. Acknowledgements

The Authors wish to thank Dr A. Relini, University of Genoa, for AFM analyses and Dr F. Guglielmi for contribution in spectroscopic analyses.

5. References

Abedini, A. & Raleigh, D.P. (2009). A critical assessment of the role of helical intermediates in amyloid formation by natively unfolded proteins and polypeptides. *Prot. Eng. Des. Sel.*, 22: 453-459.

Acton, S.; Rigotti, A.; Landschulz, K.T.; Xu, S.; Hobbs, H.H.; Krieger, M. (1996). Identification of scavenger receptor SR-BI as a high density lipoprotein receptor. *Science.*, 271(5248): 518-520.

Adorni, M.P.; Zimetti, F.; Billheimer, J.T.; Wang, N.; Rader, D.J.; Phillips, M.C.; Rothblat, G.H. (2007). The roles of different pathways in the release of cholesterol from macrophages. *J Lipid Res.*, 48(11): 2453-2462.

Ajees, A.A.; Anantharamaiah, G.M.; Mishra, V.K.; Hussain, M.M.; Murthy, H.M. (2006) Crystal structure of human apolipoprotein A-I: insights into its protective effect against cardiovascular diseases. *Proc. Natl. Acad. Sci. USA*, 103: 2126-2131. This paper is currently under dispute as reported in a PNAS editorial expression of concern (http://www.pnas.org/content/107/14/6551.3.full?sid=daacdccb-0537-41fb-87c3-8%2067aba380ca7)

Andreola, A.; Bellotti, V.; Giorgetti, S.; Mangione, P.; Obici, L.; Stoppini, M.; Torres, J.; Monzani, E.; Merlini, G.; Sunde, M. Conformational switching and fibrillogenesis in the amyloidogenic fragment of apolipoprotein A-I. (2003). *J Biol Chem.*, 278: 2444-2451.

Arciello, A.; De Marco, N.; Del Giudice, R.; Guglielmi, F.; Pucci, P.; Relini, A.; Monti, D.M.; Piccoli, R. (2011). Insights into the fate of the N-terminal amyloidogenic polypeptide of ApoA-I in cultured target cells. *J. Cell. Mol. Med.*, DOI: 10.1111/j.1582-4934.2011.01271.x

Barbaras, R.; Collet, X.; Chap, H.; Perret, B. (1994). Specific binding of free apolipoprotein A-I to a high-affinity binding site on HepG2 cells: characterization of two high-density lipoprotein sites. *Biochemistry*, 33: 2335-2340.

Bateman, D.A. & Chakrabartty, A. (2011). Cell surface binding and internalization of aβ modulated by degree of aggregation. *Int J Alzheimers Dis.*, 2011: 962352.

Bennett, M.C.; Bishop, J.F.; Leng, Y.; Chock, P.B.; Chase, T.N.; Mouradian, M.M. (1999). Degradation of α-Synuclein by Proteasome *J. Biol. Chem.* 274: 33855-33858.

Borhani, D.W.; Rogers, D.P.; Engler, J.A.; Brouillette, C.G. (1997). Crystal structure of truncated human apolipoprotein A-I suggests a lipid-bound conformation. *Proc Natl Acad Sci U S A.*, 94(23): 12291-12296.

Brouillette, C.G.; Anantharamaiah, G.M.; Engler, J.A.; Borhani, D.W. (2001). Structural models of human apolipoprotein A-I: a critical analysis and review. *Biochim Biophys Acta*, 1531:4-46.

Carulla, N.; Caddy, G.L.; Hall, D.R.; Zurdo, J.; Gairí, M.; Feliz, M.; Giralt, E.; Robinson, C.V.; Dobson, C.M. (2005). Molecular recycling within amyloid fibrils. *Nature,* 436(7050): 554-558.

Casarejos, M.J.; Solano, R.M.; Gómez, A.; Perucho, J.; de Yébenes, J.G., Mena, M.A. (2011). The accumulation of neurotoxic proteins, induced by proteasome inhibition, is reverted by trehalose, an enhancer of autophagy, in human neuroblastoma cells. *Neurochem Int.*, 58(4): 512-520.

Cavelier, C.; Lorenzi, I.; Rohrer, L.; von Eckardstein, A. (2006). Lipid efflux by the ATP-binding cassette transporters ABCA1 and ABCG1. *Biochim Biophys Acta,* 1761: 655-666.

Cavigiolio, G.; Geier, E.G.; Shao, B.; Heinecke, J.W.; Oda, M.N. (2010). Exchange of apolipoprotein A-I between lipid-associated and lipid-free states: a potential target for oxidative generation of dysfunctional high density lipoproteins. *J Biol Chem.*, 285(24): 18847-18857.

Cecchi, C.; Baglioni, S.; Fiorillo, C.; Pensalfini, A.; Liguri, G.; Nosi, D.; Rigacci, S.; Bucciantini, M.; Stefani, M. (2005). Insights into the molecular basis of the differing susceptibility of varying cell types to the toxicity of amyloid aggregates. *J. Cell Sci.*, 118 (Pt 15): 3459-3470.

Chen, W.; Sun, Y.; Welch, C.; Gorelik, A.; Leventhal, A.R.; Tabas, I.; Tall, A.R. (2001). Preferential ATP-binding cassette transporter A1-mediated cholesterol efflux from late endosomes/lysosomes. *J Biol Chem.*, 276: 43564-43569.

Chen, W.; Wang, N.; Tall, A.R. (2005). A PEST deletion mutant of ABCA1 shows impaired internalization and defective cholesterol efflux from late endosomes. *J Biol Chem.*, 280: 29277-29281.

Chiti, F. & Dobson, C. M. (2006). Protein misfolding, functional amyloid, and human disease. *Annu. Rev. Biochem.*, 75: 333 - 366.

Chou, P.Y. & Fasman, G.D. (1978). Prediction of the secondary structure of proteins from their amino acid sequence. *Adv Enzymol Relat Areas Mol Biol.*, 47: 45-148.

Clay, M.A.; Newnham, H.H.; Forte, T.M.; Barter, P.I. (1992). Cholesteryl ester transfer protein and hepatic lipase activity promote shedding of apo A-I from HDL and subsequent formation of discoidal HDL. *Biochim. Biophys. Acta*, 1124(1): 52-58.

Denis, M.; Landry, Y.D. & Zha, X. (2008). ATP-binding cassette A1-mediated lipidation of apolipoprotein A-I occurs at the plasma membrane and not in the endocytic compartments. *J Biol Chem.*, 283: 16178-16186.

Di Gaetano, S.; Guglielmi, F.; Arciello, A.; Mangione, P.; Monti, M.; Pagnozzi, D.; Raimondi, S.; Giorgetti, S.; Orrù, S.; Canale, C.; Pucci, P.; Dobson, C.M.; Bellotti, V.; Piccoli R. (2006). Recombinant amyloidogenic domain of ApoA-I: analysis of its fibrillogenic potential. *Biochem Biophys Res Commun.*, 351(1): 223-228.

Duong, P. T.; Weibel, G. L.; Lund-Katz, S.; Rothblat, G. H.; Phillips, M. C. (2008). Characterization and properties of pre beta-HDL particles formed by ABCA1-mediated cellular lipid efflux to apoA-I. *J. Lipid Res.*, 49(5): 1006–1014.

Ehahalt, R.; Keller, P.; Haass, C.; Thiele, C.; Simons, K. J. (2003). Amyloidogenic processing of the Alzheimer beta-amyloid precursor protein depends on lipid rafts. *Cell Biol.*, 160: 113-123.

Eriksson, M.; Schönland, S.; Yumlu, S.; Hegenbart, U.; von Hutten, H.; Gioeva, Z.; Lohse, P.; Büttner, J.; Schmidt, H.; Röcken, C. (2009). Hereditary apolipoprotein AI-associated amyloidosis in surgical pathology specimens: identification of three novel mutations in the APOA1 gene. *J Mol Diagn.*, 11: 257-262.

Fantini, J. & Yahi, N. (2010). Molecular insights into amyloid regulation by membrane cholesterol and sphingolipids: common mechanisms in neurodegenerative diseases. *Expert Rev Mol Med.*, doi: 10.1017/S1462399410001602.

Fernandez-Escamilla, A.M.; Rousseau, F., Schymkowitz, J.; Serrano, L. (2004) Prediction of sequence-dependent and mutational effects on the aggregation of peptides and proteins. *Nat Biotechnol.*, 22(10): 1302-1306.

Fielding, C.J. & Fielding, P.E. (1995). Molecular physiology of reverse cholesterol transport. *Lipid Res.* 36(2): 211-228.

Frank, P.G. & Marcel, Y.L. (2000). Apolipoprotein A-I: structure-function relationships.*J. Lipid Res.* 41: 853–872.

Gast, K.; Damaschun, H.; Eckert, K.; Schulze-Forster, K.; Maurer, H.R.; Müller-Frohne, M.; Zirwer, D.; Czarnecki, J.; Damaschun, G. (1995). Prothymosin alpha: a biologically active protein with random coil conformation. *Biochemistry*, 34(40): 13211-13218.

Gaus, K.; Kritharides, L.; Schmitz, G.; Boettcher, A.; Drobnik, W.; Langmann, T.; Quinn, C.M.; Death, A.; Dean, R.T.; Jessup, W. (2004). Apolipoprotein A-1 interaction with plasma membrane lipid rafts controls cholesterol export from macrophages. *FASEB J.*, 18: 574-576.

Glass, C.K.; Pittman, R.C.; Keller, G.A.; Steinberg, D. (1983). Tissue sites of degradation of apoprotein A-I in the rat. *J. Biol Chem.*, 258(11): 7161-7167.

Guruprasad, K.; Reddy, B.V. & Pandit, M.W. (1990) Correlation between stability of a protein and its dipeptide composition: a novel approach for predicting in vivo stability of a protein from its primary sequence. *Protein Eng.*, 4(2): 155-161.

Hou, X.; Richardson, S.J.; Aguilar, M.I.; Small, D.H. (2005). Binding of amyloidogenic transthyretin to the plasma membrane alters membrane fluidity and induces neurotoxicity. *Biochemistry*, 44(34): 11618-11627.

Kakio, A.; Nishimoto, S.-L.; Kozutsumi, Y.; Matsuzaki, K. (2003). Formation of a membrane-active form of amyloid beta-protein in raft-like model membranes. *Biochim. Biophys. Res. Commun.*, 303(2): 514-518.

Kakio, A.; Yano, Y.; Takai, D.; Kuroda, Y.; Matsumoto, O.; Kozutsumi, Y.; Matsuzaki, K. (2004). Interaction between amyloid beta-protein aggregates and membranes. *J Pept Sci.*, 10(10): 612-621.

Kazlauskaite, J.; Sanghera, N.; Sylvester, I.; Vénien-Bryan, C.; Pinheiro, T.J. (2003). Structural changes of the prion protein in lipid membranes leading to aggregation and fibrillization. *Biochemistry*, 42(11): 3295-3304.

Lee, H.J.; Suk, J.E.; Bae, E.J.; Lee, J.H.; Paik, S.R.; Lee, S.J. (2008). Assembly-dependent endocytosis and clearance of extracellular alpha-synuclein. *Int J Biochem Cell Biol.*, 40(9): 1835-1849.

Lee, S.J.; Liyanage, U.; Bickel, P.E.; Xia, W.; Lansbury, P.T. Jr; Kosik, K.S. (1998). A detergent-insoluble membrane compartment contains A beta in vivo. *Nat Med.*, 4(6): 730-734.

Liang, H.Q.; Rye, K.A.; Barter, P.J. (1995). Cycling of apolipoprotein A-I between lipid-associated and lipid-free pools. *Biochim Biophys Acta.*, 1257(1): 31-37.

Liang, H.Q.; Rye, K.A.; Barter, P.J. (1996). Remodelling of reconstituted high density lipoproteins by lecithin: cholesterol acyltransferase. *J Lipid Res.*, 37(9): 1962-1970 .

Lusa, S.; Jauhiainen, M.; Metso, J.; Somerharju, P.; Ehnholm, C. (1996). The mechanism of human plasma phospholipid transfer protein-induced enlargement of high-density lipoprotein particles: evidence for particle fusion. *Biochem. J.*, 313 (Pt 1): 275-282.

Luzio, J.P.; Pryor, P.R. & Bright, N.A. (2007). Lysosomes: fusion and function. *Nat Rev Mol Cell Biol.*, 8: 622-632.

Martinez, Z.; Zhu, M.; Han, S.; Fink, A.L. (2007). GM1 specifically interacts with alpha-synuclein and inhibits fibrillation. *Biochemistry*, 46: 1868-1877.

Martins I.C.; Kuperstein I.; Wilkinson H.; Maes E.; Vanbrabant M.; Jonckheere W.; Van Gelder P.; Hartmann D.; D'Hooge R.; De Strooper B.; Schymkowitz J.; Rousseau F. (2008). Lipids revert inert Abeta amyloid fibrils to neurotoxic protofibrils that affect learning in mice. *EMBO J.*, 27(1): 224-233.

Mason, R.P.; Shoemaker, W.J.; Shajenko, L.; Chambers, T.E.; Herbette, L.G. (1992). Evidence for changes in the Alzheimer's disease brain cortical membrane structure mediated by cholesterol. *Neurobiol. Aging*, 13: 413-419.

Maurer-Stroh, S.; Debulpaep, M.; Kuemmerer, N.; Lopez de la Paz, M.; Martins, I.C.; Reumers, J.; Morris, K.L.; Copland, A.; Serpell, L.; Serrano, L.; Schymkowitz, J.W.; Rousseau, F. (2010). Exploring the sequence determinants of amyloid structure using position-specific scoring matrices. *Nat Methods*, 7(3): 237-242.

McNaught, K.S.; Mytilineou, C.; Jnobaptiste, R.; Yabut, J.; Shashidharan, P.; Jennert, P.; Olanow, C.W. (2002). Impairment of the ubiquitin-proteasome system causes dopaminergic cell death and inclusion body formation in ventral mesencephalic cultures. *J. Neurochem.*, 81: 301-306.

Monti, D.M.; Guglielmi, F.; Monti, M.; Cozzolino, F.; Torrassa, S.; Relini, A.; Pucci, P.; Arciello, A.; Piccoli R. (2010). Effects of a lipid environment on the fibrillogenic pathway of the N-terminal polypeptide of human apolipoprotein A-I, responsible for in vivo amyloid fibril formation. *Eur Biophys J.*, 39(9): 1289–1299.

Mukherjee, S.; Zha, X.; Tabas, I.; Maxfield, F.R. (1998). Cholesterol distribution in living cells: fluorescence imaging using dehydroergosterol as a fluorescent cholesterol analog. *Biophys J.*, 75: 1915-1925.

Mulya, A.; Lee, J.Y.; Gebre, A.K.; Thomas, M.J.; Colvin, P.L.; Parks, J.S. (2007). Minimal lipidation of pre-beta HDL by ABCA1 results in reduced ability to interact with ABCA1. *Arterioscler Thromb Vasc Biol.*, 27(8): 1828-1836.

Obici, L.; Bellotti, V.; Mangione, P.; Stoppini, M.; Arbustini, E.; Verga, L.; Zorzoli, I.; Anesi, E.; Zanotti, G.; Campana, C.; Viganò, M.; Merlini, G. (1999). The new apolipoprotein A-I variant Leu^{174}→Ser causes chardiac amyloidosis, and the fibrils are constituted by the 93-residue N-terminal polypeptide. *Am J Pathol.*, 155(3): 695-702.

Obici, L.; Franceschini, G.; Calabresi, L.; Giorgetti. S.; Stoppini, M.; Merlini, G.; Bellotti, V. (2006). Structure, function and amyloidogenic propensity of apolipoprotein A-I. *Amyloid.*, 13(4): 191-205.

Oram, J.F. (2008). The ins and outs of ABCA. *J Lipid Res.*, 49: 1150-1151.

Pastore, L.; Belalcazar, L.M.; Oka, K.; Cela, R.; Lee, B.; Chan, L.; Beaudet, A.L. (2004). Helper-dependent adenoviral vector-mediated long-term expression of human apolipoprotein A-I reduces atherosclerosis in apo E-deficient mice. *Gene*, 327(2): 153-60.

Raimondi, S.; Guglielmi, F.; Giorgetti, S.; Di Gaetano, S.; Arciello, A.; Monti, D.M.; Relini, A.; Nichino, D.; Doglia, S.M.; Natalello, A.; Pucci, P.; Mangione, P.; Obici, L.; Merlini, G.; Stoppini, M.; Robustelli, P.; Tartaglia, G.G.; Vendruscolo, M.; Dobson, C.M.; Piccoli, R.; Bellotti, V. (2011). Effects of the known pathogenic mutations on the aggregation pathway of the amyloidogenic peptide of apolipoprotein A-I. *J Mol Biol.*, 407(3): 465-476.

Rohrer, L.; Cavelier, C.; Fuchs, S.; Schlüter, M.A.; Völker, W.; von Eckardstein, A. (2006). Binding, internalization and transport of apolipoprotein A-I by vascular endothelial cells. *Biochim Biophys Acta.*, 1761: 186-194.

Ryan, R.O.; Yokoyama, S.; Liu, H.; Czarnecka, H.; Oikawa, K.; Kay, C.M. (1992). Human apolipoprotein A-I liberated from high-density lipoprotein without denaturation. *Biochemistry*, 31(18): 4509-4514.

Rye, K.A.; Hime, N.J.; Barter, P.J. (1997). Evidence that cholesteryl ester transfer protein-mediated reductions in reconstituted high density lipoprotein size involve particle fusion. *J Biol Chem.*, 272(7): 3953-3960.

Rye, K.A. & Barter, P.J. (2004). Formation and metabolism of prebeta-migrating, lipid-poor apolipoprotein A-I. *Arterioscler. Thromb. Vasc. Biol.* 24(3): 421–428.

Sacks, F.M.; Rudel, L.L.; Conner, A.; Akeefe, H.; Kostner, G.; Baki, T.; Rothblat, G.; de la Llera-Moya, M.; Asztalos, B.; Perlman, T.; Zheng, C.; Alaupovic, P.; Maltais, J.A.; Brewer, H.B. (2009). Selective delipidation of plasma HDL enhances reverse cholesterol transport in vivo. *J. Lipid Res.* 50(5): 894-907.

Sanghera N. & Pinheiro, T.J. (2002) Binding of prion protein to lipid membranes and implications for prion conversion. *J Mol Biol.*, 315(5): 1241-1256.

Sarnataro, D.; Campana, V.; Paladino, S., Stornaiuolo, M.; Nitsch, L.; Zurzolo, C. (2004). PrP(C) association with lipid rafts in the early secretory pathway stabilizes its cellular conformation. *Mol Biol Cell.*, 15(9): 4031-4042.

Shanmugam, G. & Jayakumar, R. (2004). Structural analysis of amyloid beta peptide fragment (25-35) in different microenvironments. *Biopolymers*. 76: 421-434.

Silva, R.A.; Hilliard, G.M.; Fang, J.; Macha, S.; Davidson, W.S. (2005). A three-dimensional molecular model of lipid-free apolipoprotein A-I determined by cross-linking/mass spectrometry and sequence threading. *Biochemistry.*, 44(8): 2759-2769.

Sorci-Thomas, M.G. & Thomas M.J. (2002). The effects of altered apolipoprotein A-I structure on plasma HDL concentration. *Trends Cardiovasc. Med.*, 12: 121-128.

Sreerama, N. & Woody, R.W. (2000). Estimation of protein secondary structure from circular dichroism spectra: comparison of CONTIN, SELCON, and CDSSTR methods with an expanded reference set. *Anal Biochem.*, 287(2): 252-260.

Steward, A.; Adhya S.; Clarke, J. (2002) Sequence conservation in Ig-like domains: the role of highly conserved proline residues in the fibronectin type III superfamily. *Mol. Biol*, 318(4): 935-940.

Tanaka, M.; Dhanasekaran, P.; Nguyen, D.; Ohta, S.; Lund-Katz, S.; Phillips, M.C.; Saito, H. (2006). Contributions of the N- and C-terminal helical segments to the lipid-free structure and lipid interaction of apolipoprotein A-I. *Biochemistry*, 45: 10351-10358.

Taraboulos, A.; Scott, M.; Semenov, A; Avrahami, D.; Laszlo, L.; Prusiner, S.B. (1995). Cholesterol depletion and modification of COOH-terminal targeting sequence of the prion protein inhibit formation of the scrapie isoform. *J Cell Biol.*, 129(1):121-32.

Tartaglia, G.G.; Pawar, A.P.; Campioni, S.; Dobson, C.M.; Chiti, F.; Vendruscolo, M. (2008). Prediction of aggregation-prone regions in structured proteins. *J. Mol. Biol.*, 380: 425-436.

Tofaris, G.K.; Layfield, R. & Spillantini, M.G. (2001). alpha-synuclein metabolism and aggregation is linked to ubiquitin-independent degradation by the proteasome. *FEBS Lett.*, 509: 22-26.

Tseng, B.P.; Green, K.N.; Chan, J.L.; Blurton-Jones, M.; Laferla, F.M. (2008). Abeta inhibits the proteasome and enhances amyloid and tau accumulation. *Neurobiol Aging.*, 29(11): 1607-1618.

Uversky, V.N. (2002). Natively unfolded proteins: a point where biology waits for physics. *Protein Science*, 11(4): 739-756.

Vedhachalam, C.; Duong, P.T.; Nickel, M.; Nguyen, D.; Dhanasekaran, P.; Saito, H.; Rothblat, G.H.; Lund-Katz, S.; Phillips, M.C. (2007). Mechanism of ATP-binding cassette transporter A1-mediated cellular lipid efflux to apolipoprotein A-I and formation of high density lipoprotein particles. *J. Biol. Chem.*, 282: 25123-25130.

Wang, N.; Silver, D.L.; Costet P.; Tall, A.R. (2000). Specific binding of ApoA-I, enhanced cholesterol efflux, and altered plasma membrane morphology in cells expressing ABC1. *J Biol Chem.*, 275(42): 33053-33058.

Weinreb, P.H.; Zhen, W. ; Poon, A.W. ; Conway, K.A. ; Lansbury, P.T. Jr. (1996). NACP, a protein implicated in Alzheimer's disease and learning, is natively unfolded. *Biochemistry*, 35(43): 13709-13715.

Wootton, J.C. & Federhen, S. (1996). Analysis of compositionally biased regions in sequence databases. *Methods Enzymol*, 266: 554-571.

Zampagni, M.; Cascella R.; Casamenti F.; Grossi C.; Evangelisti E.; Wright D.; Becatti M.; Liguri G.; Mannini B.; Campioni S.; Chiti F.; Cecchi C. (2010). A comparison of the biochemical modifications caused by toxic and nontoxic protein oligomers in cells. *J Cell Mol Med.*, doi: 10.1111/j.1582-4934.2010.01239.x.

Zha, X.; Genest, J. Jr & McPherson, R. (2001). Endocytosis is enhanced in Tangier fibroblasts: possible role of ATP-binding cassette protein A1 in endosomal vesicular transport. *J Biol Chem.* 276(42): 39476-39483.

Zhang, NY, Tang Z, Liu CW. (2008). alpha-Synuclein protofibrils inhibit 26 S proteasome-mediated protein degradation: understanding the cytotoxicity of protein protofibrils in neurodegenerative disease pathogenesis. *J Biol Chem.*, 283(29): 20288-20298.

Zhu, M. & Fink, A.L. (2003). Lipid binding inhibits alpha-synuclein fibril formation. *J Biol Chem.*, 278(19): 16873-16877.

5

Interaction and Aggregation of Amyloid β Peptide with Multivalent Sulfonated Sugar

Yoshiko Miura and Tomohiro Fukuda
Kyushu University
Japan

1. Introduction

Proteins have native functional states but can also form amyloid fibrils (Fowler et al .,2007, Maji et al., 2009, Dobson et al., 2003). In the amyloid state, proteins are denaturated and aggregated with β-sheet-rich structures. Accumulation of amyloids can result in protein amyloidosis, which has attracted much attention. Amyloidosis is associated with many serious neurodegenerative diseases, such as Alzheimer's disease (Sipe et al., 1992), dialysis-related amyloidosis (Rochet et al., 2000), prion disease (Prusiner, 1998), and type II diabetes (Ahmad et al., 2004). Consequently, it is important to clarify the mechanism of amyloidosis, so that it can be inhibited or controlled. Amyloid structures have been analyzed by various methods including nuclear magnetic resonance (NMR) spectroscopy, electron microscopy, X-ray spectroscopy and Fourier transform infrared (FTIR) spectroscopy. Theoretical calculations of amyloidosis have also been conducted (Miller et al., 2010).

Protein amyloidosis is affected by environmental conditions such as the temperature (Kusumoto et al., 1998), pH (Petkova et al., 2004), and ionic strength (Zidar et al., 2011), and by nucleation (Kanji et al., 2008). Because amyloidosis occurs at the cell surface, the interaction between the protein and cell interface is also important (Xu et al., 2005). Therefore, the amyloidosis of proteins can be controlled by manipulating the environmental conditions. However, it has been reported that artificial additives, such as metal ions (Chanki et al., 2007), peptides (Suzuki et al., 2010), sugars (Anubhav et al., 2004) and nanoparticles (Saraiva et al., 2010), can alter the environmental conditions and affect amyloidosis.

Because amyloidosis occurs *in vivo*, the molecules on the cell surfaces are of interest as additives to control amyloidosis. It has been reported that protein amyloidosis with Amyloid beta (Aβ) (Alzheimer's disease) (McLaurin et al., 1996), β2-microglobulin (dialysis-related amyloidosis) (Bourgault et al., 2011), and prion protein (Pan et al., 2002) formation is affected by interactions with glycosaminoglycans (GAGs) on the cell surfaces. This affects all these proteins, even though they have different amino acid sequences and native protein structures. GAGs are long unbranched polysaccharides of repeating disaccharide subunits of hexosamines (glucosamine and galactosamine) and uronic acid (glucuronic acid and iduronic acid) (Rudd et al., 2010). Well-known GAGs are heparin, chondroitin sulfate, keratin sulfate, dermatan sulfate and hyaluronic acid. Most GAGs are highly sulfonated. The interaction of proteins with GAGs is important in amyloidosis, but it is difficult to analyze the detail of this interaction because GAGs have complex structures and high molecular weights.

Synthetic model molecules are useful to clarify the biological function of GAGs. Suda et al. used a synthetic pentasaccharide that bound antithrombin III to study the function of heparin, and produced a biochip with the synthetic GAG (Suda et al., 1993, 2006). Although a number of studies have been reported the compositions of oligosaccharides in GAGs (Jose et al., 2006) and syntheses for GAGs (Jeroen et al., 2005), these investigations did not consider the effect of the molecular weight of GAGs even though they have high molecular weights (5,000-30,000). It is difficult to account for the physical properties and multivalent effects of saccharides within the oligosaccharide following polymerization.
We previously investigated the biological functions using multivalent glycoclusters, and applied these results to production of materials (Miura et al., 2007). Multivalency is important in the biological function of saccharides because it increases the affinity between the saccharides and proteins when the saccharide interaction is weak (Mammen et al., 1998). Glycoclusters include glycopolymers, glycodendrimers (Aoi et al., 1995), and glyco-thin layers (Lang et al., 2008), which all increase the protein–saccharide interactions. Among these types of glycoclusters, glycopolymers with pendant saccharides showed the strongest amplification effect. In this work, we investigated the interaction between GAG models and Aβ to examine the function of GAGs in amyloidosis. The saccharide used was 6-sulfo-*N*-acetyl-glucosamine (6S-GlcNAc), which is frequently present in heparin (Uchimura et al., 1998, Sasaki et al. 2003). An artificial glycocluster of glycopolymer and a glyco-thin layer was prepared, and its interaction with Aβ was investigated.

2. Inhibition of aggregation of amyloid β with sulfonated glycopolymers

In this section, synthetic glycopolymers were produced to mimic GAGs and used to investigate control of aggregation of Aβ. Although the saccharide–protein interaction is generally weak, the glycopolymer increases this interaction through its multivalency. The multivalency can be easily altered by adjusting the initial feed ratio in the polymerization. It is difficult to complete the total synthesis of GAGs. In the present study, GAGs were mimicked using a glycopolymer (Figure 1) that was an acrylamide derivative of the saccharide 6S-GlcNAc.

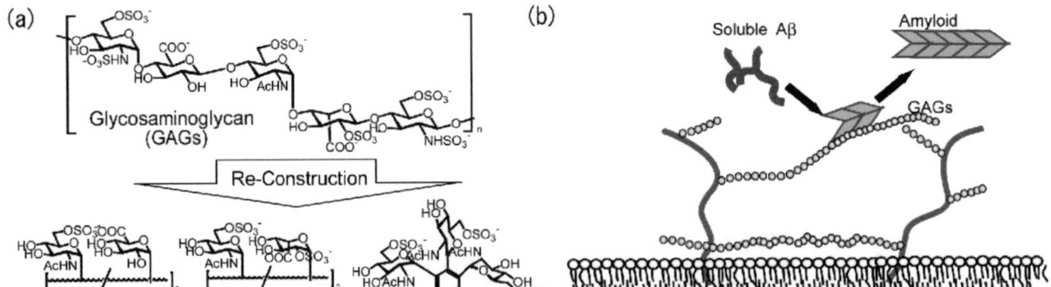

Fig. 1. The GAGs in amyloidosis and this chapter's study. (a)The design of GAGs mimic compounds. (b) The role of GAGs in amyloidosis.

The monomer was synthesized from *N*-acetyl-glucosamine (GlcNAc) by modification with *p*-nitrophenyl-GlcNAc. The obtained acrylamide derivative was polymerized using a radical initiator. The saccharide contents were varied in the copolymerization of glycopolymer and acrylamide. The sugar contents of the polymers were 10–100 %, and the molecular weights of the polymers were in the order of 10^5. The reference polymers were the glycopolymer of GlcNAc without sulfonated GlcNAc, polyacrylamide, and monomeric 6S-GlcNAc (Figure 2). The interactions of Aβ with the glycopolymers were evaluated by a Thioflavin T (ThT) fluorescence assay, observation of the morphology by atomic force microscopy (AFM), circular dichroism (CD) spectroscopy, and *in vitro* neutralization of an MTT assay. The protein used in this section was Aβ(1-42).

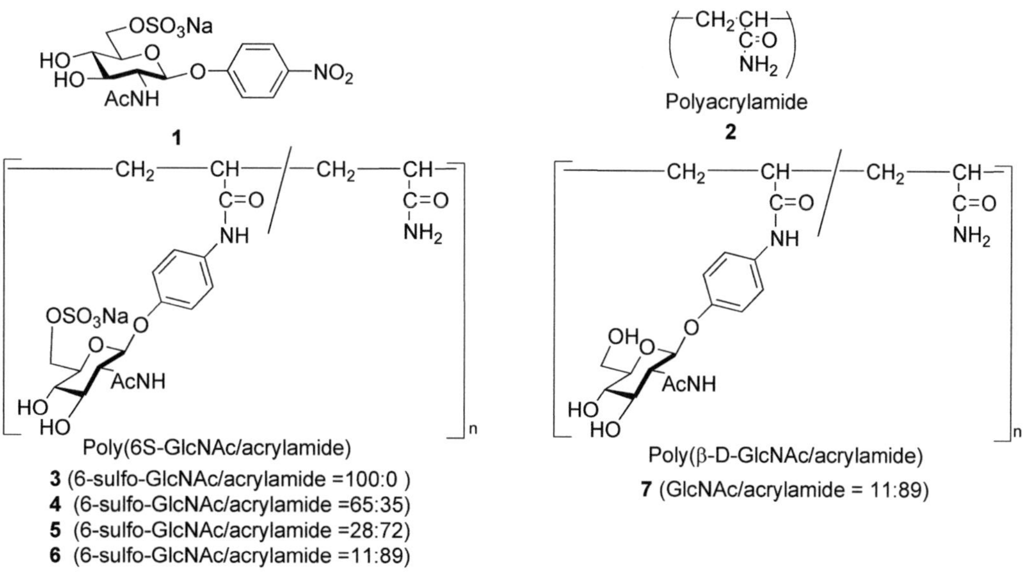

Fig. 2. Chemical structure of GAGs mimic polymers used in section 2

2.1 ThT fluorescence assay of Aβ aggregation in the presence of glycopolymers

The aggregation of Aβ was monitored with ThT in the presence of different glycopolymers (Figure 3). ThT binds to β-sheet aggregates. The ThT fluorescence of Aβ in the absence of any additive increased for 8 h to a final fluorescence of 100. When the monomeric sulfonated GlcNAc (pNP-6S-GlcNAc, **1**) was added to the Aβ solution, no remarkable change was observed in the time-course ThT fluorescence. To improve the weak interaction between 6S-GlcNAc and Aβ, multivalent compounds were then investigated. The addition of glycopolymers of 6S-GlcNAc (**3–6**) resulted in inhibition of Aβ aggregation. Interestingly, the inhibition effect was dependent on the sugar content of the polymer. While the glycopolymers with low sugar contents, **5** (28 %) and **6** (12 %), showed strong inhibition of Aβ aggregation, the glycopolymers with high sugar contents, **3** (100 %) and **4** (65 %), did not show strong inhibition. The glycopolymer of GlcNAc without the sulfonate did not change the time-course of ThT fluorescence, and polyacrylamide without the saccharide or sulfonate did not inhibit aggregation.

These data suggest that the sulfonate in the glycopolymer is essential for Aβ aggregation, and that the level of inhibition is also related to the sugar content the glycopolymer. This indicates that the degree of sulfonation in GAGs and their physical properties are important in the formation of Aβ deposits. It has been reported that GAGs induce and also inhibit the aggregation of Aβ, which is related to the degree of sulfonation and the physical properties.

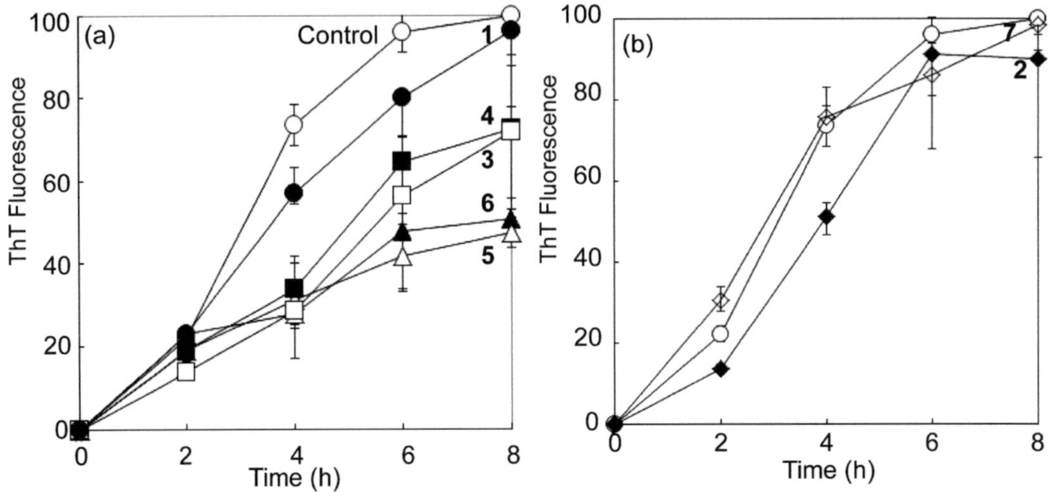

Fig. 3. Time-course of the fluorescence change in ThT at 37°C with Aβ (1-42) and sugar additives (a) with sulfonated GlcNAc of **1**, **3**, **4**, **5**, and **6**, (b) with polymers of **2** and **7**. The concentration of Aβ and sugar was 20 μM and 200mM

2.2 Changes in morphology and neutralization of Aβ by glycopolymers

The morphology of aggregated Aβ was observed in the presence of glycopolymers by AFM (Figure 4). Aβ readily formed amyloid fibrils 15–50 nm wide, 5–15 nm high, and a few micrometers in length. While the addition of monomeric saccharide (**1**) reduced the size of the amyloid fibrils, fibril formation still occurred. The addition of the glycopolymers with 6S-GlcNAc acid (**3–6**) changed the morphology. The addition of the glycopolymer with a low sugar content (**5** and **6**) changed the Aβ into spheres with diameters of 10–250 nm. By contrast, the glycopolymers with a high sugar content (**3** and **4**) did not inhibit fibril formation, and the fibrils increased in size (width 60–300 nm). These morphology observations suggest that Aβ interacted strongly with the sulfonated glycopolymers. These changes were interesting because of the relationship of Aβ's morphology to cytotoxicity (Hoshi et al., 2003, Hardy et al., 2002, Kayed et al., 2003). The cytotoxity Aβ relates the amount of accumulated Aβ, and the morphology, where the oligomeric Aβs with nm order and round morphology has been reported to show the cytotoxity. The results of AFM observation suggest that the development of Alzheimer's disease is related to the degree of sulfonation of GAGs. Control of Aβ's morphology was investigated with specific sulfonated glyco-clusters in a later section.

The neutralization of the cytotoxicity of Aβ was investigated using HeLa cells. When the cells were incubated with Aβ, Aβ reduced the cell survival rate by about 50 %, but the addition of sulfonated glycopolymer (**6**) restored the cell survival rate. Glycopolymer **6** alone did not show any cytotoxicity. The interaction between Aβ and the the glycopolymer ihibitied the accumulation or oligomer formation. Therefore, this glycopolymer, and perhaps GAGs, could safely be used as polymer medicines.

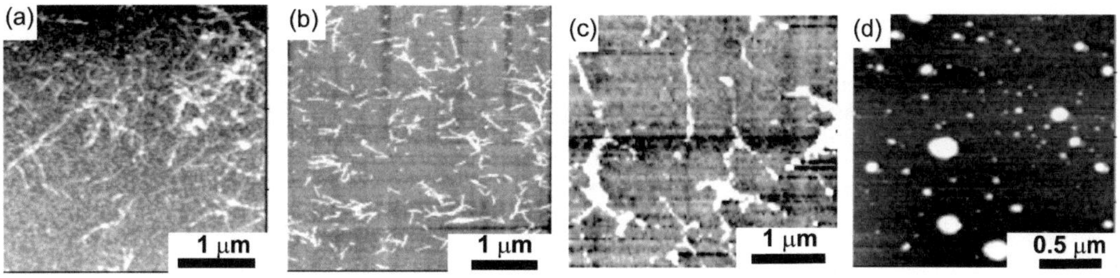

Fig. 4. AFM observations of Aβ(1-42) (a) without glycopolymer, (b) in the presence of **1**, (c) **3** and (d) **6**.

3. The inhibition of amyloid β aggregation by the glycopolymer with precise molecular weight via living radical polymerization

In section 2, glycopolymers with 6S-GlcNAc were shown to bind to Aβ, inhibit Aβ aggregation, and neutralize the cytotoxicity of Aβ. Because of the structural diversity of GAGs, the glycopolymer library is useful to analyze the function of GAGs in Aβ amyloidosis. This could be used to develop a glycopolymer that acts as a better inhibitor of Aβ aggregation. Although it is difficult to analyze the GAGs, the fabrication of glycopolymers is easily achieved by facile radical polymerization. Other polymerization techniques, such as living radical polymerization and graft polymerization, can also be used for this. In this section, a library of glycopolymers with different molecular weights and saccharide structures was prepared to analyze the interaction of Aβ with various glycopolymer. Because natural GAGs are copolymer with hexosamines and uronic acids, the glycopolymers were synthesized using 6S-GlcNAc and glucuronic acid (GlcA).

3.1 Glycopolymer library via living radical polymerization

The glycopolymer library was designed using acrylamide derivatives of 6S-GlcNAc and GlcA (Figure 5). The glycopolymers with 6S-GlcNAc were polyanionic, and were mimics of heparin, while the glycopolymers with GlcA were mimics of hyaluronic acid. The terpolymer of 6S-GlcNAc and GlcA was better mimic of general GAGs in terms of the sugar structure. The sugar contents of the polymers were set at about 10 % based on the results from section 2.1, and the monomer structures were investigated.

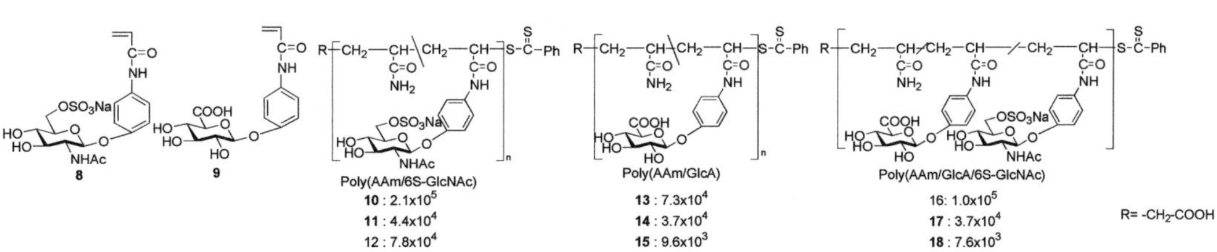

Fig. 5. Chemical structure and molecular weight (M_n) of GAGs mimic polymers in section 3.

Because the molecular weight of GAG affects its biological function, the impact of the molecular weight of the glycopolymer was also investigated. Low molecular GAGs have been reported to show therapeutic effects (Walzer et al., 2002, Zhu et al., 2001) in protein

amyloidosis. Glycopolymers with various molecular weights were synthesized by reversible addition–fragmentation chain transfer (RAFT) living radical polymerization (Moad et al 2008). The living radical polymerization can be used to synthesize well-defined polymers with various molecular weights. Compared with other methods like atom transfer radical polymerization (ATRP), it is easier to synthesize bulky complicated monomers using RAFT living radical polymerization. Dithioesters and trithiocarbonates can be used as reagents in RAFT polymerization. In this study, (thiobenzoyl)thioglycolic acid was used as the RAFT reagent in glycopolymer syntheses.
Glycopolymers with 6S-GlcNAc (**10–12**), GlcA(**13–15**), and terpolymer (**16–18**) were synthesized, and the molecular weights of these polymers were in the order of 10^5 (**10, 13**, and **16**), 10^4 (**11, 14** and **17**) and 10^3 (**12, 15**, and **18**) (Figure 5).

Sample	k_n (s^{-1})	k_e ($L\ mol^{-1}\ s^{-1}$)
Aβ (control)	1.3×10^{-6}	3.4
8	1.4×10^{-6}	3.7
10	7.3×10^{-9}	6.6
11	2.5×10^{-8}	5.9
12	5.1×10^{-10}	7.9
9	3.4×10^{-6}	3.0
13	4.2×10^{-6}	2.5
14	2.5×10^{-6}	4.2
15	6.7×10^{-6}	2.5
16	1.3×10^{-6}	4.3
17	6.7×10^{-7}	3.4
18	6.8×10^{-7}	3.1
Heparin	3.1×10^{-6}	3.7
Hyaluronic acid	1.5×10^{-6}	3.4

Table 1. Nucleation and elongation rate constants calculated by fitting ThT data.

The protein Aβ(1-40) was used to analyze the inhibition effect and kinetics. Aβ(1-40) is the main component of amyloid deposits, and has lower ability to aggregate than Aβ(1-42). Because Aβ(1-40) is less likely to aggregate, the amyloid fibril formation was measured with fast shaking (400 rpm) after monomerization by hexafluoro-2-propanol.

3.2 Kinetic analyses of the inhibition of Aβ aggregation in the presence of glycopolymers

Aggregation of Aβ(1-40) was monitored in detail using its ThT fluorescence, which showed a sigmoidal curve (Figure 6). The addition of glycopolymers changed the time-course of ThT fluorescence. The glycopolymers with 6S-GlcNAc (**10–12**) extended the lag phase, which is the time taken for the fluorescence to increase initially, and the final fluorescence intensity was lower than that of control. However, the glycopolymers with GlcA (**13–15**) did not change the lag phase, which suggests these polymers had a weak interaction with Aβ. The ter-glycopolymer with both of 6S-GlcNAc and GlcA showed the best inhibition of Aβ aggregation. The level of inhibition was largely dependent on the sugar structure.

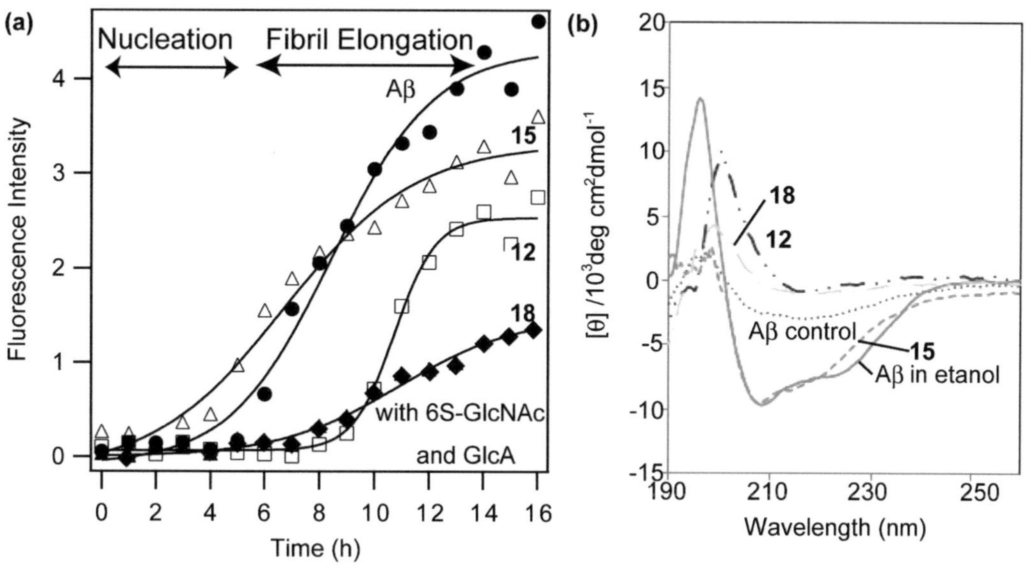

Fig. 6. The time courses of aggregation and the secondary structures of Aβ. (a) Time course of fibril formation with 400 rpm shaking at 37°C. The concentrations of Aβ and sugar were 23 and 200μM. The sugar additives were poly(AAm/6S-GlcNAc)(**12**), poly(AAm/GlcA) (**15**) and poly(AAm/6S-GlcNAc/GlcA) (**18**). (b) The CD spectra of Aβ in the presence of glycopolymers (**12**, **15** and **18**).

The level of inhibition was also dependent on the molecular weight of the polymer. The final fluorescence intensity changed with the molecular weight of the polymer even if the sugar content was the same. Glycopolymers with lower molecular weights produced a lower fluorescence intensity and the longer lag phase than glycopolymers with higher molecular weights.

The aggregation properties were analyzed in detail by fitting of the fluorescence curve. The aggregation of Aβ was analyzed using the processes of nucleation and elongation of the amyloid as follows:

$$nM \rightarrow P_n \qquad \text{(nucleation process, } k_n\text{)}$$

$$M + P_n \rightarrow P_{n+1} \qquad \text{(elongation process, } k_e\text{)}$$

where M and P are the monomeric and polymeric peptides, respectively. The kinetics data are summarized in Table 1. The results were analyzed in terms of the nucleation (k_n) and elongation (k_e) rate constants compared with the control. The glycopolymers with 6S-GlcNAc showed smaller k_n and larger k_e in comparison to the glycopolymers with GlcA, which induced larger k_n and smaller k_e. The 6S-GlcNAc monomer inhibited the nucleation of Aβ, and the GlcA unit inhibited the elongation of the fibril. Among the glycopolymers, the terpolymer with both 6S-GlcNAc and GlcA showed the best inhibition of Aβ aggregation and had the smallest k_n and moderate k_e. The effect of the molecular weight on Aβ aggregation was analyzed using the kinetic parameters. With the 6S-GlcNAc polymer, the polymer with lower molecular weight had a smaller k_n, which gave better inhibition of nucleation. With the glycopolymer of both 6S-GlcNAc and GlcA, that with the lowest molecular weight was the best inhibitor (**18**). The molecular weight of a polymer affects various physical properties such as mobility, and low molecular weight polymers should have better binding to Aβ. These results were corresponding to those for heparin, which has a low molecular weight.

		19 (monovalent)	**20** (divalent)	**21** (trivalent)
Aggregate Pattern		Fibril	Fibril, Globule	Globule
Fibril	Width Length Height	8-12nm 1-2μm 4-6nm	8-12nm 1-2μm 4-6nm	
Globule	Height Diameter		7-9nm 200-500nm	10-20nm 500-600nm

Table 2. Aggregate patterns and sizes of Aβ (1–42) on **19**, **20** and **21**.

3.3 The conformation and morphology of Aβ aggregation in the presence of various glycopolymers

The AFM results were consistent with the ThT assay. The Aβ aggregates without additives formed amyloid fibrils that were 1–3.5 μm long, 160–230 nm wide, and 15–45 nm high. The Aβ fibrils in the presence of the glycopolymer with 6S-GlcNAc (**12**) were 0.19–2.0 μm long, 110–180 nm wide, and 1–8 nm high. The Aβ fibrils in the presence of the terpolymer (**18**) were 0.10–1.7 μm long, 80–120 nm wide and 1.5-4.0 nm high (Table 2).

The glycopolymer additives induced a specific conformation in Aβ (Figure 7). Aβ(1–40) without additives showed a β-sheet structure with a negative Cotton effect around 220 nm in the CD spectra. The glycopolymer with 6S-GlcNAc gave a β-sheet structure, and the Cotton effect was smaller than for the control Aβ. With the ter-glycopolymers, the spectra showed broad negative Cotton effects with weak intensity. Interestingly, the glycopolymers with GlcA induced a different conformation, with the CD spectra showing negative Cotton effects around 208 nm and 220 nm, which suggests a partial α-helical structure.

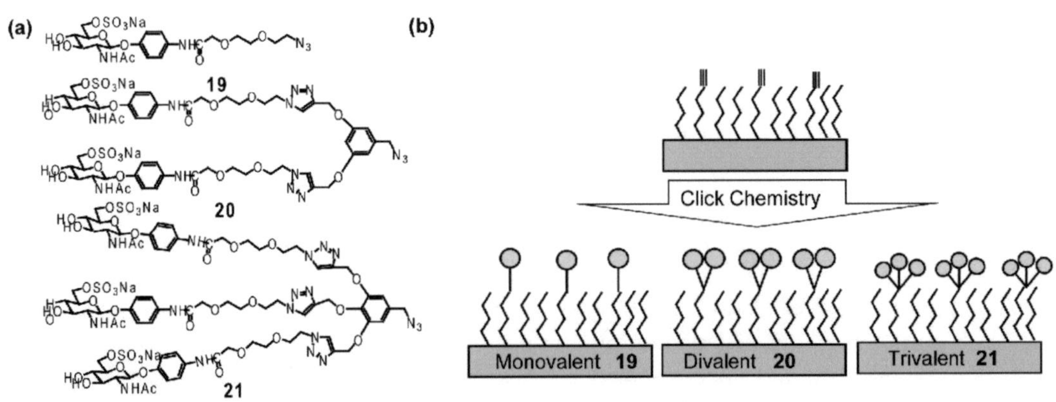

Fig. 7. (a) Chemical structures of glyco-cluster and (b) the schematic illustration of the glyco-cluster at the interface.

The conformation of Aβ was also examined with addition of the natural GAGs heparin (containing 6S-GlcNAc) and hyaluronic acid (containing GlcA). The addition of heparin induced a β-sheet structure with a negative Cotton effect at 218 nm, which was consistent with the CD spectra in the presence of the 6S-GlcNAc glycopolymer. The addition of hyaluronic acid induced a broad negative Cotton effect at 208 nm, which suggests the conformation is not β-sheet. When comparing the sulfonated GAGs like heparin, the roles of uronic acid and hyaluronic acid were not considered because of their weak interactions. If the polyvalent uronic acid or hyaluronic acid can operate as a molecular chaperon in amyloidosis, they will be useful bioactive compounds.

3.4 Mechanism of inhibition of Aβ aggregation

Because the sulfonic acid in the GlcNAc was essential to inhibit Aβ aggregation, this indicates the electrostatic interaction was the driving force behind the inhibition. Both Aβ(1–40) and Aβ(1–42) have a net negative charge, but the proteins of Aβ also contained cationic residues (Arg15, His6, His13, His14, Lys16, and Lys28). The anionic region of 13-HHQK-16 was considered to play an important role, and the HHQK region has been reported to be important in determining the conformation of Aβ (Giulian et al. 1998).

The sugar content of the polymer and the molecular weight effect were interesting for molecular design of an inhibitor. The glycopolymers of 6S-GlcNAc with a high sugar contents did not inhibit Aβ aggregation. The conformation of this glycopolymer was stiff because of the bulky side chain of the polymer, which weakened the interaction with Aβ. The cluster of anionic groups also inhibited the interaction because of electrostatic repulsion that occurred with the net negative charge of Aβ. The role of GlcA was not clear but it provided the hydrogen bonding section and inhibited elongation of the fibrils.

In this section, the effects of the glycopolymer, GAGs, and saccharides were investigated using the glycopolymer technique. The glycopolymer approach clearly showed the role of each saccharide, where sulfonated GlcNAc inhibited nucleation and induced fibril formation and β-sheet formation, and uronic acid induced formation of a partial α-helical structure. The library of glycopolymers with various molecular weights indicated the importance of the physical and chemical properties of GAGs, and suggested low molecular weight polymers were better for inhibition of Aβ aggregation than high molecular weight polymers.

4. The control of Aβ amyloidosis with precise manipulation of the glyco-interface

In section 2 and 3, sulfonated GlcNAc was determined to be a key monomer for Aβ aggregation and protein amyloidosis. The results showed the effect a glycopolymer mimic of a GAG had on the amyloidosis was based on the interaction between Aβ and sulfonated GlcNAc or Aβ and sulfate group. We investigated the control of amyloidosis of Aβ by manipulating the glyco-cluster interface with 6S-GlcNAc. The experiments were conducted on a gold interface for interaction analysis by surface plasmon resonance (SPR), FTIR, and AFM. The protein used was Aβ(1–42), which can have various morphologies because of its self-assembly properties.

4.1 Molecular design of the glyco-interface

Self-assembled monolayers (SAMs) of 6S-GlcNAc were prepared for fabrication of the glyco-cluster interface. An alkyl-disulfide with an acetylenyl group was modified via click chemistry, because an alkyl-disulfide with an oligoethylene glycol has been shown to be bioinert to inhibition of protein adsorption by non-specific interaction (Kolb et al. 2001) (Figure 8). Glyco-clusters with 6S-GlcNAc were synthesized using hydroxyl-benzene templates, and glyco-clusters with mono- (**19**), di- (**20**) and tri- (**21**) valent 6-S-GlcNAc with an azide-group were also synthesized. To modify the substrate, the reactive functional surface was prepared using SAMs. The alkyl-disulfide with an acetylene group was synthesized, and mixed SAMs were prepared using the alkyl-disulfide with acetylene and oligoethylene groups on the gold substrate. The ratio of the acetylene terminal was 20 %. The acetylene group was immobilized by click chemistry.

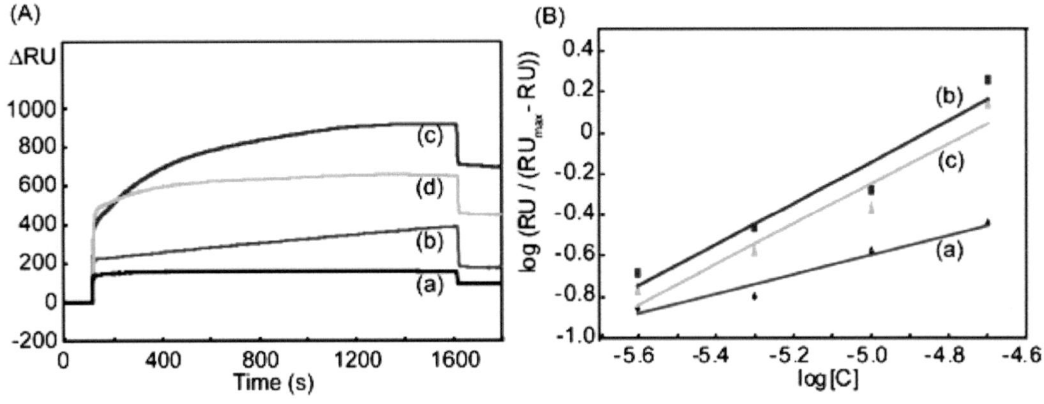

Fig. 8. (A) Time courses of RU change on (a) no-sugar SAM, (b) **19**, (c) **20** and (d) **21**. (B) Hill plot analysis using the RU_{eqmax} on (a) **19**, (b) **20** and (c) **21**.

The glyco-cluster of 6S-GlcNAc was prepared on the gold substrate. Gold substrates have advantages in biological analyses for surface plasmon resonance (SPR), quartz crystal microbalance (QCM), and electrochemistry. The interaction between 6S-GlcNAc and Aβ was analyzed by SPR. The amount of bound Aβ(1–42) (RU_{max}) changed with the valency, and for the different valency glycoclusters was in the order mono- (**19**)<<tri- (**21**)<di-valent (**20**). This suggests that multivalency is important for Aβ binding to the glycocluster. The amount of Aβ bound to the substrate was plotted to calculate the binding constants. The SPR results for the glycoclusters and Aβ were fitted using a Hill plot, not by a Langmuir plot. The multivalent binding was quantitatively analyzed as follows:

$$\log\left(\frac{[RU_{eq\max}]_{C[\mu M]}}{[RU_{eq\max}]_{40[\mu M]}-[RU_{eqmzx}]_{C[\mu M]}}\right)=n\log[C[\mu M]]-n\log K_D$$

where n and K_D represent the Hill coefficient (cooperativity) and apparent binding constant, respectively. The equilibrium constants from the SPR results were 1.49 x 10^{-4}, 1.16 x 10^{-5} and 1.89 x 10^{-5} M for the mono-, di- and tri-valent saccharides, respectively. The Hill coefficients indicated the binding ratios (sugar/Aβ) of the mono-, di-, and tri-valent glycoclusters were 2:1, 1:1 and 1:1, respectively. This shows that multivalent binding is essential even for the monovalent cluster of **19** (binding with an adjacent sugar). The multiple sugar binding was accomplished by the two sugars binding to 13-HHQK-16 or to 13-HHQK-16 and Lys28.

4.2 The morphology of Aβ on the sugar interface

The morphology on the glyco-substrate was investigated by AFM (Figure 9). Interestingly, the morphology of Aβ was dependent on the type of glyco-cluster at the interface. The results are summarized in Table 2. When Aβ(1-42) was incubated on the monovalent 6S-GlcNAc (**19**), fibrils formed that were 4-6 nm high, 8-12 nm wide, and 1-2 μm long. For di-valent 6S-GlcNAc (**20**), both fibrils and spherical aggregates were observed. Furthermore, the incubation of Aβ with trivalent 6S-GlcNAc (**21**) induced formation of only the spherical aggregates with inhomogeneous sizes. The spheres were a mixture of those 10-20 nm and 500-600 nm in diameter.

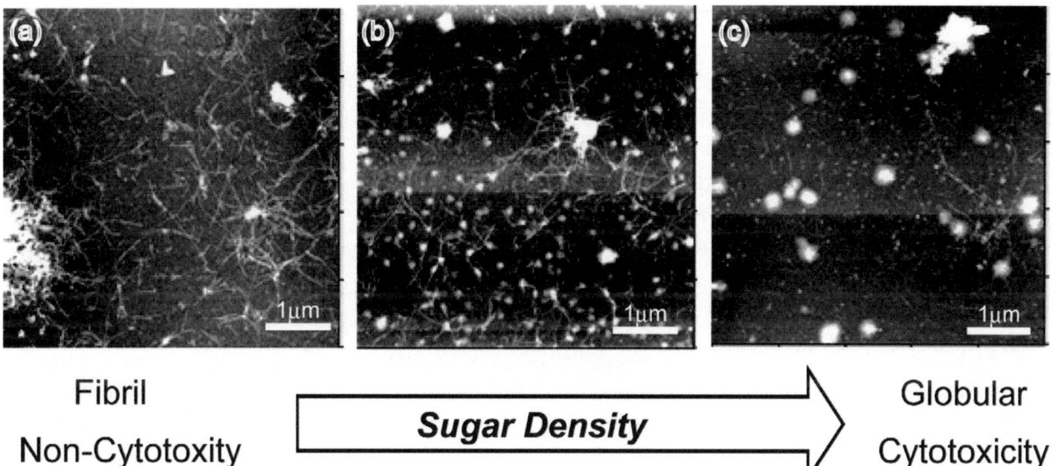

Fig. 9. Morphologies observed by AFM with 6S-GlcNAc glyco-cluster of (a) monovalent (**19**), (b) divalent (**20**) and (c) trivalent (**21**).

The AFM observation of the glycocluster substrate suggested that Aβ(1–42) had a tendency to form fibrils with the low valency 6-S-GlcNAc, and spherical aggregates with higher valency glycoclusters. The densely packed sulfonated or acidic sugars induced a strong morphological change in the Aβ(1-42) aggregates. The morphological change of the amyloid aggregates from fibrils to spheres is consistent with the report of Ban et al.(Ban et al., 2006). The valency of the sulfonated GlcNAc determined the affinity to Aβ, which induced specific morphologies and secondary structures.

The secondary structure of Aβ was measured on the glyco-cluster interface by FTIR in the amide region. The amide I band (C=O stretching) at 1670 cm^{-1} was the main peak in all cases, and corresponded to a β-turn or unknown structure. The band at 1632 cm^{-1} indicated an antiparallel β-sheet structure, which was dependent on the valency of 6S-GlcNAc. Remarkably, that band was the least intense in the spectrum of the trivalent interface (**21**), and the strongest in the spectrum of the monovalent interface (**19**). Taking into account the AFM observations, these results indicated that the fibrils on **19** had predominantly β-sheet structure and the spheres on **21** had little β-sheet structure. The strong binding of Aβ to the 6S-GlcNAc interface suppressed the interaction with each peptide, which reduced the content of β-sheet structure on **21**. The secondary structure revealed that the structure with anti-parallel β-sheet resulted in the fibril formation, and that with less β-sheet structure resulted in the spheres. The negatively charged surface also contributed to the formation of the spherical morphology because of the electrostatic repulsion.

The cytotoxicity of Aβ(1–42) to HeLa cells was evaluated by MTT assay on the substrate. The cell viabilities with Aβ(1–42) on the mono- (**19**), di- (**20**) and tri-(**21**) valent glycoclusters were 104 %, 84 %, 76 %, respectively. These results indicate that the cytotoxicity of Aβ(1–42) varied because of the aggregation process. Aggregation of Aβ(1-42) on the trivalent glycocluster of 6S-GlcNAc formed globular objects, where the small spherical aggregates have been reported to show the high cytotoxity. Though the size of the aggregates were much smaller than that of toxic oligomers (Hoshi et al 2003, Hardy et al 2002, Kayed et al 2003), the observed globular objects on trivalent 6S-GlcNAc had similar round morphology and had the high cytotoxicity. By contrast, aggregation on monovalent 6-S-GlcNAc showed no cytotoxicity. It has been reported that the spherical Aβ exhibit strong cytotoxicity.

The specific morphology of Aβ was induced by the glycocluster on the substrate, which affect the secondary conformation, morphology and finally the cytotoxicity.

5. Conclusion

These studies using artificial glycoclusters revealed the role of sugars in GAGs in amyloidosis. Inhibition and control of amyloidosis of Aβs was accomplished using glycoclusters of glycopolymers and a glycointerface with 6-sulfo-GlcNAc. The glycopolymer with 6-sulfo-GlcNAc inhibited the aggregation of Aβ(1–40) and Aβ(1–42). The appropriate valency of the polymer was essential to aggregation. The glycopolymers of 6-sulfo-GlcNAc with low sugar contents efficiently inhibited the Aβ aggregation and neutralized its cytotoxicity. Kinetic analyses indicated that the sulfonated GlcNAc inhibited the nucleation, and that GlcA of uronic acid inhibited the fibril elongation. The molecular weight of the polymers was also important, and the glycopolymer with a low molecular weight provided strong inhibition. The low molecular weight glycopolymer with both 6-sulfo-GlcNAc and GlcA showed the strongest inhibition.

With specific glycocluster interfaces, the amyloidosis of Aβ was dependent on the valency and the distance of the 6-sulfo-GlcNAc. High valent 6-sulfo-GlcNAc showed stronger interaction with Aβ than mono valent 6-sulfo-GlcNAc. The dense tri-valent 6-sulfo-GlcNAc induced formation of spheres of Aβ with less β-sheet structure than with the other valencies of 6-sulfo-GlcNAc, and this structure showed cytotoxicity. By contrast, the non-dense monovalent saccharide induced fibril formation with a β-sheet-rich structure without cytotoxicity.

It is difficult to investigate the function of GAGs because of their complex structures, and this method using glycoclusters can be used to clarify their functions. In this investigation, only 6-sulfo-GlcNAc was used as a representative sugar of GAGs. Although wild type GAGs contain various and complicated sulfonated saccharides, this study of GAGs mimics provides useful information on the GAGs functions using precise control of the 6-sulfo-GlcNAc cluster. To extend on this, glycocluster of other sulfonated saccharides are being synthesized in our laboratory.

6. References

Ahmad, A.; Millett, I. S.; Doniach, S.; Uversky, V. N.& Fink, A. L. (2004) Stimulation of Insulin Fibrillation by Urea-induced Intermediates. *J. Biol. Chem.* 279(15), 14999-15013.

Aoi, K.; Itoh, K. & Okada, M. (1995) Globular Carbohydrate Macromolecules „Sugar Balls".1. Synthesis of Novel Sugar-Persubstututed Poly(amidoamine) Dendrimers. *Macromolecules* 28(15), 5391-5392.

Arora, A.; Ha, C. & Park, C. B.(2004) Inhibitiono f Insulin Amloid Formation by Small Stress Molecules. *FEBS Lett.* 564(1-2), 121-125.

Bourgalt, S.; Solomon, J. P.; Reixach, N. & Kelly, J. W. (2011) Sulfated Glycosaminoglycans Accelerate Transthyretin Amyloidogenesis by Quaternary Structural Conversion. *Biochemistry*, 50(6), 1001-1015.

Codée, J. D.; Stubba, B.; Schiattarella, M.; Overkleeft, H. S.; van Boeckel, C. A.; van Boom J. H.& van der Marel G. A. (2005) A Modular Strategy Toward the Synthesis of Heparin-like Oligosaccharides using Monomeric Building Blocks in a Sequential Glycosylation Strategy. *J. Am. Chem. Soc.* 127(11), 3767-3773.

dePaz, J. L.; Noti, C. & Seeberger, P. H. (2006) Microarrays of Synthetic Heparin Oligosaccharides. *J. Am. Chem. Soc.* 128(9), 2766-2777.

Dobson, C. M. (2003) Protein Folding and Misfolding. *Nature*,884-890.

Fowler, D.M.; Koulov, A. V.; Balch, W. E.& Kelly, J. W. (2007)Functional Amyloid-from Bacteria to Humans. *Trends Biochem Sci.* 32(5), 217-224.

Kolb, H. C.; Finn, M. G. & Sharpless, K. B. (2001) Click Chemistry: Diverse Chemical Function From a Few Good Reactions. *Angew. Chem. Int. Ed.* 40(11), 2004-2021.

Kusumoto, Y.; Lomakin, A.; Teplow, D. B.& Benedek, G. B. (1998)Temeprature Dependence of Amyloid beta-Protein Fibrillization, *Proc. Natl. Acad. Sci. USA*, 95(21), 12277-12282.

Giulian, D.; Haverkamp, L. J.; Yu, J.; Karshin, W.; Tom, D.; Li, J.; Kazanskaia, A.: Kirkpatrick, J., & Roher, A. E. (1998) The HHQK Domain of β-Amyloid Provides a Structural Basis for the Immunopathology of Alzheimer's Disease *J. Biol. Chem.* 273(6), 29719–29726.

Ha, C.; Ryu, J. & Park, C. B. (2007) Metal Ions Differentially Influence the Aggregation and Deopsition of Alzheimer's Beta-Amyloid on a Solid Template. *Biochemistry*, 46(20), 6118-6125.

Hardy, J. & Selkoe, D. J. (2002) The Amyloid Hypothesis of Alzheimer's Disease: Progress and Problems on the Road to Therapeutics. *Science* 297(5580), 353-356.

Hou, X.; Richardson, S. J.; Aguilar, M. I. & Small, D. H. (2005) Binding of Amyloidogenic Transthyretin to the Plasma Membrane Alters Membrane Fluidity and Induces Neurotoxicity. *Biochemistry*, 44(34), 11618-11627.

Hoshi, M.; Sato, M.; Matsumoto, S.; Noguchi, A.; Yasutake, K.; Yoshida, N. & Sato, K. (2003) Spherical Aggregates of beta-Amyloid (Amylospheroid) Show High Neurotoxicity and Activate Tar Protein Kinase I/Glycogen Synthase Kinase-3β. *Proc. Natl. Acad. Sci. USA*, 100(11), 6370-6375.

Kayed, R.; Head, E.; Thompson, J. L.; McIntire, T. M.; Milton, S. C.; Cotman, C. W. & Glabe, C. G. (2003) Common Structure of Soluble Amyloid Oligomers Implies Common Mechanism of Pathogenesis. *Science*, 300(5618), 486-489.

Liang, P.H.; Wu, C. Y.; Greenberg, W. A. & Wong,C. H. (2008) Glycan Arrays: Biological and Medical Applications. *Curr. Opin. Chem. Biol.* 12(1), 86-92.

Maji, S. K.; Perrin, M. H.; Sawaya, M. R.; Jessberger, S.; Vadodaria, K.; Rissman, R. A.; Singru, P. S.; Nilsson; K. P.; Simon, R.; Schubert, D.; Eisenberg, D.; Rivier, J.; Sawchenko, P.; Vale, W.& Riek, R. (2009) Functional Amyloids as natural Storage of Peptide Hromones in Pituitary Secretory Granules. *Science* 325(5938), 328-332.

McLaurin, J.; Franklin, T.; Zhang, X.; Deng, J. & Fraser, P. E. (1999) Interactions of Alzheimer Amyloid-Beta Peptides with Glycosaminoglycans. *Eur. J. Biochem.* 266(3), 1101-1110.

Mammen, M.; Choi, S. K. & Whitesides, G. M. (1998), Polyvalente Wechselwirkungen in Biologischen Systemen: Auswirkungen auf das Design und die Verwendung Multivalenter Liganden und Inhibitoren. *Angewante Chem* 110(20), 2908-2953.

Miller, Y.; Ma, B.& Nussinov, R.(2010) Polymorphism in Alzheimer A beta Amyloid Organization Reflects Conformational Selection in a Rugged Energy Landscape. *Chem. Rev.* 110(8), 4820-4838.

Miura, Y. (2007) Synthesis and Biological Application of Glycopolymers. *J. Polym. Sci. Part A. Polym. Chem.* 45(22), 5031-5036.

Moad, G.; Rizzardo, E. & Thang, S. H. (2008) Toward Living Radical Polymerization. *Acc. Chem. Res.* 41(9), 1133-1142.

Pan, T.; Wong, B. S.; Liu, T.; Li, R.; Petersen, R. B. & Sy, M. S. (2002) Cell-Surface Prion Protein Interacts with Glcosaminoglycans. *Biochem. J.* 368(1), 81-90.

Petkova, A. T.; Buntkowsky, G.; Dyda, F.; Leapman, R. D.; Yau, W. M.&Tycko, R. (2004) Solid State NMR Reveals a pH-Dependent Antiparallel Beta-Sheet Registry in Fibrils Formed by a Beta-Amyloid Peptide. *J. Mol. Biol.* 335 (1), 247-260.

Prusiner, S. B. (1998) Prions, *Proc. Natl. Acad USA*, 95(23), 13363-13383.

Rochet, J. C., & Lansbury, P. T. Jr (2000), Amyloid Fibrillogenesis: Themes and Variations. *Curr. Opin. Struct. Biol.* 10(1), 60-66.

Rudd, T. R.; Skidomore, M. A.; Guerrini, M.; Hricovini, M.; Powell, A. K. Siligardi, G. & Yates, E. A. (2010) The Conformation and Structure of GAGs: Recent Progress and Perspectives. *Curr. Opin. Struct. Biol.*20(5), 567-574.

Saahara, K.; Yagi, H.; Sakai, M.; Naiki, H. & Goto, Y. (2008) Amyloid Nucleation Triggered by Agitation of Beta-2 Microglobulin Under Acidic and Neutral pH Conditions. *Biochemistry*, 47(8), 2650-2660.

Saraiva, A. M.; Cardoso, I.; Saraiva, M. J.; Tauer, K.; Pereira, M. C.; Coelho, M. A.; Mőhwald, H. & Brezesinski, G. (2010) Randomization of Amyloid beta Peitde(1-42) Conformation by Sulfonated and Sulfated Nanoparticles Reduces Aggregation and Cytotoxity. *Macromol. Biosci.* 10(10), 1152-1163.

Sasaki, K.; Nishida, Y.; Uzawa, H.& Kobayashi, K.(2003) N-Acetyl-6-Sulfo-D-glucosamine as a Promising Mimic of N-Acetyl Neuraminic Acid. *Bioorg. Med. Che. Lett.* 13(17), 2821-2823.

Sipe, J. D.(1992) Amyloidosis, *Annu. Rev. Biochem*, 61,947-975.

Suda, Y.; Marques, D.; Kermode, J. C.; Kusumoto, S. & Sobel,M (1993) Structural Characterization of Heparin's Binding Domain for Human Platelets. *Thromb Res.* 69(6), 501-508.

Suda, Y.; Arano, A.; Fukui, Y.; Koshidai, S.; Wakao, M.; Nishimura, T.; Kusumoto, S.& Sobel, M. (2006) Immobilization and Clustering of Structurally Defined Oligosaccharides for Sugar Chips: An Improved method for Surface Plasmon Resonance Analysis of Protein-Carbohydrate Interactions. *Bioconjugate Chem.* 17(5), 1125-1135.

Suzuki, M.; Takahashi, T.; Sato, J.; Mie, M.; Kobatake, E. & Mihara, H.(2010) Designed Short Peptides that Form Amyloid-Like Fibrils in Coassembly with Amyloid Beta Peptide (Abeta) Decrease the Toxicity of Abeta to Neuronal PC12 Cells. *ChemBioChem* 11(11), 1525-1530.

Uchimura, K.; Muramatsu, H.; Kadomatsu, K.; Fan, Q.-W.; Kurosawa, N.; Mitsuoka, C.; Kannnagi, R.; Habuchi, O.& Muramatsu, T. (1998) Molecular Cloning and Characterization of an N-acetylglucosamine-6-O-sulfotransferase. *J. Biol. Chem.* 273(35), 22577-22583.

Walzer, M.; Lorens, S.; Heina, M.; Fareed, J.; Hanin, I.; Cornelli, U. & Lee, J. M. (2002) Low Molecular Weight Glycosaminoglycan Blockade of Beta-Amyloid Induced Neuropathology, *Eur. J. Pharmacol*, 445(3), 211-220.

Zhu, H.; Yu, J. & Kindy M. S. (2001) Inhibition of Amyloidosis using Low-Molecular-Weight Heparins. *Mol. Med.* 7(8), 517-522.

Zidar, J.& Merzel, F. (2011) Probing Amyloid-Beta Fibril Stability by Increasing Ionic Strength. *J. Phys. Chem.* 115(9), 2075-2081.

6

Laboratory Methods for the Diagnosis of Hereditary Amyloidoses

S. Michelle Shiller, Ahmet Dogan and W. Edward Highsmith, Jr.
Department of Laboratory Medicine and Pathology, Mayo Clinic College of Medicine, Rochester, Minnesota
United States of America

1. Introduction

The majority of systemic amyloid disorders are acquired in nature and are most often secondary to plasma cell dyscrasias (AL amyloid), age-related accumulation of transthyretin (senile ATTR amyloid) or chronic inflammation (AA amyloid). A smaller, though significant, fraction of cases are due to inherited mutations in one of several amyloidogenic proteins. As described elsewhere in this volume, amyloid consists of fibrils composed of stacked proteins which have adopted a beta pleated sheet conformation. The mechanism by which a protein which has substantial alpha helical character refolds into a configuration with it's primarily beta pleated sheet is unclear and is the subject of much ongoing research. It is clear, however, that specific amino acid substitutions in a small number of circulating proteins can accelerate or facilitate this process.

All of the hereditary amyloidoses (also known as familial or systemic amyloidoses) are inherited in an autosomal dominant manner, as is the case for other "gain of function" mutations in disorders such as Huntington disease, myotonic dystrophy, or the spinocerebellar ataxias. The dominant inheritance of the familial amyloidoses has implications for family members of an affected individual. First, careful attention to the family history will often reveal symptoms in one parent, which may or may not have come to medical attention. However, even in the setting of a thorough family history, hereditary amyloidosis can be missed and attributed to more common diseases. It is important to understand that siblings and children of an affected individual have a 1 in 2 chance of being affected themselves. Thus, after the identification of an amyloidogenic mutation in an individual, it is important to offer testing for at-risk family members so that appropriate monitoring can be carried out for mutation positive family members.

The hereditary amyloidoses involve deposition of amyloid in a variety of tissues. Typically, there is a proclivity for the vascular tree, particularly the microvasculature, and it can be a cause of cerebral hemorrhage. The kidneys and the heart are the most commonly involved organs. However, virtually any organ can become involved, with liver, spleen, thyroid, larynx, gastric wall, and salivary glands all described. Further, amyloid deposition can also occur in the soft tissue adjacent to the salivary gland, tracheobronchial tree, the tongue, and in the skin.. On physical examination this diverse distribution manifests with a similar broad spectrum of features including macroglossia, peripheral edema, peripheral neuropathy, hypertension, papular rash, and waxy papules. Patients may demonstrate congestive heart failure as part of the restrictive cardiomyopathy conferred due to the amyloid deposition within cardiac muscle. Additionally, gastric dysmotility occurs, and cerebral hemorrhage is documented, as previously mentioned.

Clinically, it may be difficult to distinguish amyloidosis that is secondary to overproduction of immunoglobulin light chains (AL amyloid), age-related ATTR amyloidosis or serum amyloid A (AA amyloid) from an amyloidosis that is hereditary in nature. As the treatment for the underlying cause of amyloidosis is drastically different for the different etiologies, it is critical that the amyloid be properly classified. Therapy for plasma cell disease can include chemotherapy and/or bone marrow transplant, and the therapy for AA amyloid involves addressing the underling cause of inflammation, while the curative treatment for two varieties of familial amyloidosis, including the most common form due to mutant transthyretin (ATTR amyloid) is liver transplant.

To make a diagnosis, including identification of the protein being deposited as amyloid fibrils, it is typically necessary to obtain biopsy material from an affected organ or site. Most often, biopsies are obtained from either the bone marrow, subcutaneous fat (often of the abdomen), or the rectum. Following tissue acquisition, a variety of methods are used in identifying and characterizing amyloid protein. These include Congo Red staining, immunoperoxidase staining of histological tissue, mass spectrometry and genetic evaluation in cases of familial disease.

While the majority of systemic amyloidosis is due to transthyretin (TTR) mutations, identification of other genes involved in conferring aberrant protein folding with subsequent amyloid deposition have been identified. These additional genes have been documented in a substantially smaller number of individuals than TTR mutations and include ApoA1, ApoA2, gelsolin, lysozyme, and fibrinogen alpha (FGA). By and large, the most common symptom of these genetic variants is nephropathy. However, the gelsolin variant of disease does not involve the kidneys, rather it displays a predisposition for cranial nerve tissue, lattice corneal dystrophy, and cutis laxa of the facial skin. As gelsolin amyloidosis was originally identified in a large Finnish family , and is more common, but not limited to individuals of Finnish descent, it is often referred to as Finnish amyloidosis.

The differential diagnosis of systemic amyloidosis includes light chain disease, Sjögren's syndrome, rheumatoid arthritis, other inflammatory conditions, β2-microglobulinemia, and Familial Mediterranean Fever, as well as other similar conditions. A discussion of a thorough diagnostic evaluation for these conditions is beyond the scope of this chapter. However, a few key laboratory tests can expedite the process: serum protein electrophoresis (assists in the diagnosis of light chain disease or β2-microglobulinemia), the presence of antinuclear antibody and SSBLa>SSBRo by immunofluoresence for Sjögren's syndrome. The presence of rheumatoid factor points towards Rheumatoid Arthritis. Detection of serum amyloid A in amyloid deposits by immunohistochemistry elicits a definitive diagnosis of AA amyloid, or amyloid deposition of an inflammatory origin.

With respect to AL amyloidosis, while serum protein electrophoresis is the classical method of working up this diagnosis, ruling out hereditary amyloidosis through DNA interrogation is pivotal. Studies have demonstrated that individuals with hereditary amyloidosis may also demonstrate monoclonal immunoglobulins on serum protein electrophoresis in as many as 24% of patients. In the study by Lachmann et al., all of the patients had less than 0.2 g/dL of immunoglobulins in the serum, and none of the patients had kappa or lambda free light chains by urine protein electrophoresis. Comenzo et al. had similar findings, with six percent of patients with a hereditary amyloidosis presenting definitive monoclonal gammopathies in a subject population of similar size. The differences between these two studies is that the patients with monoclonal gammopathy in the Lachmann et al. study demonstrated mutations in a variety of genes for hereditary amyloidosis, whereas in the Comenzo et al. study, all patients had TTR mutations. In the absence of DNA analysis, these patients with hereditary amyloidosis masquerading with a monoclonal gammopathy would be misdiagnosed, and the improper clinical management could be implemented.

2. Methods used for the evaluation of tissue amyloid

2.1 Congo red staining

The gold standard for the detection of the presence of amyloid is Congo Red staining (Figure 1). A paper by Cooper compared Congo Red staining against other techniques to detect amyloid at the time, and his findings demonstrated that the green birefringence demonstrated under polarized light was completely specific for the presence of amyloid. A positive Congo Red stain on a biopsy or fat aspirate does not give the specific precursor protein causing the amyloid deposition. It does, however, define the presence of amyloid, setting the stage for further diagnostic evaluation.

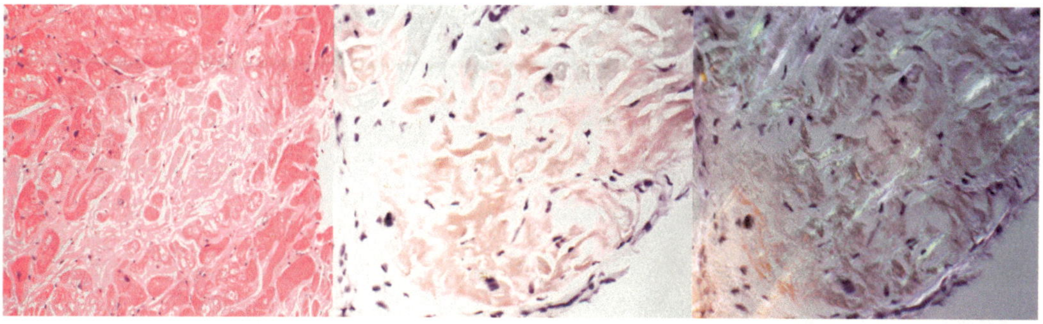

Fig. 1. Cardiac biopsy from a patient with TTR amyloidosis by hematoxylin and eosin (left), Congo Red (middle), Congo Red under polarized light with apple green birefringence (right). (Courtesy of Ahmet Dogan, MD, PhD; Mayo Clinic, Rochester, MN).

2.2 Immunohistochemistry

Immunohistochemistry (IHC) has been in use for many years to identify the specific protein involved in amyloid deposits identified by Congo red staining. In principle, IHC can differentiate the most common types of amyloid, light chain, serum amyloid A, and transthyretin (Figure 2). However, it is the authors' experience that, with the exception of serum amyloid A, the results can be equivocal and difficult to interpret. One of the problems is that the epitopes that specific antisera recognize can be partially or even completely buried in the insoluble amyloid fibril. There is a lack of high affinity antibodies specific for amyloidogenic proteins in the beta pleated sheet conformation. Further, a trained eye for interpretation of the results is required, with the ability to discern a poor staining pattern (such as that seen with serum leakage into amyloid plaques), and to recognize nonspecific or non-contributory background staining (low specificity and sensitivity). In addition, the adverse effects of changing protein structure by crosslinking due to formalin fixation limits the utility of immunohistochemistry in detecting amyloid deposition (demonstration of this phenomena thus far has been limited to TTR). If TTR is identified, IHC is unable to distinguish between a mutant TTR protein in a case of familial amyloid and a wild-type protein in case of senile amyloid (see the discussion of TTR and ApoA2 amyloid below). Finally, typical IHC panels consisting of antibodies to kappa and lambda light chains, serum amyloid A, and TTR, cannot identify the presence of less common amyloids consisting of lysozyme, gelsolin, fibrinogen alpha, or apolipoproteins 1, or 2.

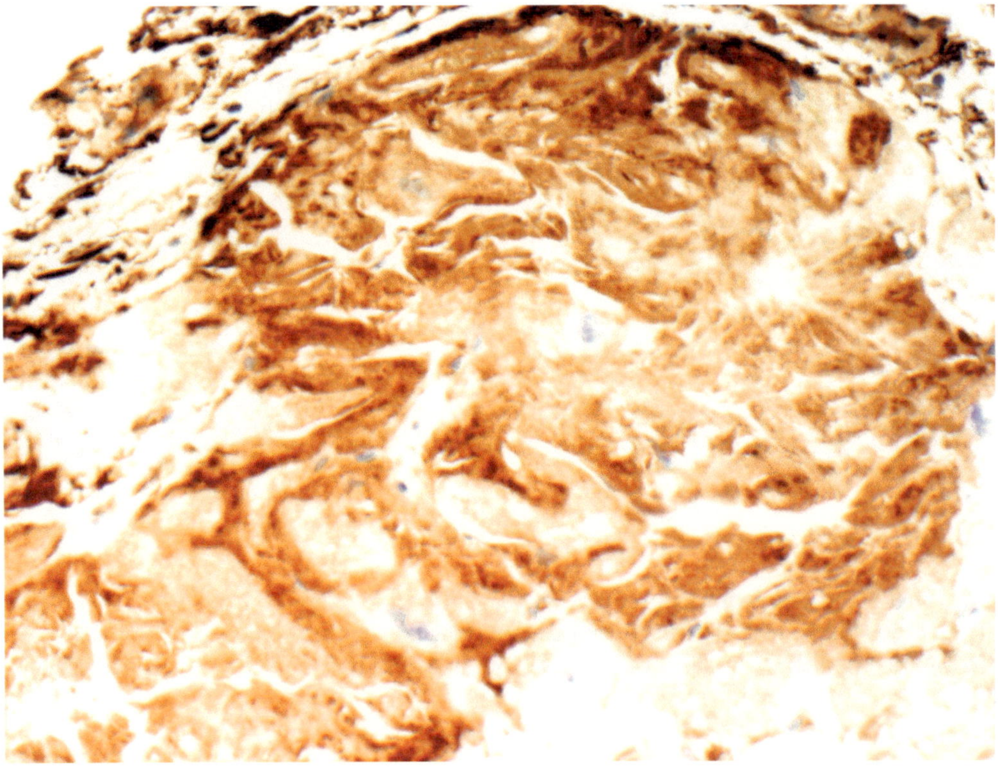

Fig. 2. Cardiac biopsy with TTR amyloid, positive for TTR by immunohistochemistry (photograph courtesy of Ahmet Dogan, MD, PhD; Mayo Clinic, Rochester, MN).

2.3 Electron microscopy

Ultrastructural examination (electron microscopy) of amyloid is not a common method of identifying this pathology. However, on ultrastructural examination, amyloid has a fibrillar pattern (Figure 3). Of note, there are several other fibrillary diseases of the kidney such as fibrillary glomerulonephritis and immunotactoid glomerulopathy, both of which are completely different entities than hereditary amyloid. Thus, fibrillary glomerular deposits by electron microscopy are non-specific, and additional studies are warranted to determine their etiology.

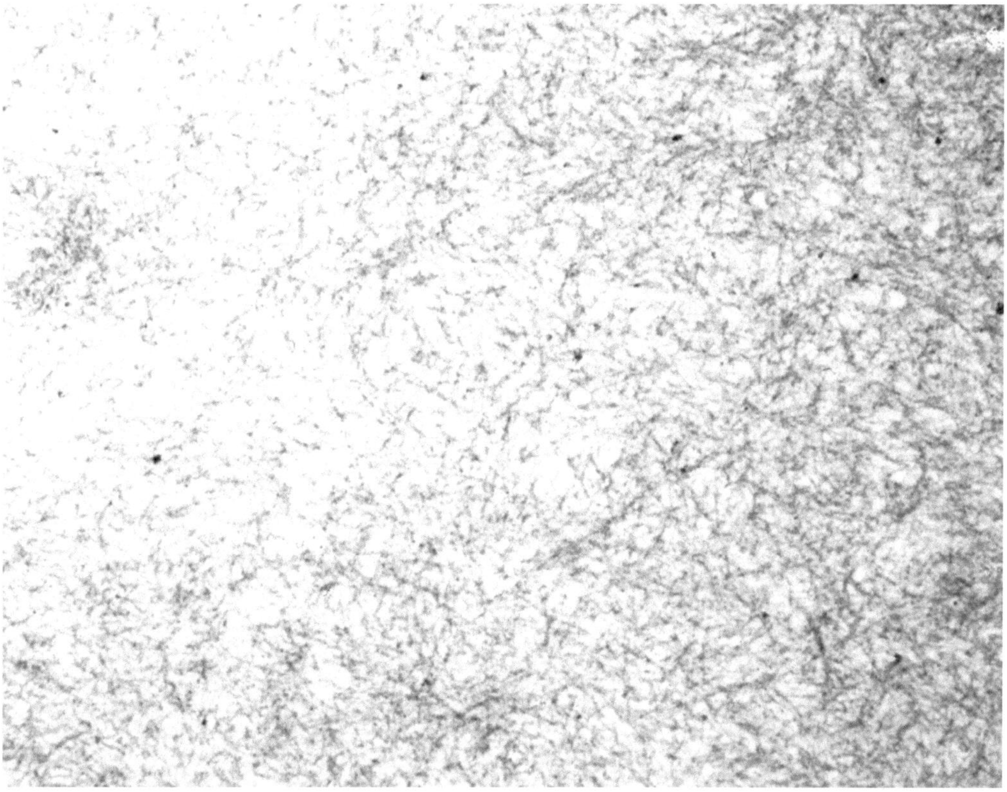

Fig. 3. Electron microscopy of amyloid fibrils measuring 6-10 nanometers in a patient with cardiac amyloidosis (photograph courtesy of Ahmet Dogan, MD, PhD; Mayo Clinic, Rochester, MN).

2.4 Mass spectrometry

More recently with new technological developments, mass spectrometry (MS) based proteomic methodologies have been applied to subtype amyloidosis. Initial studies using MS, similar to amino acid sequencing approaches, required large quantities of fresh or frozen tissue with a heavy amyloid load. However, in recent years, the sensitivity of MS based technologies has significantly improved and methods to extract proteins and peptides from small amounts of clinical biopsy specimens have been developed. This has led to development of a highly sensitive and specific clinical test for typing of amyloid deposits in paraffin embedded tissues. The approach incorporates laser capture microdissection (LCM) of amyloid plaques up front which dramatically increases the amount of proportion signal coming from the amyloidogenic protein compared to the signal coming from the background tissue (Figure 4).

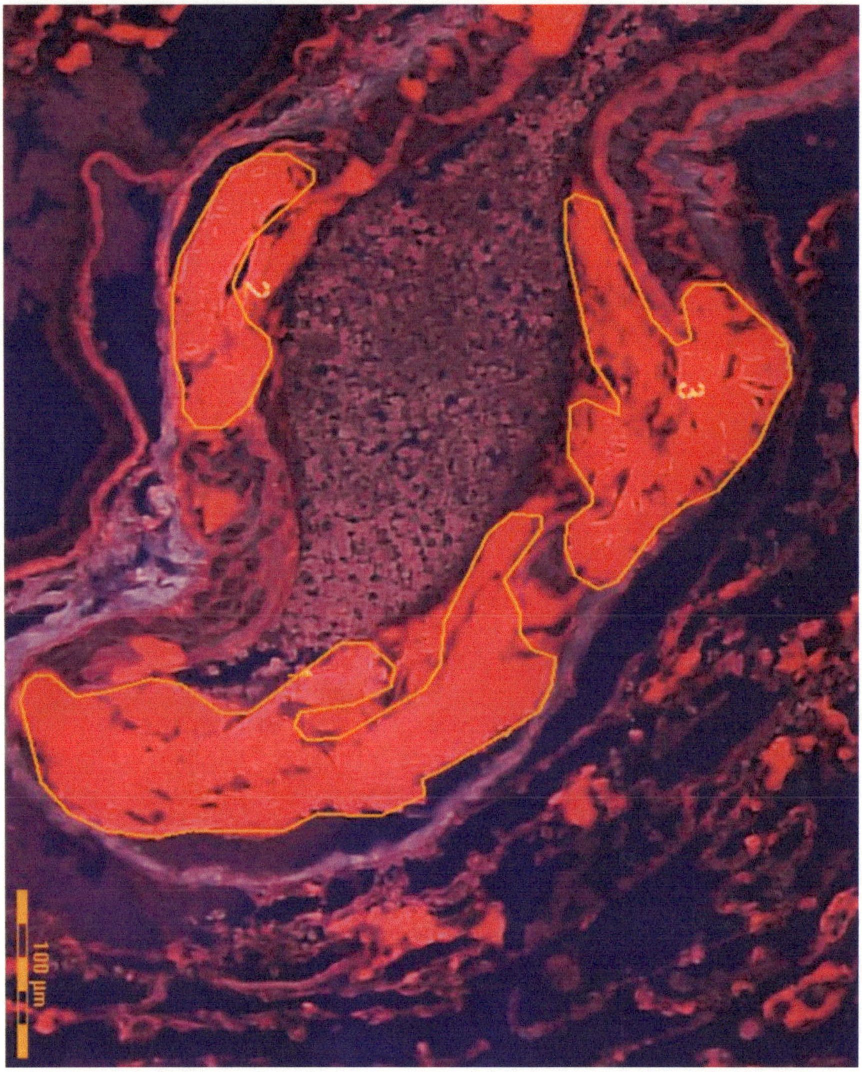

Fig. 4. AA amyloidosis showing predominantly vascular deposition with Congo red staining. For mass spectrometry based proteomic analysis, the areas circled by yellow lines are microdissected with laser and the microdissected fragments are collected in the tube cap ready for protein extraction and digestion into peptides suitable for tandem mass spectrometry (courtesy of Ahmet Dogan, MD, PhD; Mayo Clinic, Rochester, MN).

Once the amyloid plaques are captured, they are fragmented by heating and sonication to reverse crosslinking caused by formalin fixation, followed by digestion into peptide fragments by trypsin. Trypsin specifically cleaves the proteins following lysine and arginine residues and generates a peptide "soup." For each protein a specific and reproducible set of peptides is generated. The peptide solution is fractionated by high performance liquid chromatography and peptides are introduced into the mass spectrometer by a process called electrospray ionization (ESI). ESI provides the interface between the liquid environment of the HPLC and the high vacuum environment of the MS. It also adds charges to the peptides so that they can be detected and manipulated by MS. After ESI, the peptides are analyzed by tandem MS/MS. The first MS detects mass/charge ratio (m/z) of each peptide (precursor ion) as they are focused in the mass spectrometer. Based on relative abundance and other preset criteria, a subset of the charged peptides are selected for collision-induced dissociation. This leads to fragmentation of the peptides into smaller charged particles (product ions). Mass/charge ratio of these fragments is captured by the second MS (tandem mass spectrometry, MS/MS). This raw MS data is then interrogated by bio-informatic algorithms which match the fragmentation pattern of each peptide to one of the theoretical tryptic peptides present in human proteome. In this way, amino acid sequence of each peptide analyzed by MS/MS is predicted with high specificity. Proteins are identified and displayed in order of relative abundance based on the total number of peptide spectra identified for each protein (Figure 5). Using this approach amyloid deposits can be subtyped by very high sensitivity and specificity (100% for both in the published validation set) (Vrana et al., 2009).

Probability Legend:
over 95%
80% to 94%
50% to 79%
20% to 49%
0% to 19%

#	Bio View: Identified Proteins (463)	Accession Number	Molecular Weight	1	2	3	4
1	Serum albumin OS=Homo sapi...	ALBU_HUMAN	69 kDa	58	79	59	52
2	Transthyretin OS=Homo sapie...	TTHY_HUMAN	16 kDa	26	26	26	25
3	Apolipoprotein E OS=Homo sa...	APOE_HUMAN	36 kDa	30	31	25	19
4	Serum amyloid P-component ...	SAMP_HUMAN	25 kDa	33	27	25	19
5	Apolipoprotein A-IV OS=Homo...	APOA4_HUMAN	45 kDa	24	28	17	18
6	Collagen alpha-1(I) chain OS...	CO1A1_HUMAN	139 kDa	14	16	24	22
7	Vitronectin OS=Homo sapiens...	VTNC_HUMAN	54 kDa	22	17	13	11
8	TTR Val30Met GTG --> ATG "A...	TTHY_Val30...	1 kDa	19	13	13	12
9	Complement C3 OS=Homo sap...	CO3_HUMAN	187 kDa	15	15	8	6
10	Collagen alpha-2(I) chain OS...	CO1A2_HUMAN	129 kDa	9	13	18	14
11	Complement factor H-related ...	FHR1_HUMAN	38 kDa	12	13	8	7
12	Ig gamma-1 chain C region O...	IGHG1_HUMAN	36 kDa	9	7	9	8
13	Fibulin-1 OS=Homo sapiens G...	FBLN1_HUMAN	77 kDa	8	10	9	6
14	Vimentin OS=Homo sapiens G...	VIME_HUMAN	54 kDa	6	12	6	7
15	Collagen alpha-3(VI) chain OS...	CO6A3_HUMAN	344 kDa	5	11	5	3
16	Ig kappa chain C region OS=...	IGKC_HUMAN	12 kDa	5	6	5	7
17	Katanin p60 ATPase-containin...	KATL1_HUMAN	55 kDa	2	3	4	
18	Trypsin-3 OS=Homo sapiens ...	TRY3_HUMAN	33 kDa	5	5	4	5
19	Midkine OS=Homo sapiens GN...	MK_HUMAN	16 kDa	6	5	2	1
20	Collagen alpha-1(III) chain O...	CO3A1_HUMAN	139 kDa	2	4	2	4

Fig. 5. Mass spectrometry based proteomic analysis of hereditary amyloidosis. Transthyretin (red arrow) is the most dominant amyloidogenic protein in all four microdissections studied. Gene sequencing confirmed Val50Met in this case. (courtesy of Ahmet Dogan, MD, PhD; Mayo Clinic, Rochester, MN).

3. Genetic evaluation of familial amyloidosis

3.1 Genetic evaluation

Gene sequencing is the gold standard to detect aberrations such as substitutions, and small deletions and insertions at the nucleotide level. Sequencing is particularly useful when heterogeneity occurs in a disease, as with amyloidosis. The familial amyloidoses display both genetic heterogeneity (multiple genes being involved in a disease) and allelic heterogeneity (multiple mutations in the sample gene being able to cause the disease).

The first step in any DNA sequencing is the extraction, or purification, of DNA, typically from a peripheral blood sample. Many platforms are available for DNA extraction, the authors use the MagNaPure® LC (Roche Diagnostics). Following DNA extraction, the samples are prepared for PCR with primers specific to the gene of interest, and the standard PCR constituents (Taq polymerase, buffer, magnesium chloride and PCR-grade water). The authors perform a gel electrophoresis next to confirm the PCR reaction prior to proceeding with the sequencing assay. Next, the PCR product is treated, or "cleaned" to remove unincorporated primers and nucleotides. Again, there are multiple ways that this can be accomplished. The authors utilize shrimp alkaline phosphatase (to convert unincorporated deoxynucleotide triphosphates (dNTP's) into dephosphorylated products that will not interfere with the downstream sequencing reaction) and exonuclease (to digest unextended PCR primers into nucleotides to prevent unwanted extension during the sequencing reaction). The cleaned PCR product is next combined with a mixture of fluorescently labeled di-deoxynucleotide triphosphates and dNTP's (ex: BigDye® terminators [Applied Biosystems]), sequencing buffer, PCR grade water, and a thermostabile DNA polymerase. After carrying out the sequencing reaction by thermal cycling and another purification step, this time removing unincorporated fluorescent material, the sample is analyzed by capillary electrophoresis. There are multiple software programs commercially available for base calling, alignments, and mutation detection. The authors use Mutation Surveyor® (Soft Genetics) (Figure 6).

4. Genes involved in hereditary amyloidosis

4.1 Notes on nomenclature

The Human Genome Variation Society (HGVS) has proposed standard nomenclature for variation both at the nucleotide and the protein level (www.hgvs.org/mutnomen/). In this chapter, all mutations and variants will be discussed referring to protein sequence, or amino acid changes. The HGVS recommends that proteins be numbered starting with the initiator methionine as amino acid number one. Older literature often uses a different convention. Previously, the standard nomenclature was to number the first amino acid of the mature, processed protein as amino acid number one. For secreted proteins (such as those involved in familial amyloidoses), this numbering system neglected the signal peptides and propeptides that are cleaved from the amino terminus after translation as the protein is being processed by the cell for secretion. All of the amino acid changes discussed here will use the HGVS standard nomenclature.

For example, the signal peptide of the TTR protein is 20 amino acids in length. One mutation seen in TTR amyloid is Cys30Arg (new nomenclature). Using historical nomenclature, the mutation is termed Cys10Arg (subtract 20 amino acids that account for the signal peptide in

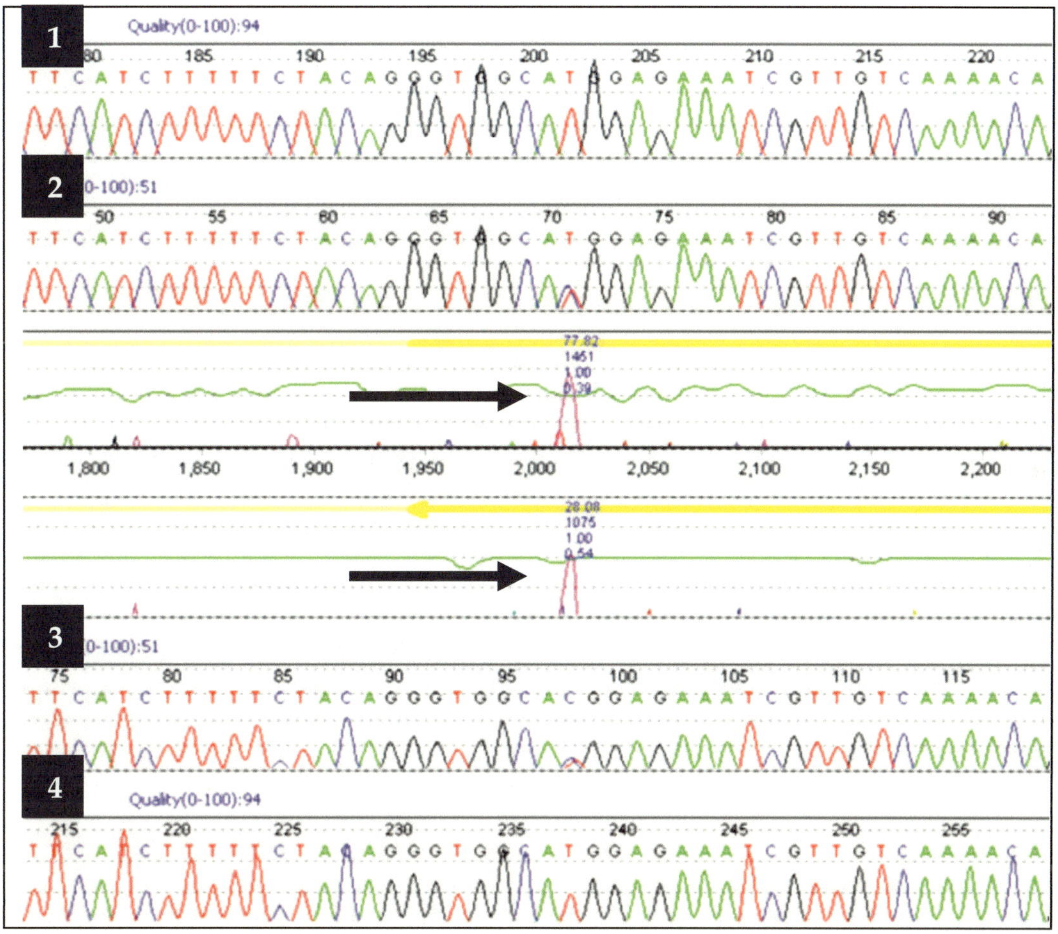

Fig. 6. Gene sequencing for lysozyme showing c. 388T>A, p. W130R, a pathogenic mutation. The top and bottom sequences (1 and 4) are the reference sequences against which the sample is compared. Sequences 2 and 3 are the patient sample. The top trace (1, 2) are sequenced in the forward direction, and the bottom trace (3, 4) in the reverse. The two middle traces are the subtraction plots between the reference sequence and the patient sample. The intronic region is indicated by the tan line, the yellow line indicates the exon. The pink peak is the location of the mutation (arrows), indicating substitution of a cytosine for a thymine. This nucleotide substitution alters the tryptophan (W) codon TGG to CGG, which codes for arginine (R).

the new nomenclature to derive this). Apolipoprotein A1 (ApoA1) is an example of a protein with a signal peptide and a propeptide. The signal peptide is 18 amino acids in length, and the propeptide is 6. Hence, to extrapolate the historical nomenclature from the new nomenclature for a mutation in ApoA1, Gly50Arg would be Gly26Arg. Please refer to Table 1 for a listing of all genes and the conversions.

Protein	Signal Peptide/Propeptide	Example (historical→new)
TTR	20	Cys10Arg→Cys30Arg
ApoA1	18/6	Gly26Arg→Gly50Arg
ApoA2	18/5	Stop78S→Stop101S
Gelsolin A	27	Asp187Tyr→Asp214Tyr
Fibrinogen Alpha	19	Arg554Leu→Arg573Leu
Lysozyme	18	W112R→W130R

Table 1. Table depicting nomenclature conversion from historical to new. The primary difference is that the new nomenclature includes all codons beginning with the initiating methionine, and the historical nomenclature utilizes only the mature protein. Hence, to convert to the new nomenclature requires adding the appropriate number of codons acting as signal peptides and propeptides, as indicated.

4.2 Transthyretin (TTR)

Transthyretin (TTR) was the first protein identified in hereditary amyloidosis with amyloid deposition due to coding sequence missense mutations was transthyretin. Notably, it is by far the most common protein and gene involved in familial amyloidosis, accounting for between 95-98% of reported familial amyloid cases, and often presenting after the age of 50. TTR is a transport protein that has four exons, 127 amino acids and weighs 55kDa, and is synthesized predominantly in the liver. The function of TTR is to carry thyroxine (T4) and to participate in the thyroxine-retinol binding protein complex. Consequently, when TTR is mutated, aberrant protein folding results with deposition as described above with the clinical sequelae including most predominantly peripheral polyneuropathy, and/or cardiomyopathy (with or without eye and brain involvement).

Due to its predominantly hepatic synthesis, liver transplantation is the treatment of choice for patients with TTR amyloidosis. Since this treatment is vastly different than the cytotoxic chemotherapeutic regimens and/or bone marrow transplant indicated for AL amyloidosis, the correct diagnosis of these two disorders with supporting laboratory data is paramount. Also, senile amyloid deposition is often composed of wild-type TTR protein. In this case, the conversion of TTR into amyloid fibrils is not driven by pathogenic mutations. Gene sequencing is necessary to distinguish TTR type senile amyloid from a hereditary disorder.

Though more than 100 mutations have been reported in TTR, almost all of them are due to single base substitutions in the gene, located on chromosome 18. Common single base substitutions include V50M, L75P, L78H, T80A, and Y134H. A common three-nucleotide/single codon deletion is ΔVal142. Moreover, ethnic propensities exist such as the association of V142I with African Americans. Further, M33I is seen in the German population, A45T, Y89I, and Q112K segregate amongst the Japanese. Variants common in the United States are D38N, A45S, F53C, W61L, T69P, L75Q, A101T, and R123S. Phenotypic clustering is seen in some codon changes (Table 2), and Tyr89Ile is the only double nucleotide substitution documented to date. Specifically, Tyr89Ile is seen in the Japanese population, with cardiac and connective tissue involvement, and autonomic neuropathy.

Mutation	Clinical Features	Geographic kindreds
Phe53Ile	Peripheral Neuropathy, Eye	Israel
Phe53Leu	Peripheral Neuropathy, Heart	USA
Phe53Val	Peripheral Neuropathy	UK, Japan, China
Ala65Thr	Heart	USA
Ala65Asp	Heart, Peripheral Neuropathy	USA
Ala65Ser	Heart	Sweden
Ile104Asn	Heart, Eye	USA
Ile104Thr	Heart, Peripheral Neuropathy	Germany, UK
Glu109Gln	Peripheral Neuropathy, Heart	Italy
Glu109Lys	Peripheral Neuropathy, Heart	USA
Val142Ile	Heart	USA
ΔVal142	Heart, Peripheral Neuropathy	USA
Val142Ala	Heart, Eye, Peripheral Neuropathy	USA

Table 2. Phenotypic correlations of TTR mutations along with segregation among particular geographic kindreds (adapted from Benson 2003).

4.3 Apolipoprotein A1 (ApoA1)

Apolipoprotein A1 (ApoA1), another protein involved with hereditary amyloidosis, contains four exons, 243 amino acids, weighs 28kDa, and is located on chromosome 11q23-q24. ApoA1 is synthesized in the liver and small intestine, conferring a plasma protein that is the main protein of high-density lipoprotein particles and has a key role in lipoprotein metabolism. As such, ApoA1 is important for the formation of high-density lipoprotein cholesterol esters, promoting efflux of cholesterol from cells. Mutations in ApoA1 can lead to one of two rare disease of lipoprotein metabolism, primary hypoalphalipoproteinemia or Tangier's disease; or, ApoA1 amyloidosis, depending on the mutation. Thirteen mutations are associated with ApoA1 amyloidosis, predominantly nucleotide substitutions. However, two are deletions, and one is a deletion/insertion mutation. Most of the deletionss are in-frame, with the exception of Asn122fs and eAla202fs. Hence, the mechanism of amyloid production for all of the ApoA1 mutations involve aberrant folding, the unstable species produced with the Asn122fs and Ala202fs mutations is a truncated protein rather than a full length one.

The clinical presentation of amyloidosis consistent with ApoA1 involves the liver, kidney, larynx, skin and myocardium most commonly; rarely the testes and adrenal glands. The most common mutations to date include G50R, L99P, A197P, A199P, and L198S. Most of these mutations are present in Northern Europeans. Specifically, G50R is common among British, Scandinavians and North Americans, L99P in Italians, Germans, and North Americans, A197P in Americans and British, and L198S in Italian and Dutch individuals (Table 3).

Mutation	Clinical Features
Gly50Arg	Peripheral neuropathy, Nephropathy
Glu58Lys	Nephropathy
Leu84Arg	Nephropathy
Glu94_Trp96del	HTN, Nephropathy
Trp74Arg	Nephropathy
Del84-85insVal/Thr	Hepatic
Leu88Pro	Nephropathy
Del94-96	Nephropathy
Phe95Tyr	Palate
Asn98fs	Nephropathy, gastrointestinal
Leu99Pro	Hepatic
Leu114Pro	Cardiomyopathy, cutaneous
Lys131del	Aortic intima
Ala178fs	Nephropathy
Leu194Pro	Laryngeal
Arg197Pro	Cardiomyopathy, cutaneous, laryngeal
Leu198Ser	Cardiomyopathy
Ala199Pro	Laryngeal
Leu202His	Cardiomyopathy, laryngeal

Table 3. Common ApoA1 mutations (adapted from Benson, 2003; Eriksson, et al., 2009; Rowczenio, et al., In Progress).

4.4 Apolipoprotein A2 (ApoA2)

Apolipoprotein A2 (ApoA2), similar to ApoA1, is an amyloidogenic protein involved with lipid metabolism. ApoA2, unlike ApoA1, can be found in senile amyloidosis. As is the case with TTR, gene sequencing is required to determine if ApoA2 deposition in a given case is due to deposition of a wild-type protein (senile amyloid) or a mutant one (familial amyloidosis). Structurally, it is a 77 amino acid, 17.4kDa protein located on chromosome 1p21-1qter. While comprised of four exons, three exons in ApoA2 are coding: exons 2, 3 and the 5′ end of exon 4 (Alamut). The Apo A2 gene is one of the more recently described forms of hereditary amyloid, with a clinical picture of early adult-onset, rapidly progressive renal failure. The abrupt renal failure occurs in the absence of proteinuria and has no associated neuropathy. Mutations in the stop codon are the common genetic change resulting in a 21-amino acid extension at the carboxy terminus of the mature protein. All of these changes occur at codon 101 in exon 4 as follows: Stop101G, Stop101S, and Stop101R (Table 4). Geographically, these mutations are seen in North Americans, with the exception of Stop101R, which is also seen in Russians.

Protein	Mutation	Clinical Features
ApoA2	Stop78Gly	Nephropathy
	Stop78Ser	Nephropathy
	Stop78Arg	Nephropathy
Gelsolin A	Asp214Asn	PN, LCD
	Asp214Tyr	PN
Fibrinogen Alpha	Arg573Leu	Nephropathy
	Glu545Val	Nephropathy
	1629delG	Nephropathy
	1622delT	Nephropathy
Lysozyme	Ile74Thr	Nephropathy, petechiae
	Asp85His	Nephropathy
	Trp82Arg	Nephropathy
	Phe75Ile	Nephropathy

Table 4. Listing of common mutation for other amyloidogenic proteins. PN = Peripheral Neuropathy, LCD = lattice corneal dystrophy.

4.5 Gelsolin A (GSN)

Gelsolin protein is associated with actin metabolism. Also known as brevin, or, actin-depolymerizing factor, it acts to prevent toxicity due to the release of actin into the extracellular space in the presence of cell necrosis. The gene is comprised of 17 exons and is located on chromosome 9q34 (centromeric to ABL); the protein weighs 82kDa. In the setting of familial/hereditary amyloidosis presents with unique features of neuropathy, particularly of the cranial nerves. Additionally, Gelsolin A has distinguishing clinical features that merit clinical, not genetic, subclassification of the disease. For example, some patients may have lattice corneal dystrophy, the "Meretoja" subtype, and cutis laxia of facial skin. Known pathogenic mutations include D214N in individuals from Finland, North America, Denmark and Japan, and D214Y (c. 654G>C), in individuals from Finland, Denmark, and the Czech Republic. The D214N and D214Y mutations permit exposure of an otherwise masked cleavage site, and is the initial step of amyloid formation. Both of these mutations result in the production of an aberrant, 68-kD fragment, likely a carboxy-terminal part of the protein which is suggested to be amyloidogenic.

The Meretoja subtype is associated with the D214N mutation, a single base mutation c. 654G>A (GAC>GAA), p. D214N (Asp214Asn). The pathogenic protein is comprised of 71 amino acids. Individuals that are heterozygous for this mutation may be asymptomatic early in life, with possibly only lattice corneal dystrophy (in their thirties); those who are homozygous may have significant manifestations of visceral involvement, specifically renal, including proteinuria and amyloid nephropathy with nephrotic syndrome by their twenties. Regardless of the genotype, the gelsolin variant of amyloid is classically associated with cranial neuropathy, possibly even bilateral, with additional phenotypic features rendering subclassification as described herein (Table 4).

4.6 Fibrinogen alpha (FGA)

Synthesized in the liver, fibrinogen is a plasma glycoprotein with three structural subunits: alpha (FGA), beta (FGB), and gamma (FGG). Most research regarding fibrinogen has been in the context of hemostasis, where it has a primary functional role. Two rare diseases due to mutations in fibrinogen alpha confer bleeding disorders: afibrinogenemia and dysfibrinogenemia. Afibrinogenemia has an absence of fibrinogen due to a truncating mutation, and dysfibrinogenemia has decreased fibrin production due to a mutation at the cleavage site for thrombin to convert inactive fibrinogen to fibrin. The mutations seen with bleeding are different than those seen in FGA amyloid. Fibrinogen alpha is located on chromosome 4q28, with 6 exons, and varying amino acid lengths as determined by alternative splicing.

Phenotypically, FGA amyloidosis is associated with visceral involvement, specifically renal, with the manifestations including hypertension, proteinuria, and subsequent azotemia. Importantly, renal involvement in amyloid of this genetic origin is associated with rapidly progressive renal failure. Hence, detection of amyloid with a FGA mutation, like TTR, permits consideration of liver transplant for curative treatment, and, perhaps, could avoid the negative consequences of renal disease. Historically, renal transplantation, which has also been performed, has not had long-term success, thus, this paradigm-shift to hepatic transplantation, especially in light of the ability to detect the mutation, is a promising alternative for patients. Neuropathy has not been seen in this type of amyloidosis, and cardiomyopathy is reported in one case, thus far. Hence, neurologic and cardiac involvement would be the exception rather than the rule at this early phase of diagnosing FGA amyloid.

To date, there are four common mutations associated with FGA amyloidosis: two point mutations with pathogenic single amino acid substitutions, and two single nucleotide deletions yielding a frameshift in DNA transcription, with subsequent premature termination of protein synthesis. One point mutation, c. 4993 G>T, p. R573L has been identified in a Peruvian family, and another, c. 1674 A>T, p. E545V has been detected in individuals of American and Irish descent. Specifically, the E545V mutation is the one example of cardiac manifestations of FGA amyloid. One mutation, 1629delG, a deletion of the third base in codon 543, was detected in an American family with hereditary renal amyloidosis. Due to this mutation, a premature stop codon is created at codon 567. Individuals with the 1629delG mutation had a later onset of disease (later thirties and early forties) when compared to those with the R573L mutation . Finally, early renal disease with terminal renal failure has been documented in French kindred with a single nucleotide deletion c.1622T, with subsequent frameshift mutation at codon 541 and, similar to 1629delG, premature termination of protein synthesis at codon 567 (Table 4). This particular subtype, with its inherently aggressive sequelae, is particularly relevant to consideration of liver transplantation early in the course of disease.

4.7 Lysozyme (LYZ)

Lysozyme is an enzyme that catalyzes the hydrolysis of certain mucopolysaccharides of bacterial cell walls. Specifically, it catalyzes the hydrolysis of the beta (1-4) glycosidic linkages between N-acetylmuramic acid and N-acetylglucosamine. Lysozyme is found in the spleen, lung, kidney, white blood cells, plasma, saliva, milk and tears. The gene is located on chromosome 12q15 and contains 4 exons. The 14.6kDa protein contains 130 amino acids.

In the same vein with regard to management, early detection of this amyloid variant alters the course of treatment in that individuals with this mutation experience a very early onset of renal disease, with rapid decline (this is similar, in some regards, to some variants of FGA). However, unlike FGA, benefit from renal transplantation has proven effective. Other manifestations include gastrointestinal involvement (peptic ulcer), cardiac disease, Sicca syndrome, and propensity towards petechiae, hemorrhage and hematoma, including hepatic hemorrhage. Uniquely, neuropathy is not a component of this type of amyloid, and in fact, might suggest a different variant, such as gelsolin, depending on the presentation.

The mutations documented thus far with lysozyme amyloid have their ancestral roots associated with the United Kingdom, France, America, and Italy (specifically, Piedmont, Italy). The D85H (Asp85His) mutation regionalizes to the United Kingdom, renal disease is the predominant symptom associated with this mutation. A tryptophan-to-arginine substitution at codon 82 (W82R) has been documented with a French family, with Sicca syndrome contributing to the phenotype in addition to renal manifestations. Two other mutations, Phe75Ile (F75I), and Trp82Arg (W82R), are described in an Italian-Canadian family, and an Italian family (Piedmont, Italy), respectively. The W82R variant had predominant gastrointestinal involvement; however, the same mutation in an English man presented with dramatic bleeding and rupture of abdominal lymph nodes (Table 4).

4.8 LECT2: A new hereditary amyloidosis gene?

The most recently described gene in systemic amyloidosis is LECT2. LECT2 is a leukocyte chemotactic factor whose synthetic origin is uncertain at this time (Benson 2010). Some studies indicate a hepatic origin as LECT2 is expressed in the adult and fetal liver, but follow-up immunohistochemical studies have detected LECT2 in many tissues of the body. LECT2 weighs 16.4kDa, is comprised of 133 residues (after cleavage of the 18 amino acid signal peptide), and is located on chromosome 5q31.1-q32.

Functionally, LECT2 can serve as a cartilage growth factor (chondromodulin II), as well as in neutrophil chemotaxis, as the name implies. With its role in neutrophilic chemotaxis, LECT2 has a presumable role in cell growth and repair after damage. Further, LECT2 has also been detected in hepatocellular carcinoma cell lines, suggesting a role in neoplasia, and also supporting its potential origin within hepatic tissue.

To date, LECT2 amyloidosis has been seen primarily in individuals of Mexican American ancestry. A study by Murphy et al. reported a series of 21,985 consecutive renal biopsies, of which 285 had positive Congo Red staining. Seven of ten cases with LECT2 renal amyloidosis were of Mexican descent. In some cases (typically reported in smaller studies), the amyloid was detected after longstanding, slowly progressive renal disease.

The case reported by Benson is a patient with a long history or slowly progressive renal failure, without a diagnosis of amyloidosis including its specific subtype until nephrectomy due to renal-cell carcinoma. Moreover, since its recent discovery, there is suggestion by Larsen et al. that the incidence of LECT2 amyloid might actually exceed TTR. While a polymorphism has been detected in all of the cases affected with LECT2 amyloid (Ile58Val), no pathogenic mutations are present to date. Thus, whether or not LECT2 will emerge under the category of systemic or hereditary amyloidosis is yet to be determined.

5. Conclusion

In summary, many laboratory techniques to detect and characterize the presence of amyloid are available. With these tools, the ability to detect the presence of amyloid has improved, as well as our ability to better understand the varying presentations and pathologic processes associated with the presence of amyloid.

While the understanding of amyloid continues to evolve, so does our ability to detect, diagnose, and treat the varying etiologies. Two techniques pivotal this progress are tissue mass spectrometry and gene sequencing. The refined finesse available utilizing mass spectrometry and gene sequencing continues to unravel the amyloid puzzle, and reveal more patients, with more unique phenotypic expression of disease. As our ability to identify and characterize systemic amyloidosis improves, and genotype-phenotype correlations become more clear, it will likely be possible in the future to explain seemingly unique manifestations of the disease, such as the cardiac specific presentation seen with the V142I TTR mutation.

The ultimate beneficiary of the utility of the refined laboratory diagnosis of amyloidosis is, of course, the patient. However, the information gathered due to test results is best handled in a multidisciplinary practice with well-established genetic counseling to educate the patient and family regarding the disease process, screening, and treatment considerations. At present, no direct pharmacologic therapy "cures" for the amyloid disease. However, understanding the origin of the proteins involved in the subtypes has achieved better control of this process in some types (TTR, FGA).

6. Acknowledgments

The authors would like to thank Steven R. Zeldenrust, MD, PhD Consultant, Division of Hematology, Mayo Clinic, Rochester, Minnesota for his critical review of the manuscript and clinical support; Jason Theis and Karen Schowalter for their assistance in the mass spectrometry and molecular genetics laboratories respectively, at Mayo Clinic, Rochester, Minnesota; Tad Holtegaard and Cindy McFarlin for their technical support, and Debbie Johnson for her administrative support; Mayo Clinic, Rochester, Minnesota.

7. References

Lysozyme; Lyz, In: *GeneTests*: Medical Genetics Information Resource (database online), 1993-2011. University of Washington, Seattle. Accessed March 10, 2011. Available from: <http://www.genetests.org>

Alamut®. Version 2.5.2011. Computer Software by Interactive Biosoftware, Rouen, France.

Fibrinogen, a Alpha Polypeptide; Fga, In: *GeneTests*: Medical Genetics Information Resource (database online), 1993-2011. University of Washington, Seattle. Accessed March 10, 2011. Available from: <http://www.genetests.org>

Gelsolin; Gsn, In: *GeneTests*: Medical Genetics Information Resource (database online), 1993-2011. University of Washington, Seattle. Accessed March 10, 2011. Available from: <http://www.genetests.org>

Benson, M. D., Liepnieks, J., Uemichi, T., Wheeler, G., & Correa, R. (1993). Hereditary Renal Amyloidosis Associated with a Mutant Fibrinogen Alpha-Chain. *Nature Genetics*, Vol. 3, No. 3, pp. 252-255

Benson, M. D. (2003). The Hereditary Amyloidoses. *Best Practice & Research. Clinical Rheumatology,* Vol. 17, No. 6, pp. 909-927

Benson, M. D., James, S., Scott, K., Liepnieks, J. J., & Kluve-Beckerman, B. (2008). Leukocyte Chemotactic Factor 2: A Novel Renal Amyloid Protein. *Kidney International,* Vol. 74, No. 2, pp. 218-222

Benson, M. D. (2010). Lect2 Amyloidosis. *Kidney International,* Vol. 77, No. 9, pp. 757-759

Brill, A. K., Woelke, K., Schadlich, R., Weinz, C., & Laier-Groeneveld, G. (2007). Tracheobronchial Amyloidosis--Bronchoscopic Diagnosis and Therapy of an Uncommon Disease: A Case Report. *Journal of Physiology and Pharmacology,* Vol. 58 Suppl 5, No. Pt 1, pp. 51-55

Cendron, L., Trovato, A., Seno, F., Folli, C., Alfieri, B., Zanotti, G., & Berni, R. (2009). Amyloidogenic Potential of Transthyretin Variants: Insights from Structural and Computational Analyses. *Journal of Biological Chemistry,* Vol. 284, No. 38, pp. 25832-25841

Coelho, T., Ericzon, B. G., Falk, R., Grogan, D. R., Ikeda, S., Maurer, M., Plante-Bordeneuve, V., Suhr, O. B., & Trigo, P. (2008). A Physician's Guide to Transthyretin Amyloidosis. Publication from Amyloidosis Foundation, Inc., Clarkston, Michigan.

Comenzo, R. L., Zhou, P., Fleisher, M., Clark, B., & Teruya-Feldstein, J. (2006). Seeking Confidence in the Diagnosis of Systemic Al (Ig Light-Chain) Amyloidosis: Patients Can Have Both Monoclonal Gammopathies and Hereditary Amyloid Proteins. *Blood,* Vol. 107, No. 9, pp. 3489-3491

Connors, L. H., Lim, A., Prokaeva, T., Roskens, V. A., & Costello, C. E. (2003). Tabulation of Human Transthyretin (Ttr) Variants, 2003. *Amyloid,* Vol. 10, No. 3, pp. 160-184

Cooper, J. H. (1969). An Evaluation of Current Methods for the Diagnostic Histochemistry of Amyloid. *Journal of Clinical Pathology,* Vol. 22, No. 4, pp. 410-413

de la Chapelle, A., Tolvanen, R., Boysen, G., Santavy, J., Bleeker-Wagemakers, L., Maury, C. P., & Kere, J. (1992). Gelsolin-Derived Familial Amyloidosis Caused by Asparagine or Tyrosine Substitution for Aspartic Acid at Residue 187. *Nature Genetics,* Vol. 2, No. 2, pp. 157-160

Eriksson, M., Schonland, S., Yumlu, S., Hegenbart, U., von Hutten, H., Gioeva, Z., Lohse, P., Buttner, J., Schmidt, H., & Rocken, C. (2009). Hereditary Apolipoprotein Ai-Associated Amyloidosis in Surgical Pathology Specimens: Identification of Three Novel Mutations in the Apoa1 Gene. *Journal of Molecular Diagnostics,* Vol. 11, No. 3, pp. 257-262

Fu, X., Koremaga, T., Fu, L., Xing, Y., Guo, Z., Matsushita, T., Hosokawa, M., Naiki, H., Baba, S., Kawata, Y., Ikeda, S.-i., Ishihara, T., Mori, M., & Higuchi, K. (2004). Induction of Aapoaii Amyloidoisis by Various Heterogeneous Amyloid Fibrils. *FEBS Letters,* Vol. 563, No., pp. 179-184

Granel, B., Serratrice, J., Valleix, S., Grateau, G., Droz, D., Lafon, J., Sault, M. C., Chaudier, B., Disdier, P., Laugier, R., Delpech, M., & Weiller, P. J. (2002). A Family with Gastrointestinal Amyloidosis Associated with Variant Lysozyme. *Gastroenterology,* Vol. 123, No. 4, pp. 1346-1349

Granel, B., Serratrice, J., Disdier, P., Weiller, P. J., Valleix, S., Grateau, G., & Droz, D. (2005). Underdiagnosed Amyloidosis: Amyloidosis of Lysozyme Variant. *American Journal of Medicine,* Vol. 118, No. 3, pp. 321-322

Hamidi Asl, L., Liepnieks, J. J., Uemichi, T., Rebibou, J. M., Justrabo, E., Droz, D., Mousson, C., Chalopin, J. M., Benson, M. D., Delpech, M., & Grateau, G. (1997). Renal Amyloidosis with a Frame Shift Mutation in Fibrinogen Aalpha-Chain Gene Producing a Novel Amyloid Protein. *Blood,* Vol. 90, No. 12, pp. 4799-4805

Jacob, E., Edwards, W., Zucker, M., D'Cruz, C., Seshan, S., Crow, F., & Highsmith, W. (2007). Homozygous Transthyretin Mutation in an African American Male. *Journal of Molecular Diagnostics,* Vol. 9, No. 1, pp. 127-131

Kitagawa, K., Wang, J., Mastushita, T., Kogishi, K., Hosokawa, M., Fu, X., Guo, Z., Mori, M., & Higuchi, K. (2003). Polymorphisms of Mouse Apolipoprotein a-Ii: Seven Alleles Found among 41 Inbred Strains of Mice. *Amyloid,* Vol. 10, No. 4, pp. 207-214

Labro, H., Al-Kadhimi, Z., Djmil, M., Oghlakian, R., & Alshekhlee, A. (2009). Brain Amyloidoma with Cerebral Hemorrhage. *Journal of the American Osteopathic Association,* Vol. 109, No. 7, pp. 372-375

Lachmann, H. J., Booth, D. R., Booth, S. E., Bybee, A., Gilbertson, J. A., Gillmore, J. D., Pepys, M. B., & Hawkins, P. N. (2002). Misdiagnosis of Hereditary Amyloidosis as Al (Primary) Amyloidosis. *New England Journal of Medicine,* Vol. 346, No. 23, pp. 1786-1791

Lackner, K. J., Law, S. W., & Brewer, H. B., Jr. (1985). The Human Apolipoprotein a-Ii Gene: Complete Nucleic Acid Sequence and Genomic Organization. *Nucleic Acids Research,* Vol. 13, No. 12, pp. 4597-4608

Larsen, C. P., Walker, P. D., Weiss, D. T., & Solomon, A. (2010). Prevalence and Morphology of Leukocyte Chemotactic Factor 2-Associated Amyloid in Renal Biopsies. *Kidney International,* Vol. 77, No. 9, pp. 816-819

Lee, W. M., & Galbraith, R. M. (1992). The Extracellular Actin-Scavenger System and Actin Toxicity. *New England Journal of Medicine,* Vol. 326, No. 20, pp. 1335-1341

Mainenti, P. P., Segreto, S., Mancini, M., Rispo, A., Cozzolino, I., Masone, S., Rinaldi, C. R., Nardone, G., & Salvatore, M. (2010). Intestinal Amyloidosis: Two Cases with Different Patterns of Clinical and Imaging Presentation. *World Journal of Gastroenterology,* Vol. 16, No. 20, pp. 2566-2570

Maury, C. P., & Baumann, M. (1990). Isolation and Characterization of Cardiac Amyloid in Familial Amyloid Polyneuropathy Type Iv (Finnish): Relation of the Amyloid Protein to Variant Gelsolin. *Biochimica et Biophysica Acta,* Vol. 1096, No. 1, pp. 84-86

Maury, C. P. (1991). Gelsolin-Related Amyloidosis. Identification of the Amyloid Protein in Finnish Hereditary Amyloidosis as a Fragment of Variant Gelsolin. *Journal of Clinical Investigation,* Vol. 87, No. 4, pp. 1195-1199

Meretoja, J. (1973). Genetic Aspects of Familial Amyloidosis with Corneal Lattice Dystrophy and Cranial Neuropathy. *Clinical Genetics,* Vol. 4, No. 3, pp. 173-185

Mourad, G., Delabre, J. P., & Garrigue, V. (2008). Cardiac Amyloidosis with the E526v Mutation of the Fibrinogen a Alpha-Chain. *New England Journal of Medicine,* Vol. 359, No. 26, pp. 2847-2848

Murphy, C. L., Eulitz, M., Hrncic, R., Sletten, K., Westermark, P., Williams, T., Macy, S. D., Wooliver, C., Wall, J., Weiss, D. T., & Solomon, A. (2001). Chemical Typing of Amyloid Protein Contained in Formalin-Fixed Paraffin-Embedded Biopsy Specimens. *American Journal of Clinical Pathology,* Vol. 116, No. 1, pp. 135-142

Murphy, C. L., Wang, S., Williams, T., Weiss, D. T., & Solomon, A. (2006). Characterization of Systemic Amyloid Deposits by Mass Spectrometry. *Methods in Enzymology,* Vol. 412, No., pp. 48-62

Murphy, C. L., Wang, S., Kestler, D., Larsen, C., Benson, D., Weiss, D. T., & Solomon, A. (2010). Leukocyte Chemotactic Factor 2 (Lect2)-Associated Renal Amyloidosis: A Case Series. *American Journal of Kidney Diseases,* Vol. 56, No. 6, pp. 1100-1107

Paunio, T., Kangas, H., Kalkkinen, N., Haltia, M., Palo, J., & Peltonen, L. (1994). Toward Understanding the Pathogenic Mechanisms in Gelsolin-Related Amyloidosis: In Vitro Expression Reveals an Abnormal Gelsolin Fragment. *Human Molecular Genetics,* Vol. 3, No. 12, pp. 2223-2229

Picken, M. M., & Herrera, G. A. (2007). The Burden of "Sticky" Amyloid: Typing Challenges. *Archives of Pathology and Laboratory Medicine,* Vol. 131, No. 6, pp. 850-851

Rodriguez, F. J., Gamez, J. D., Vrana, J. A., Theis, J. D., Giannini, C., Scheithauer, B. W., Parisi, J. E., Lucchinetti, C. F., Pendlebury, W. W., Bergen, H. R., 3rd, & Dogan, A. (2008). Immunoglobulin Derived Depositions in the Nervous System: Novel Mass Spectrometry Application for Protein Characterization in Formalin-Fixed Tissues. *Laboratory Investigation,* Vol. 88, No. 10, pp. 1024-1037

Rowczenio, D., Dogan, A., Theis, J., Vrana, J., Lachmann, H., Wechalekar, A., Gilbertson, J., Hunt, T., Gibbs, S., Sattianayagam, P., Pinney, J., Hawkins, P., & Gillmore, J. (In Progress). Five Novel Mutations of the Apolipoprotein a-I Gene with Variable Amyloidogenicity and Clinical Phenotype.

Solomon, A., Murphy, C. L., & Westermark, P. (2008). Unreliability of Immunohistochemistry for Typing Amyloid Deposits. *Archives of Pathology and Laboratory Medicine,* Vol. 132, No. 1, pp. 14; author reply 14-15

Uemichi, T., Liepnieks, J. J., & Benson, M. D. (1994). Hereditary Renal Amyloidosis with a Novel Variant Fibrinogen. *Journal of Clinical Investigation,* Vol. 93, No. 2, pp. 731-736

Uemichi, T., Liepnieks, J. J., Alexander, F., & Benson, M. D. (1996). The Molecular Basis of Renal Amyloidosis in Irish-American and Polish-Canadian Kindreds. *Quarterly Journal of Medicine,* Vol. 89, No. 10, pp. 745-750

Uemichi, T., Liepnieks, J. J., Yamada, T., Gertz, M. A., Bang, N., & Benson, M. D. (1996). A Frame Shift Mutation in the Fibrinogen a Alpha Chain Gene in a Kindred with Renal Amyloidosis. *Blood,* Vol. 87, No. 10, pp. 4197-4203

Vrana, J. A., Gamez, J. D., Madden, B. J., Theis, J. D., Bergen, H. R., 3rd, & Dogan, A. (2009). Classification of Amyloidosis by Laser Microdissection and Mass Spectrometry-Based Proteomic Analysis in Clinical Biopsy Specimens. *Blood,* Vol. 114, No. 24, pp. 4957-4959

Yamagoe, S., Kameoka, Y., Hashimoto, K., Mizuno, S., & Suzuki, K. (1998). Molecular Cloning, Structural Characterization, and Chromosomal Mapping of the Human Lect2 Gene. *Genomics,* Vol. 48, No. 3, pp. 324-329

Yazaki, M., Liepnieks, J. J., Barats, M. S., Cohen, A. H., & Benson, M. D. (2003). Hereditary Systemic Amyloidosis Associated with a New Apolipoprotein Aii Stop Codon Mutation Stop78arg. *Kidney International,* Vol. 64, No. 1, pp. 11-16

7

Electron Microscopy in the Diagnosis of Amyloidosis

Tosoni A., Barbiano di Belgiojoso G. and Nebuloni M.
*Pathology Unit and *Nephrology Unit, L.Sacco Dept. Clinical Sciences, University of Milan, Milan, Italy*

1. Introduction

Amyloidosis defines a pathological condition in which organ and tissue damage is related to the extracellular deposition of amyloid fibrils, deriving from specific proteins, the amyloid precursor proteins. More than 25 different precursor proteins are associated with different forms of amyloidosis, which are summarized in Tables 1 and 2. The modern nomenclature is based on the type of amyloid protein involved (Sipe et al., 2010). A subdivision into systemic and localized amyloidosis is also frequently adopted and is relevant in clinical practice and histopathology (Picken, 2010). However, although certain amyloid forms are exclusively localized (e.g. neurodegenerative Aβ), others (e.g. AL) can be either systemic or localized. Prions are usually considered a distinct clinico-pathological entity in connection with their peculiar infectious nature.

2. Structural and morphological aspects of amyloid

2.1 Amyloid fibrils structure

Structural definition of amyloid differs from those used for diagnostic purpose (Fandrich, 2007; Greenwald & Riek, 2010). Pathologists define amyloid on the basis of its presentation in pathological tissues, namely: extracellular deposition of protein with characteristic fibrils appearance in electron microscopy -EM-, typical X-ray diffraction pattern and affinity for Congo red with concomitant green birefringence. Secondary components such as serum amyloid P integrate definition of amyloid deposits. By contrast, in molecular structural studies, tissue depositions are less important than structural similarities. In this context amyloid is defined on the basis of the characteristic conformational arrangement of the proteins, consisting in highly ordered cross-beta sheet aggregates. This definition of amyloid includes pathologic amyloid proteins, synthetic peptides or proteins that form amyloid fibrils *in vitro* but are not associated to clinical symptoms, such as glucagon (Pedersen et al., 2010), certain intra-cellular physiological and pathological proteins (e.g. pituitary peptide hormones, tau neurofibrillary tangles in Alzheimer's disease, α-synuclein in Lewy bodies of Parkinson's diseases), and peculiar natural functional proteins such as curli, an *E. coli* biofilm protein (Greenwald & Riek 2010; Pedersen et al., 2010). Most common high resolution structural methods for proteins, such as Nuclear Magnetic Resonance -NMR- in aqueous solution and crystals X-ray diffraction, are not feasible or limited by the intrinsic nature of the fibrils, which

Precursor	**Amyloid protein**	**Disease**	**Mainly involved organs**
Ig k or λ chain	AL	Primary Myeloma associated SA	Kidney, heart, liver, GI, peripheral nerve, soft tissues
Ig heavy chain	AH	Primary Myeloma associated SA	Kidney, heart
Serum apolipoproten A	AA	Secondary reactive SA	Kidney, GI, liver, spleen, soft tissues
β2-microglobulin	Aβ2M	Hemodialysis related SA	Osteoarticular tissue, heart, GI, lung, soft tissue
Apolipoprotein AIV	AApo AIV	SA associated with aging	Rare forms of SA
Transthyretin	ATTR	Senile SA.	Heart, vessels, soft tissues
Leukocyte chemotactic factor2	ALect2 rare	SA	Kidney, liver
Mutant fibrinogen α-chain	AFib	FSA	Kidney, liver, spleen
Mutant transthyretin	ATTR	FSA familial amyloid polyneuropathy I	Peripheral nerve, heart, GI, kidney
Mutant lysozyme	ALys	Hereditary non neuropathic SA,	Kidney, liver, spleen, GI
Mutant apolipoprotein AI	AApoAI	FSA familial amyloid polyneuropathy II	Liver, kidney, heart, spleen, peripheral nerve, GI, skin, larynx
Mutant apolipoprotein AII	AApoAII	FSA	Kidney, heart
Mutant gelsolin	AGel	Finnish hereditary SA	Cornea, cranial nerves
Mutant cystatin C	ACys	FSA Hereditary cerebral amyloid angiopathy	Cerebral vessels
Mutant protein of ABri	ABri rare	British Familial dementia	CNS

Table 1. Types of amyloid proteins associated with systemic diseases and different organ involvement. (SA=systemic amyloidosis, A=amyloidosis, FSA=familial systemic amyloidosis GI=gastrointestinal tract, NS= nervous system. Pettersoon 2010, Sipe 2010, Dember 2006)

	Precursor	Amyloid protein	Disease	Organ involved
Localized presentation of systemic form		AL	Localized primary A	Various (kidney, skin, bladder, lymph node, GI)
		AH	Localized primary A	Kidney
		AApoAI	LA	Aortic atherosclerotic plaques, meniscus
Neurodegenerative form with amyloid plaques	Aβ protein precursor AAP	Aβ	Alzheimer's disease (sporadic and familial), hereditary cerebral amyloid angiopathy, senile dementia	CNS
	Prions (transmissible amyloid proteins)	APrP	Sporadic (Kuru), new variant (alimentary) and familial CJD, GSSD	CNS
Other forms of LA	Pro-calcitonina	ACal	Tumor associated A	C-cell thyroid tumors
	Amylin - Islet amyloid polypeptide	AIAPP	Tumor associated A	Insulinoma
	Prolactin	APro	Tumor associated A	Prolactinoma
	Mutant protein of ABri and ADan	ADan	Familial dementia	CNS
	Mutant Keratoepithelin	AKer	Familial corneal amyloidosis	Cornea
	Mutant corneodesmosina	ACDSN New ^	A in hypotrichosis simplex of the scalp	Hair follicle, papillary dermis
	Lactoferrin	ALac	Corneal amyloidosis	Cornea
	Keratins	AK	Likenoid and macular A	Skin
	Lactadherin - Medin	AMed	Senile Aortic A	Aorta
	Atrial natriuretic factor	AANF	Atrial A	Cardiac atria
	Seminogelin	ASemI	LA	Vescicula seminalis
	Amylin - Islet amyloid polypeptide	AIAPP	Diabetes type II	Islets of Langerhans
	Prolactin	APro	Aging pituitary	Pituitary gland
	Insulin	AIns	Injection-localized A	Injection-localized

Table 2. Types of amyloid protein associated with localized diseases. (LA=localized amyloidosis, A=amyloidosis, CJD=Creutzfeldt-Jakob Disease, GSSD=Gerstmann-Straussler-Scheinker Disease. Sipe 2010, Merlini 2003, Furnier 2000, ^Caubet 2010, Sikorska 2009)

are insoluble in water and represent one-dimensional forms, with single translational and rotational symmetry elements. The various other technologies employed include: NMR in solid-state, circular dichroism, Fourier transform infrared spectroscopy, atomic force and EM. Currently, high resolution structural data regarding the fibrils of the different types of amyloid remain fragmentary, and frequently they depend on used technical approach (Fandrich, 2007; Sachse et al., 2006; Jimenez et al., 2001; Stromer & Serpel 2005). Most of the current structural data on amyloid fibrils derive from EM such as transmission EM –TEM-techniques, electron-diffraction microscopy, and, more recently, scanning TEM and cryo TEM, using single particle image analysis (Jimenez et al., 2001; Stromer & Serpel 2005). Reports giving models for structure of amyloid fibrils are based mainly on TEM and atomic force diffraction studies of amyloid extracted from tissue and purified (*ex vivo* studies), or synthetic short peptides from amyloid protein sequences (*in vitro* studies). Non fibrillar components of amyloid present in vivo are lost during extraction processes or normally absent in *in vitro* experiments. Globally, the data obtained so far outline the following general characteristics of amyloid fibrils (Fandrich, 2007; Jimenez et al., 2001; Makin & Serpell 2005):

- Different protein sequences form fibrils with high structural similarities.
- Amyloid fibrils extracted from tissues or assembled *in vitro*, when observed at medium magnifications, are similar in diameter and general morphology to those observed *in vivo*.
- Fibrils are long, undetermined in length, straight or moderately curved (Aβ2M), and generally not branched.
- Amyloid fibrils can appear as wavy filaments, road shaped or twisted, with a diameter ranging from 5 to 25 nm.
- Most types of amyloid fibrils are formed by assembling of fibrillar subunits named "protofilaments". In mature fibrils, protofilaments can vary in number (2-6) and can twist one another forming an hollow fibril core. Discernible periodicity can arise from twisted and ribbon-like structures of the fibrils.
- Metastable fibrils precursors include protofibrils and non fibrillar aggregate-soluble oligomers.
- Protofibrils are 2-5 nm in diameter, shorter than fibrils, curl and irregular (worm-like) in their overall structure. They contain one or more linear row of the amyloid protein molecules. Some authors use the term protofibrils also for non fibrillar aggregates.
- Mature fibrils and metastable forms of amyloid are all characterized by cross-beta-sheet conformation.
- Observed with high resolution techniques oligomers, protofibrils, protofilaments and fibrils of the amyloid are structurally heterogeneous.
- Structural characters of oligomers, protofibrils, protofilament and fibrils are influenced by: sequence of the protein, concentration, and various other fibrils growth conditions.

The most distinctive structural feature of amyloid is the structural polymorphism of their aggregates and fibrils in *in vitro* and in *ex vivo* experiments. This is found also within the tissue extracted, and even more in experiments *in vitro* under the same conditions of incubation (Pedersen et al., 2010; Fandrich, 2007, 2009). TEM images can demonstrate the variations of degree of twisting, number of protofilaments forming a fibril, and mature fibrils diameter (Fandrich et al., 2009; Greenwald & Riek 2010).

Amyloid may be considered a characteristic structural status of a protein in certain conditions. For this reason amyloidosis is defined a conformational protein disease. In amyloidosis, an amyloid precursor protein, with or without post-transcriptional modifications, sometimes favored by mutations (hereditary amyloidosis), and in particular experimental conditions *in vitro*, can lead to beta-sheet peculiar aggregation, forming insoluble fibrils. Moreover, in prion diseases, an infective prion protein can induce cross beta-sheet conformation and amyloid deposition of the constitutive protein (Pan et al, 1993; Prusiner, 1998). Understanding the structure of amyloid and their formation is the prerequisite for developing methods to rationally interfere in the mechanism of pathologic aggregation responsible for important human diseases.

2.2 Ultrastructural morphology of amyloid fibrils in tissues

In 1959 Cohen and Calkins demonstrated, for the first time, that different forms of amyloid exhibit a comparable fibrillar ultrastructure in fixed tissue sections (Sipe & Choen, 2000). This has been amply confirmed by successive studies, which evidenced that all types of amyloid deposits seen in different tissues, and regardless of the clinical/biochemical form, are mainly composed of bundle of not branched, straight fibrils, ranging from 6nm to 13nm in diameter (average 7,5-10 nm) and 100-1600 nm in length (Sipe & Choen, 2000). Ultrastructural demonstration of this peculiar fibrillar morphology was adopted as one of the criteria for the definition of amyloid. Subsequently, studies on amyloid extracted from tissues, and *in vitro* studies on amyloid proteins synthetic derivates, are the basis of the most of high-resolution structural data regarding amyloid, which are described in the previous paragraph. It must be stressed that these structural data refer to pure, purified or partially purified amyloid proteins. High resolution -HR- structural studies of amyloid in tissues (*in situ* studies) are few and consist mainly in TEM analyses at high magnification (x500000 or more) of thin sections of plastic embedded fixed tissues. Immunolabeling procedures for TEM are applied to distinguish amyloid proteins from other tissue constituents (Inoue et al., 1997, 1998, 1999). Image reconstruction techniques are used for the formulation of the structural models. Structural models deriving from *in vitro* and *ex vivo* experiments are only partially confirmed by *in situ* HR TEM analyses. In fact: amyloid fibrils in tissue appear not branched, rigid, about 10 nm in diameters, but – for example- the substructural organization in protofilaments is rarely described and can be different from that observed in *in vitro* experiments. However, immuno-labeling techniques -including immuno-electron transmission microscopy -ITEM- demonstrated that other various components are present in tissue amyloid deposits (Inoue et al., 1997, 1998, 1999; Sipe & Choen, 2000). These do not form fibrils in vitro, but are implicated in amyloid deposition and stability. Non fibrillar components, commonly present in various types of amyloid deposits, include: proteins (serum amyloid P component SAP, apolipoprotein E), proteoglycans -PG- (condroitinsulfate PG, heparansulfate PG) and lipids (Pettersson & Konttinen, 2010; Merlini et al., 2003; Gellermann et al., 2005). These are mostly or partially lost during extraction procedures, and they are not present in *in vitro* experiments. This fact could justify the structural differences of amyloid analyzed *in situ* (Sipe & Cohen, 2000; Inoue et al., 1998). At present, review of morphological studies in situ of amyloid deposits (Sipe & Cohen, 2000; Sikorska et al., 2009; Inoue et al., 1997, 1998, 1999; Bely et al., 2005) outlines the following general characteristics:

- In systemic and most of localized forms of amyloidosis, amyloid deposits contain not branched fibrils, from 6nm to 13nm in diameter (average 7,5-10 nm), and variable length.
- In neurodegenerative prion forms, amyloid fibrils diameters range form 7-8 nm –in Kuro plaques- to 17-24 nm –in variant Creutzfeldt-Jakob disease plaques- depending on the sequence mutations of amyloid precursor proteins.
- Diameters of the fibrils depend also on fixation procedure used to prepare the tissues.
- The fibrils are more frequently straight, but curved shapes were also described, especially for Aβ2M type.
- At high magnification the fibrils did not appear to be formed by protofilament sub-units. They show frequently cross bands along the axis, and a tubular appearance due to an empty core (Fig. 1), a central dense dot is described by Inoue et al. (Inoue et al., 1997, 1998, 1999).
- ITEM analyses with antibodies specific for amyloid proteins identify: non fibrillar-amorphous aggregates, filaments about 0,5-1 nm in diameter, and protofibrils 3-5 nm in diameter, which can be observed close to the fibrils or in their proximity.
- ITEM analyses show that specific antibodies to non fibrillar component of amyloid appear tight to fibrils. This fact is at the basis of Inoue models, in which SAP and PG play a structural role in the construction of the fibrils.

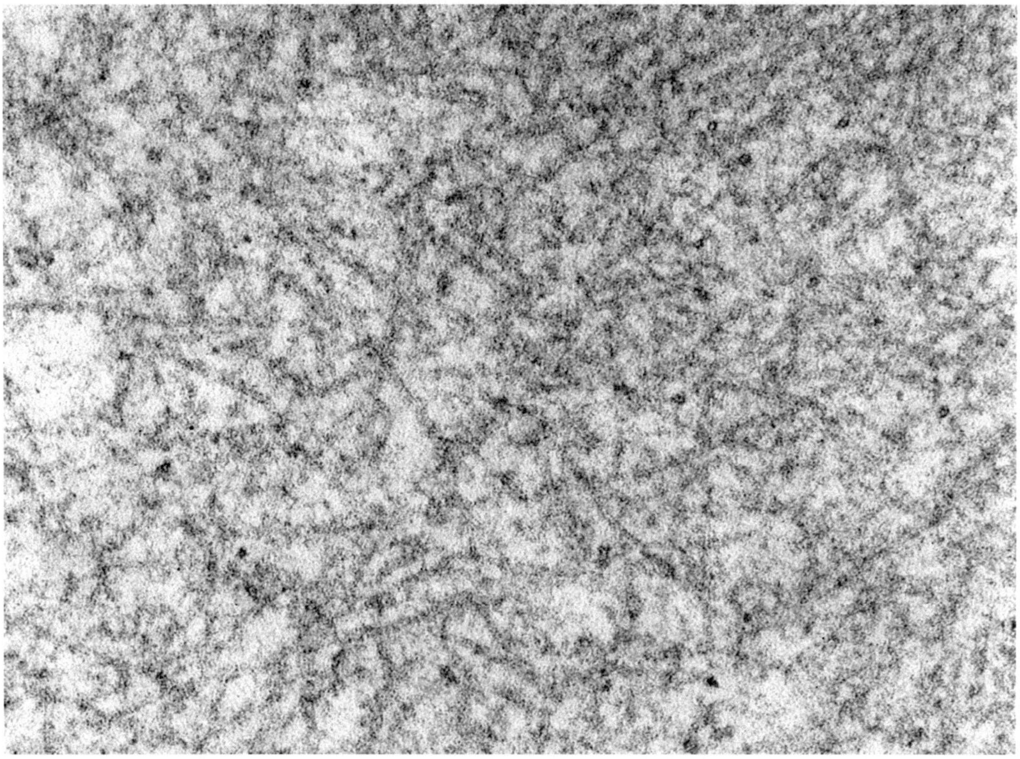

Fig. 1. Amyloid fribrils in a case with AL amyloidosis. At high magnification the fibrils appear straight and non branched. Cross band along their axis and a clear hollow centre can be seen focally. Original magnification –OM- : x50000.

Overall, the morphological definition of amyloid remains the one described by Cohen and colleagues in their first ultrastructural studies. Atypical ultrastructural presentation corresponding to Congo red stained-birefringence tissue deposits must be confirmed as amyloid using ITEM techniques. Additional studies in tissue, using new techniques, are needed to confirm the actual molecular structure of amyloid fibrils *in vivo*.

2.3 Ultrastructural morphology of amyloid deposit in tissue

Ultrastructural analyses of amyloid *in situ* provide additional information regarding arrangement and distribution of amyloid fibrils *in vivo* and their structural interaction with extracellular matrix elements and cells.

The amyloid fibrils tissues aggregates may be in sparse or dense pattern (Fig. 2).

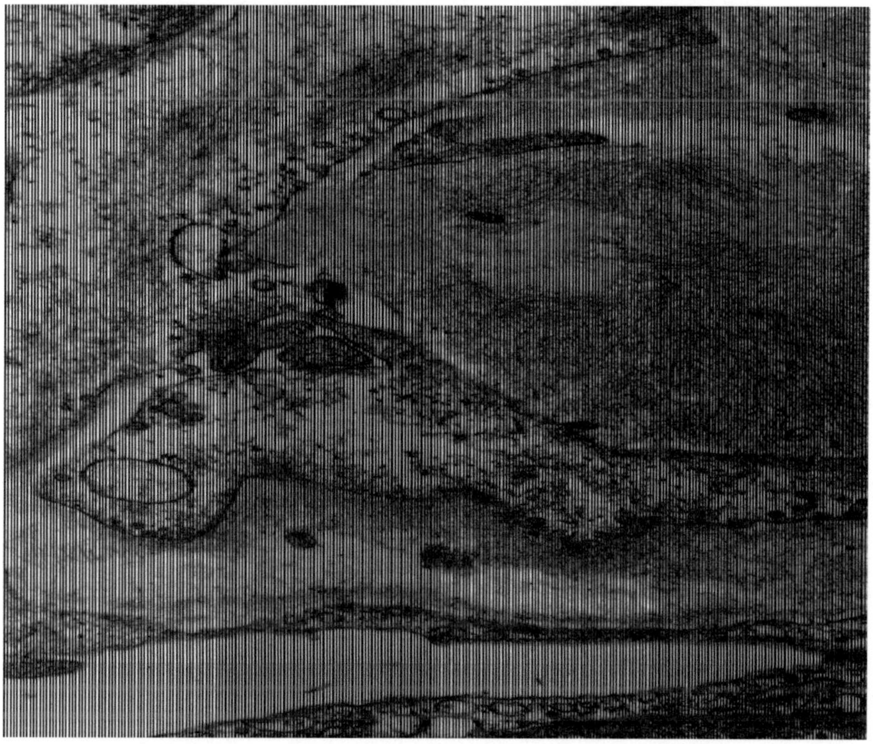

Fig. 2. Dense and few scattered aggregates of amyloid fibrils between pericytes, from a renal biopsy in a case of AL amyloidosis. OM: x7000.

Haphazard arrangement represents the more frequent and specific array of amyloid fibrils in tissues. However, star-like, parallel, and curving arrays are also frequently documented. In vivo, amyloid deposit morphology can also change after deposition. In advanced amyloidosis, older amyloid deposits, can appear as dense ovoid-globular aggregates, or inhomogeneous deposits with multifocal accumulation of densely packed short fibrils and filaments. Centre of the dense deposits may be lacking of immunoreactivity for anti-amyloid protein antibodies (Bely et al., 2005). Frequently, distinction of fibrils in dense aggregates is easier at their marginal zone (Nishi et al., 2008). Particular aggregation patterns include glomerular "spikes" and cerebral amyloid plaques.

2.3.1 Glomerular sub-epithelial "spikes"

"Spikes" are a peculiar amyloid fibrils aggregation described in glomerular AA and AL amyloidosis. They consist in fibrils in parallel spicular array, crossing the glomerular basement membrane at the right angle and pointing to the foot processes of podocytes (Fig. 3) (Dickman et al., 1981; Nishi et al., 2008).

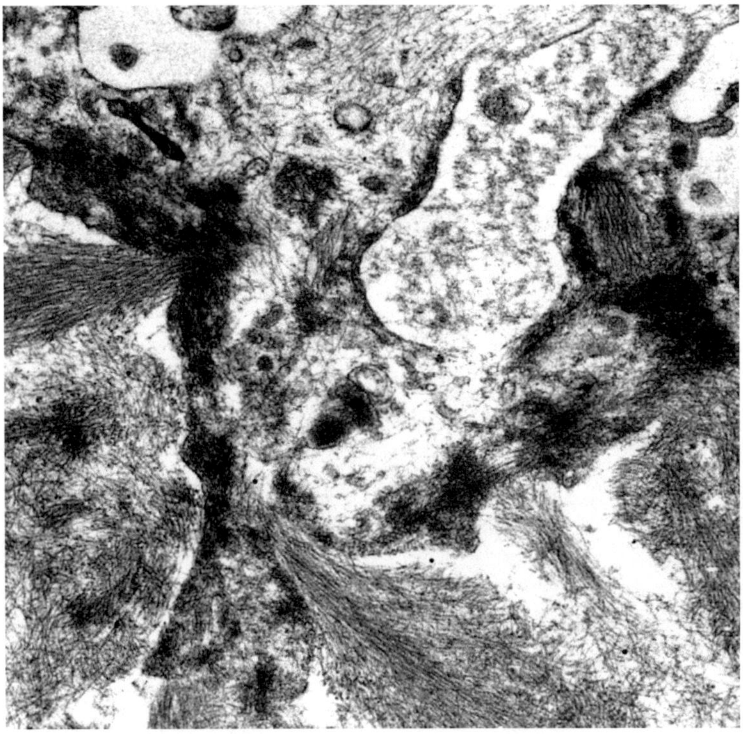

Fig. 3. Spicular array of amyloid fibrils. Under a wide foot process of a podocyte, in a case of AA amyloidosis. OM: x4400.

2.3.2 Cerebral amyloid plaques

Peculiar star-like aggregation of the fibrils are the cerebral amyloid plaques in neurodegenerative diseases due to Aβ and APr including: Alzheimer's disease (sporadic and familial), age-related or senile dementia, Sporadic (Kuru), new variant (alimentary) and familial Creutzfeldt-Jakob Disease -CJD-, Gerstmann-Straussler-Scheinker disease -GSSD-. Despite in all these forms neurotoxicity is linked mainly to oligomers of amyloid proteins, presence of amyloid plaque correlate to progression of the disease (Sikorska et al., 2009; Fiedrich et al., 2010; Merlini & Bellotti, 2003). Morphological characters and distribution of amyloid plaques, determined by light microscopy-LM-, differ in the various clinical-pathological forms, and can help the diagnosis. TEM and ITEM studies of amyloid plaques demonstrated that they are ordered aggregates with bundles of fibrils departing radially from a central core. The plaques are located at the neuropil, between glial and neural processes. The different ultrastructural characters described in the different clinical-pathological form (Serpell, 2000; Sikorska et al., 2009; Fournier et al., 2000) are summarized below:

- Classical senile plaques, present also in Alzheimer's disease, are star-like closely packed bundles of Aβ fibrils forming a generally dense fibrillar core, which is surrounded by dystrophic neuritis, activated microglia, and reactive astrocytes. In Alzheimer's diseases typically plaques are numerous, and present several dystrophic neurites and microglial cells. Senile plaques can be observed also in prion diseases, in addition to prion plaques. In Alzheimer and senile dementia another form of amyloid is present. It is the intracellular cross-beta sheet tau fibrillar aggregates forming neurofibrillary tangles.
- "Kuro" star-like plaques are relatively small, formed by bundles of fibrils mixed to electron dense material and cellular element. Dystrophic neurites are rarely identified. The plaques are surrounded by glial cells (Fig. 4). Jatrogenic CJD plaques are typically enclosed by numerous astrocytes. "Kuro" plaques are present in all forms of CJD. They are more numerous and smaller in jatrogenic CJD. Small Kuro plaques, distributed in clusters, are observed in new variant CJD (alimentary).
- Florid plaques of new variant CJD: amyloid plaques contain and are surrounded by vacuoles deriving from swelled cell processes. The radially arranged bundles of fibrils are very thick. They are loosely mixed to non fibrillar prion proteins, swollen glial and neural cell processes, and numerous dystrophic neurites with synaptic elements. Numerous microglial cells, sometimes with intracellular fibrils in vacuoles, are present around and within the plaques.
- GSSD multicentric plaques: bundles of fibrils depart radially from more than one central dense core, dystrophic neurites are mixed to fibrillar amyloid bundles. Microglial cells are also observed.

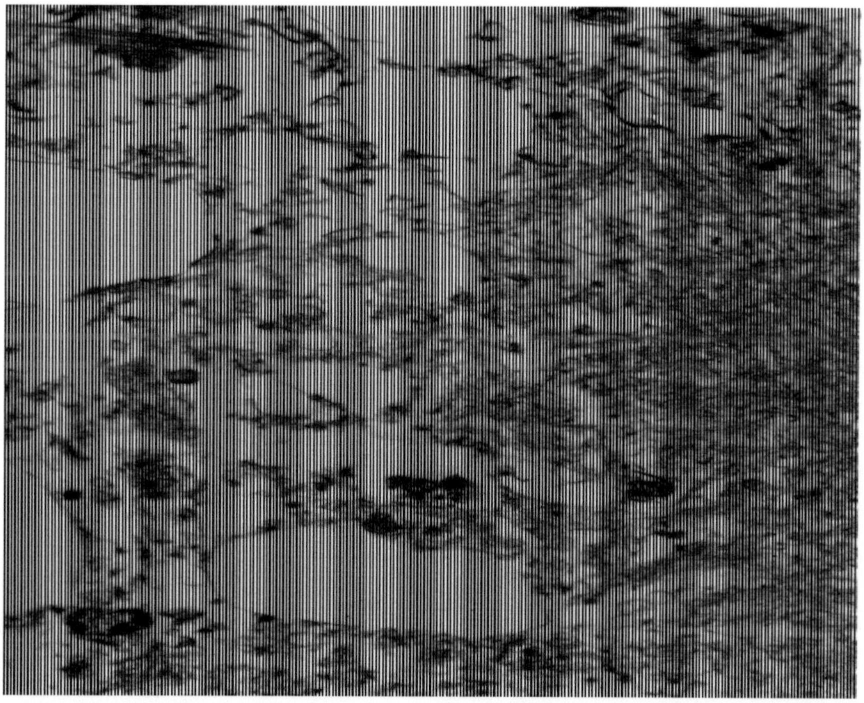

Fig. 4. A small Kuru-like PrP plaque, with bundles of filaments in a star-like array. Amyloid bundles are mixed with scattered elettrondense material. OM: x3000.

Aβ and APr fibrils are also present in haphazard arrangement in the "diffuse plaques" more frequently observed in Alzheimer's diseases associated to Down syndrome and in hereditary cerebral amyloid angiopathy (Allsop et al., 1986; Rozemulleret al., 1993; Yamaguchi et al., 1989). Diffuse plaques are not associated to neuritic alterations. They contain a scanty amount of fibrils, and can be negative at Congo red stain and birefringence. These amyloid deposits are evidenced mainly by immune-labeling, and using methenamine silver staining methods. TEM studies in Alzheimer's diseases describe also the presence of small clusters of randomly arranged fibrils associated to neurite degeneration. These are retained primitive Aβ classical plaque forms. Perivascular non ordered amyloid fibrils are frequently identified in neurodegenerative amyloidosis but they are the prevalent amyloid deposition in prion associated hereditary cerebral amyloid angiopathy. The described morphological differences of cerebral amyloid deposits in neurodegenerative amyloidosis demonstrate a different fibril distribution and different cells injury and reaction, depending from amyloid protein sequence and mutations.

2.4 Intracellular amyloid fibrils in amyloidosis

Amyloid fibrils are frequently reported within lysosomes of reticuloendothelial or macrophage system cells (including microglia and glomerular mesangial cells), in proximity to amyloid deposits (Sikorska et al., 2009; Bely et al., 2005; Santostefano et al., 2005; Keeling et al., 2004; Kluve-Beckerman et al., 1999; Morten et al., 2007). The presence of amyloid within phagocytes *in vivo* remains controversial. It can derive from the capture of extracellular amyloid by phagocytosis for degradation. This may indicate a protective role of macrophages activity. However, resistance to lysosomal proteases has been observed for Aβ2m, AAmylin, Aβ, prions, and it may be a generic feature of amyloid. Amyloid could be produced within macrophages. Phagocytes could promote fibrils self-assembling within their endosome or lysosome compartments, favoring protein precursor concentration or modifying protein conformation within acidic endolysosomal compartments. They also could be involved in proteolytic cleavages, producing protein fragments with increased amyloid propensity. Phagocytic cell lines cultured in vitro have been shown to promote the fibrillar aggregation of Ig light chains proteins and serum apolipoprotein A (Kluve-Beckerman et al., 1999; Keeling et al., 2004; Santostefano et a., l 2005; Friedrich et al., 2010; Teng et al., 2004; Yazawa et al., 2001). At present, data regarding amyloid and their biogenesis *in vivo* remain limited, especially those referred to the structural aspects in extracellular spaces and distribution within the cell compartments. Most of the data regarding fibrillogenesis derive from studies of cell lines cultured in vitro, which frequently include ITEM approach (Leonhardt et al., 2010). An increase in the knowledge on endosomal and lysosomal system involvement in amyloid genesis can guide drug discovery of new therapeutic agents.

3. Diagnostic TEM in amyloidosis

The importance of an early diagnosis of amyloid and the correct typing of fibrils have been realized in order to recent advances in the treatment of systemic amyloidosis (Picken, 2010; Pettersson & Konttinen, 2010). No diagnostic biochemical markers in body fluids are known to date. APr and Aβ neurodegenerative amyloid forms are mainly clinically diagnosed. When autopsy confirmation is required, it is relied on histochemical characterization, and immunohistochemical and biochemical typing. For the other forms of amyloidosis, the diagnosis consists in the detection and typing of deposits in tissue biopsies or needle aspirates. In the latter context, the ultrastructural analyses are used in first steps of detection of amyloid, together with polarized LM on Congo red stained sections. Congo red staining and birefringence detection are considered to be the gold standard techniques for the demonstration of amyloid deposits. However, specificity and sensitivity of this technique may depend on the experience of the observer, fixation procedure, section thickness, proper staining protocol, and appropriate optics (Picken, 2010). Ultrastructural analysis is particularly useful in early amyloid deposition. In these cases amyloidosis might not be evident at LM because fibrils deposition is minimal and Congo red staining is negative. Moreover, ultrastructural appearance of amyloid may be important in the differential diagnosis of various organized immunedeposits responsible for various forms of glomerulopathies (see upcoming paragraph) and neuropathies (Vallat et al., 2007). However, we should remember some limits of TEM analyses. These are frequently performed on a very small piece of tissue, resulting in a limitation in sensitivity when amyloid deposits are focal and irregularly distributed. The second limit of TEM is that all types of amyloid fibrils have similar morphology. A correct typing of amyloid requires the use of immunolabeling techniques. Unfortunately, the procedures used to preserve morphology at high resolution generally reduce antigens preservation, therefore, amyloid typing is preferably carried out on frozen sections or on formalin fixed paraffin embedded sections. On the other hand, some easy pretreatment of thin sections (e.g. incubation of epon-embedded sections with hydrogen peroxide or periodate solution, or embedding in hydrophilic resins) can ameliorate ITEM results (Inoue et al., 1997, 1998). Ultrastructural localization of amyloid -when possible- increases the sensitivity of the detection, and, above all, ITEM can add important informations for unusual types of amyloidosis (Arbustini et al., 2002; Inoue et al., 1997, 1998, 1999, Caubet et al., 2010). TEM techniques, in tissues and *in vitro*, are frequently included in studies defining new varieties of amyloid (Caubet et al., 2010).

3.1 Systemic amyloidosis

Systemic amyloidosis -SA- represents the most important form of amyloidosis (Pettersson & Konttinen, 2010; Picken, 2010). They comprise a biochemically heterogeneous group of potentially lethal disorders. The main types of SA include, in order of their prevalence: AL, AA, and familial forms. A more recently described form includes dialysis related Aβ2m (Jadoul et al., 2001; Bely et al., 2005). An early and specific diagnosis is crucial for the treatment and prognosis. Amyloid deposition can occur in any organ and tissue. For the detection of amyloid, the biopsy of a clinically affected organ is the most sensitive method and may also detect concomitant diseases. The most frequently involved organs correspond to the most frequent diagnostic localization of amyloid. These include kidney, gastrointestinal tract, heart and liver (Pettersson & Konttinen, 2010). Amyloid is frequently reported also in skin in systemic or localized form (Schreml et al., 2010), and in nerve biopsy in cases with neuropathies (Vallat et al., 2007). Certain symptoms in the context of chronic inflammation diseases, plasma cell dyscrasia or familial history, arouse a clinical suspicion of "amyloid syndrome"(Pettersson & Konttinen, 2010). These include mainly proteinuria or renal failure, enteropathy with malabsorption and bleeding, restrictive cardiomiopathy with thromboembolism due to neuropathy, hepatomegalia and splenomegalia. Some clinical manifestations are more common in certain types of amyloid, but a large variability of presentation is common. In the past, diagnosis of SA in clinically suspected cases was based on rectal and gingival or salivary gland biopsies examination. Currently, abdominal fat needle aspiration or, better, biopsy, are retained the gold standard to confirm the clinical suspicion of systemic amyloidosis. In most cases the samples are completely designed for histopathological analyses and typing (Picken, 2010). However, when a fragment for ultrastructural analyses is disposable, amyloid deposit can be observed in semithin blue stained sections examined by LM as extracellular accumulation of weakly stained material, more frequently in perivascular localization, similar to sclerotic changes. At TEM analysis, amyloid fibrils can be demonstrated in perivascular deposits (Fig. 5A, 5B) and in extracellular matrix deposits, with high sensitivity. It must be stressed that even in cases with a single symptomatic organ involvement with locally demonstrated amyloid deposits, a systemic form must be carefully excluded. In fact, at present the management of localized amyloidosis is mainly conservative where SA involves more radical approaches, including chemotherapy (in AL) and liver transplantation (in familial amyloidosis) (Westermark et al., 2006; Arbustini et al., 2002; Picken, 2010).

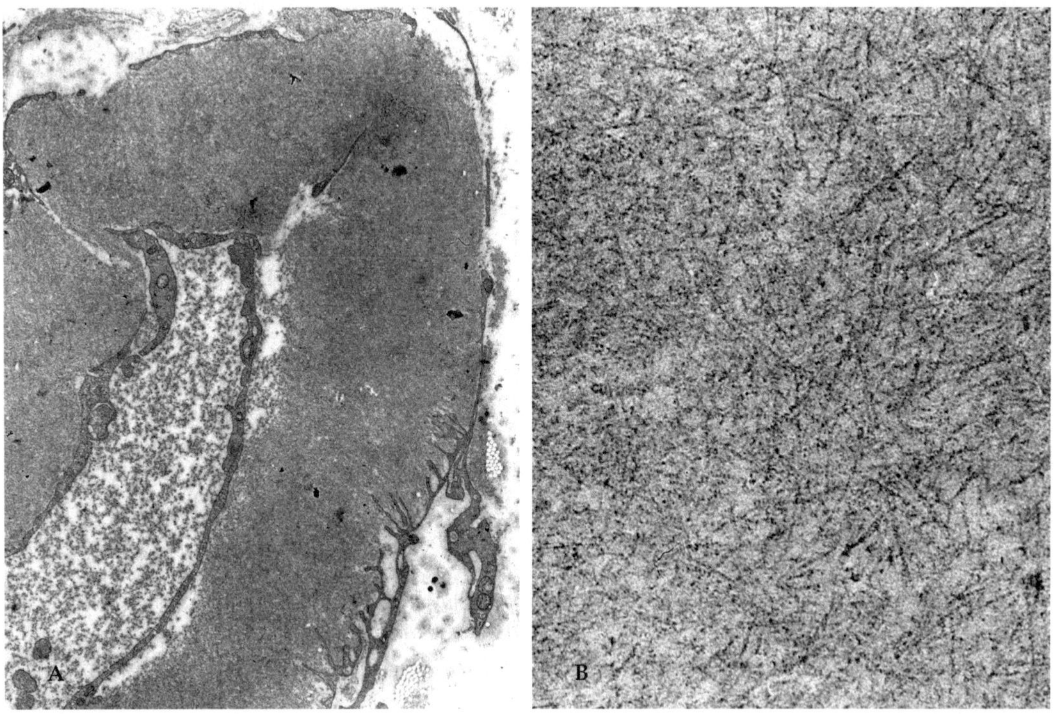

Fig. 5. A-B. Perivascular deposits (A) consisting in amyloid fibrils in haphazard arrangement (B). OM: A. x3000, B. x7000.

3.2 Renal amyloidosis

Among various involved organs in SA, kidney is the most frequently affected (Picken, 2010, Pettersson & Konttinen 2010). In the differential diagnosis of the glomerulopathies, TEM analyses are normally included. Therefore, renal amyloidosis is frequently documented by ultrastrastructural evidence of fibril deposits.

3.2.1 Clinical presentation

Proteinuria is the clinical manifestation that is present in the majority of patients with renal amyloidosis (Dember, 2006). Ranges of proteinuria are from subnephrotic to massive, with urinary protein excretion rates up to 20-30 g/day. Hypoalbuminemia can be profound, edema is often severe. The level of protein excretion in AL type has been referred to be higher than in AA type, whereas the count of red cells in the sediment significantly higher in AA type, compared to AL type. When amyloid is confined to tubulo-interstitium or vessels, proteinuria can be minimal and reduced renal function is the main clinical manifestation. Renal impairment tends to progress more rapidly when glomerular deposition predominates over tubular and interstitium involvement. Hypertension is an uncommon feature, except when amyloid deposition is relevant in vessels. An unusual manifestation of renal amyloidosis is nephrogenic diabetes insipidus, caused by amyloid deposition in the peri-collecting ducts tissue. Fanconi's syndrome is another extraglomerular manifestation, due to injury to proximal tubular cells by filtered light chains. Amyloid deposits that are isolated to renal medulla is a feature in most patients with ApoAI familial amyloidosis, and has been described in some patients with AA amyloidosis (Nishi et al., 2008; Picken & Linke, 2009). Medullary-limited disease can elude pathologic diagnosis if the biopsy specimen is limited to renal cortex. In synthesis, proteinuria, renal insufficiency, large echogenic kidneys are clinical manifestations that can suggest the suspicion for a renal amyloidosis, which prompts a kidney biopsy (Dember, 2006).

3.2.2 Diagnosis of renal amyloidosis

Amyloid can be found anywhere in the kidney, but glomerular deposition predominates. However, in a small number of cases glomerular deposits are scanty or absent and the amyloid is confined to tubuli and interstitium or vessels (Dember, 2006; Picken & Linke, 2009; Sen & Sarsik, 2010). Glomerular amyloid appears at LM eosinophilic amorphous material in the mesangium and along capillary walls. Periodic acid-Schiff -PAS- staining is weak over nodules, which can be observed in mesangial areas and represent amyloid deposition. Immunofluorescence -IF- on frozen tissue, normally used for diagnosis of immunecomplex glomerulopathy, can be positive for a single light chain isotype, more often lambda chain, in AL amyloidosis, and it can be positive for fibrinogen in cases with AFib. Nevertheless, negative kappa or lambda chain does not exclude AL disease, and a positive immunolabeling does not prove amylod deposition. The histological diagnosis of renal amyloidosis can be established using Congo red staining, and TEM. Ultrastructural analyses are very useful to identify scanty amyloid deposition in early stages of the disease. Ultrastructural main characters of renal amyloidosis are reported as follows:

- Glomerular amyloid: in the majority of amyloid forms, fibrils are localized preferentially within glomeruli, in mesangial matrix, and basal membranes. The progression of amyloid deposition is associated to mesangial matrix and basal membrane degradation and replacement by amyloid fibrils (Teng et al., 2004). Peculiar spicular aggregates under podocytes foot process, named "spikes" or "spicules" (Dickman et al., 1981; Nishi et al., 2008), are frequently associated to detachments of visceral epithelial cells (Fig. 6). Sub-epitelial "spikes", when prominent, are visualized also by LM using PAS or methenamine silver stains, which are unusual stains for amyloid. The spikes are generally considered a sign of active fibrils deposition and a bad prognostic parameter (Dickman et al., 1981).
- Extraglomerular amyloid: tubulo-interstitial and vascular deposition can accompany glomerular amyloidosis or characterize certain forms without glomerular involvement. Fibrils can be localized within tubular basal membrane (Fig. 7), in interstitial spaces, and within arteriolar walls.

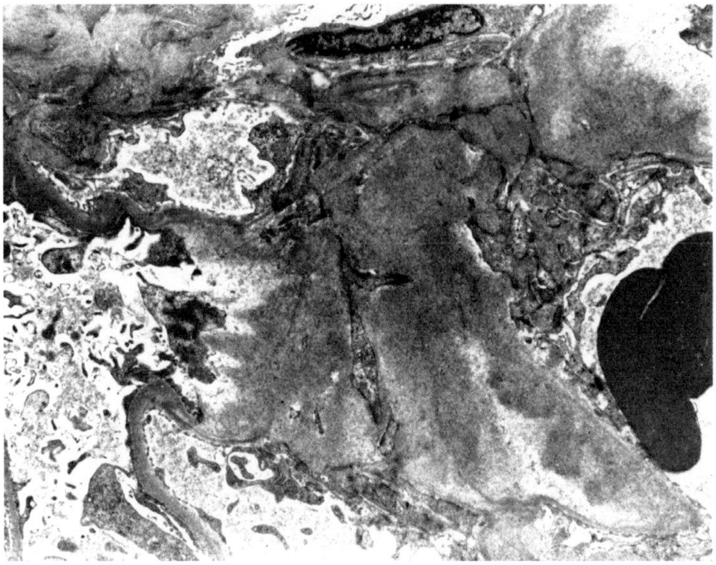

Fig. 6. Massive amyloid deposition and spicular aggregates associated with detachment of visceral epithelial cells. OM: x3000

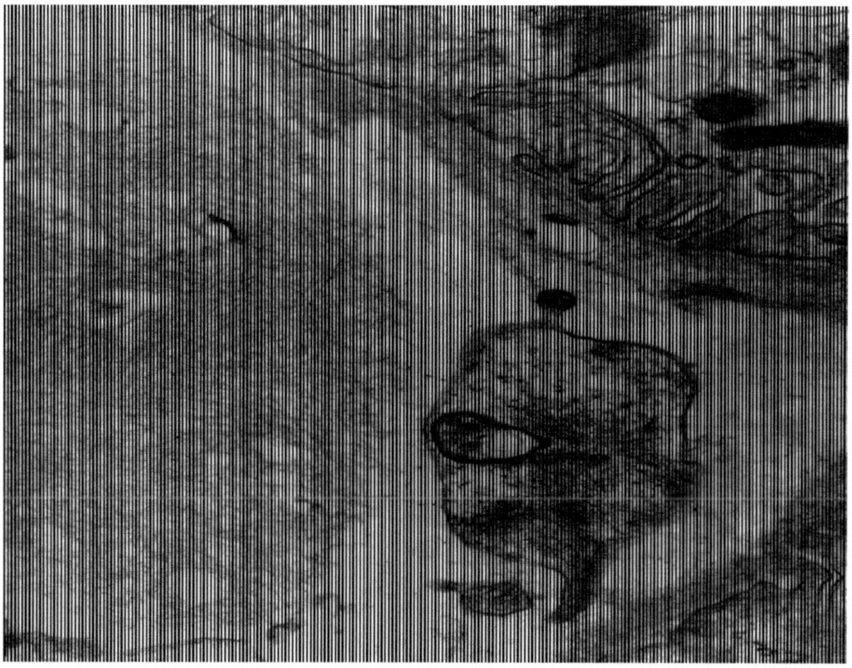

Fig. 7. Amyloid fibrils within tubular basal membrane and in extracellular matrix. OM: x12000

3.2.3 Histopathological classification and clinicopathological correlations

Though recent reports demonstrated a toxic role of amyloid precursor proteins in AL and AA, amyloid progressive accumulation play an important role in mechanism of renal dysfunction, causing glomerular disruption and also whole renal architecture alterations (Sen & Sarsik, 2010). Most patients with AA or AL disease have predominantly glomerular deposition, and therefore pathologists tried to classify different patterns of glomerular amyloid deposition, in an attempt to quantify the renal damage and to predict patient outcome, depending on severity of glomerular involvement. Dikman et al (Dikman et al., 1981) identified 4 different patterns of glomerular deposition: segmental, diffuse, nodular and mixed, nodular and diffuse. In fact, early glomerular amyloid deposits tend to be spotty and segmental, and late amyloid deposits become more uniform and diffuse. Six patterns or classes of renal amyloidosis were recently proposed by Sen and Sarsik (Sen & Sarsik, 2010), similarly to the systemic lupus erythematosus glomerulonephritis classification. Similarly, this classification of renal amyloidosis is based exclusively on glomerular pathology. Class I, is defined as minimal amyloidosis, with less than 10% extension of glomerular amyloid deposition. The minimal deposition is focal and segmental, within the vascular pole or mensangium. Congo red may not clearly identify the small amyloid deposits. TEM might be necessary for a definitive diagnosis. Definition of the classes, II, III, IV and VI, is based on extension of amyloid deposition within the glomeruli and on the total percentage of involved glomeruli. Class V, or membranous amyloid deposition, i.e. diffuse membranous pattern define a fibril deposition in glomerular basal membranes without prominent mesangial amyloid deposition. This last pattern is mostly associated with AL or non-AA amyloidosis.

Starting from class II, tubulointerstitial and vessels alteration may accompany glomerular lesions. A score of severity, or renal amyloidosis prognostic score–RAPR-, has been proposed by the same authors, taking into account the sum of above described amyloid histological classes, plus global glomerular sclerosis, inflammatory interstitial infiltration, interstitial fibrosis, and tubular atrophy. This severity score is divided into 3 grades: early, late, advanced amyloidosis. The authors applied the new classification and grading system on renal biopsy from patients with AA associated to familial Mediterranean fever, demonstrating a positive correlation between severity of glomerular amyloid deposition, interstitial fibrosis, and inflammation. However, demonstration of a correlation between RAPR and clinical presentation and prognosis are not demonstrated by the authors, and require further studies (Sen & Sarsik, 2010; Dember, 2006). In various classification systems, TEM is fundamental in the definition of class defining minimal amyloid deposition. Sen and Sarsik classification takes into account, and reviews, specific differences in fibrils distribution, depending on the amyloid form, based also on ultrastructural analysis especially for class I definition. These are briefly reported as follows:

- In early AA amyloidosis glomerular fibrils deposition are focal or segmental, within the vascular pole or mesangium. At this stage, in most cases there are no extraglomerular amyloid deposits, except rare cases with only interstitial and vascular deposition.
- In AL, glomerulopathy amyloid tends more frequently to involve capillary basal membrane, also in early stage, frequently with sub-epithelial spikes. Extraglomerular amyloid is of later onset, it is more frequently observed in medulla, and generally it is less important than glomerular deposition.
- Familial renal amyloidosis due to mutant fibrinogen α-chain -AFib – , involve strongly and exclusively the glomeruli. Tendency to amyloid deposition within the basal membrane of the capillary loops is similar to that described in AL.
- In familial renal amyloidosis due to mutant apolipoprotein AI –AApoAI-, amyloid is present only in medulla.
- In transplanted patients with recurrence, and at the same time in patients with AA and rheumatoid arthritis, amyloid may be found only in vascular wall, without glomerular involvement, causing hypertension, which is unusual in amyloidosis presentation.

It must be stressed that a negative detection of amyloid in glomeruli does not exclude a renal amyloidosis: fibrils must be searched carefully also in interstitium, in peritubular basal membranes, and arteriolar walls. Moreover, medulla should be included in the biopsy to identify AApoAI, and some cases of AA.

3.2.4 Renal amyloid typing

The difference in renal distribution of the fibrils may explain different clinical presentation (Dember, 2006), but it is not sufficiently specific to distinguish the amyloid type. IF normally used for diagnosis of glomerulopathy can identify AL light chains or AFib fibrinogen. Other amyloid forms are specifically determined mainly by immunolabeling techniques on paraffin sections and by IF on frozen sections. ITEM is a high sensitive approach to identify and typing the fibrils (Fig.8). However, in a part of cases with AL, commercially available reagents do not always detect the amyloid, because of conformational change or fragmentation of amyloidogenic light chains, which masks or deletes significant epitopes (Dember, 2006). In cases with negative immunostainimg for AL, AA, and more common familial amyloid forms (AFib, ATTR), TEM amyloid deposits demonstration can diagnose amyloidosis or confirm a positive Congo red stain and birefringence analyses. These data, including TEM, justify the demand of additional specific typing tests in specialized institutions. Molecular identification of amyloid protein using proteomic methods such as microextraction and sequencing or tandem mass spectrometry are currently being testing (Picken, 2010).

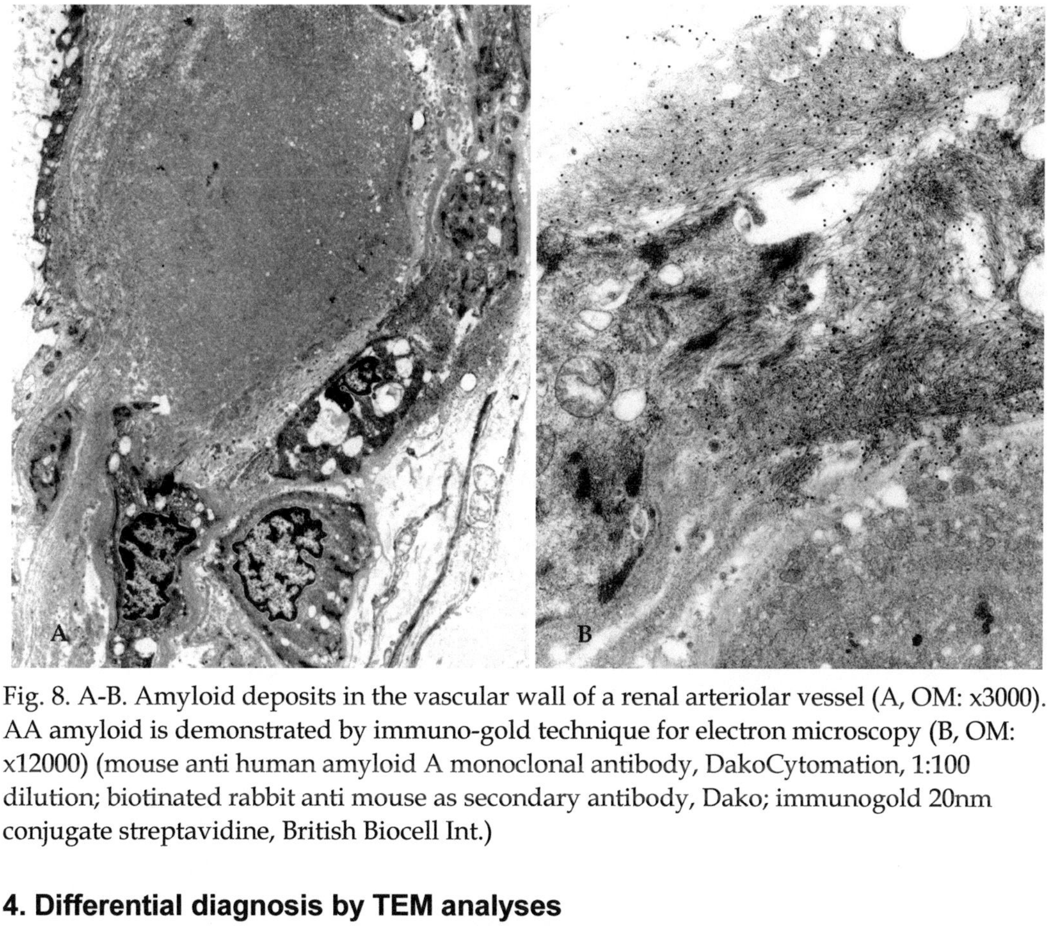

Fig. 8. A-B. Amyloid deposits in the vascular wall of a renal arteriolar vessel (A, OM: x3000). AA amyloid is demonstrated by immuno-gold technique for electron microscopy (B, OM: x12000) (mouse anti human amyloid A monoclonal antibody, DakoCytomation, 1:100 dilution; biotinated rabbit anti mouse as secondary antibody, Dako; immunogold 20nm conjugate streptavidine, British Biocell Int.)

4. Differential diagnosis by TEM analyses

4.1 Non amyloid tissue fibrils in normal and pathologic condition

Specificity and sensitivity of the TEM analyses for amyloid diagnosis are influenced by the presence of the fibrillar components of the extracellular matrix -ECM- in interstitium and basal membranes. Fibrillar ECM comprises fibrils or microfibrils, not branched, straight and with a diameter about 10 nm. These components of ECM similar to amyloid include collagen microfibrils, fibrillin, and fibronectin (Inoue et al., 1999; Kronz et al., 1998; Sherratt et al., 2001; Weber et al., 2002; Dzamba & Peters, 1991). In our experience, basically, amyloid fibrils are more frequently in haphazard arrangement, generally they appear more straight, better defined, and more electrondense than extracellular matrix fibrils (Fig. 9). The distinction of the different fibrils can be difficult in presence of fibrotic changes in various pathological conditions (e.g. trasplant glomerulopathy, focal glomerulosclerosis, hypertension, mesangiocapillary glomerulonephritis) and particularly in patients with diabetes (Inoue et al., 1999; Kronz et al., 1998). In these latter, the amount of fibrillar ECM increases, and connective fibrils appear more distinct and electrondense. However, ECM fibrils remain mostly in bundle arrays, even if random orientation is focally observed. In uncertain cases with negative Congo red and immunohistochemical staining, ITEM techniques may help a specific distinction. Glomerular normal ECM fibrils include not branched fibrils about 10 nm in diameters in mesangium and, in lesser amount, within basal membrane (Inoue et al., 1999; King et al., 2000). Congo red negative mesangial fibrils about 5-20 nm may commonly be seen in sclerosing glomerular diseases and represent a non specific reaction to glomerular injury (Kronz et al., 1998). These fibrils localize usually in a segmental fashion and are more bundle-like than random arranged. Non-amyloid fibrillar deposit has been frequently described associated to diabetic condition, phenomenon called diabetic fibrillosis. This is characterized by a large amount of not branched mesangial fibrils, and bundles of subendothelial and intramembrane fibrils, with reported diameters ranging from 7 to 16, but they are in average generally wider than amyloid fibrils (King et al., 2000; Korbet et al., 1994; Inoue et al., 1999; Kronz et al., 1998).

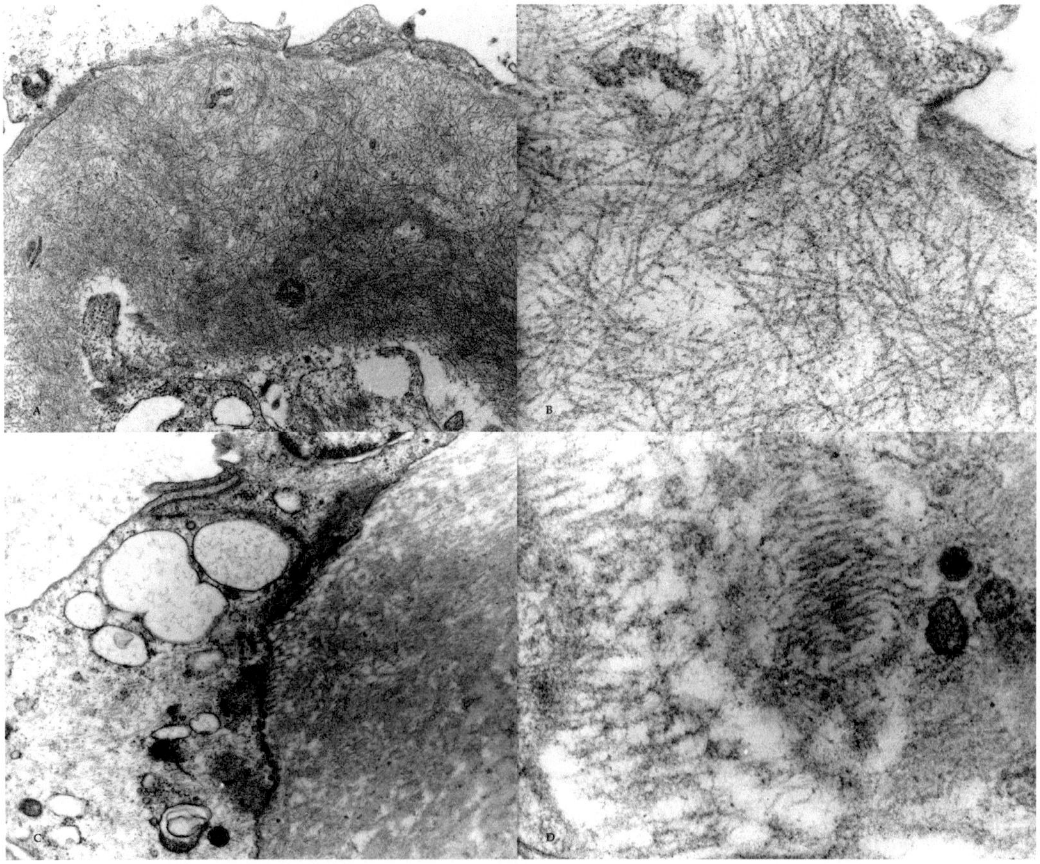

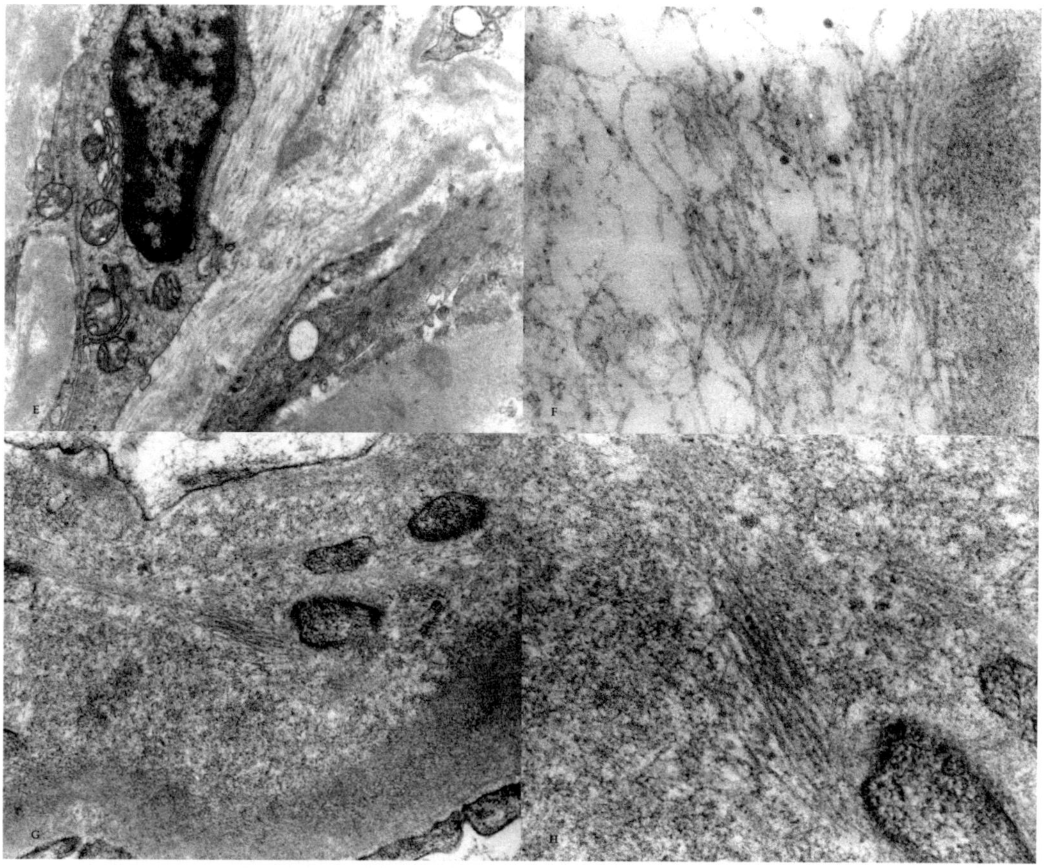

Fig. 9. A.-H. Amyloid (panels A and B) and non amyloid extracellular fibrils (panels C-H). Amyloid deposition in basal membrane of a glomerular capillary is compared with the more ordered array of fibrillin forming endothelial anchoring and stromal fibrils (panels C and D), interstitial fibrillar ECM associated with sclerotic changes (panels E and F) and glomerular sudendothelial fibrils in a case of diabetes. (Panels A, C OM: x12000; Panel E OM: x3000; Panel G OM: x20000; Panels B, D, F, H OM: 50000)

4.2 Disease with structured immunecomplex deposits

Ultrastructural demonstration of amyloid may be important in the differential diagnosis of various organized immunedeposits, responsible for various forms of glomerulopathies and neuropathies (Joh, 2007; Vallat et al., 2007). Fibrils of a wide variety of size and patterns can be seen in the kidney of patient with monoclonal immunoglobulin diseases, lupus nephritis, cryoglobulinemia, collagen III deposition glomerulophaty, hereditary fibronectin nephropaties and immunotactoid glomerulopathy. Structured immunecomplex deposits include: cryoglobulins, finger prints, and fibrillary-immunotactoid deposits (Joh, 2007; Vallat et al., 2007; King et al., 2000). Their main characters and ultrastructural morphology are summarized below:

- *Cryoglobulin deposits* consist in peculiar monoclonal or polyclonal immunoglobulin responsible of cryoglobulinemia. In tissue, their various morphological shapes include: anular, fingerprint-like, microtubular, and microfibrillar shape, with a diameter ranging from 8 to more than 60 nm. Generally, the structure appears almost indistinct and frequently associated with non-structured deposition. The more typical morphology consist in short tubules, curved and often coupled, about 25 nm in diameters (Fig. 10). These are more frequently observed in cases with mixed (IgM-IgG) essential cryoglobulinemia or type II cryoglobulinemia. They are associated to glomerulopathy (Joh, 2007) and polyneuropathy (Vallat et al., 2007). Glomerular cryoglobulin deposits localize mainly in sub-endothelial lamina rara, with a tendency to form pseudothrombi. They are frequently associated to endocapillary mononuclear infiltrates.

- *Finger-print:* are structured immunecomplex deposits consisting in curved lamelled aggregates with a finger print-like aspect (Fig. 11). They are considered highly suggestive of lupus nephritis and are present in cases with monoclonal dysglobulinemia and polyneuropathy (Joh, 2007; Vallat et al., 2007).
- *Fibrillar and microtubular immunotactoid:* immunecomplex deposition consisting in fibrillar/microtubular aggregation, containing mainly immunoglobulin IgG and complement C3, are respectively associated to fibrillary glomerulonephrites –FGN- and immunotactoid glomeulophaty –ITG- (King et al., 2000; Schwartz et al., 2002; Alpers & Kowalewska, 2008). Immunotactoid fibrillar/tubular structures have a variable diameter ranging from 9 to 60 nm or more, depending on single case (Fig.12). A lucent center, the lumen, is easily identified in microtubules with diameters of 30 nm or more, but higher magnification can demonstrate a lucent centre in all immunotactoid structures independently by their diameters. In ITG, immunotactoid is conventionally defined as deposits of microtubular structures with a diameter greater than 30 nm (mean range 30-60 nm). A larger diameter is associated to the tendency at a parallel arrangement that contribute to define tubular immunotactoid. In FGN, fibrillary form is conventionally defined by presence of Congo red negative deposits of not branched elongated fibrils, more frequently without evidence of a clear centre at median magnification, with a diameter smaller than 30nm and, in some cases, overlapping the amyloid fibrils diameter. Fibrils of FGN, as well as amyloid, typically present a random array of the fibrils.

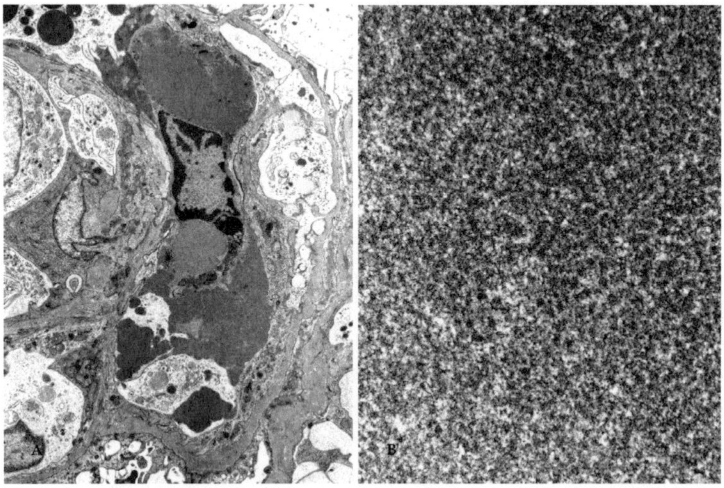

Fig. 10. A glomerular pseudo thrombus (A, OM: x3000) due to cryoglobulin deposition. At high magnification (B, OM: x30000) , the typical structure consisting in curved and often coupled short tubules is shown.

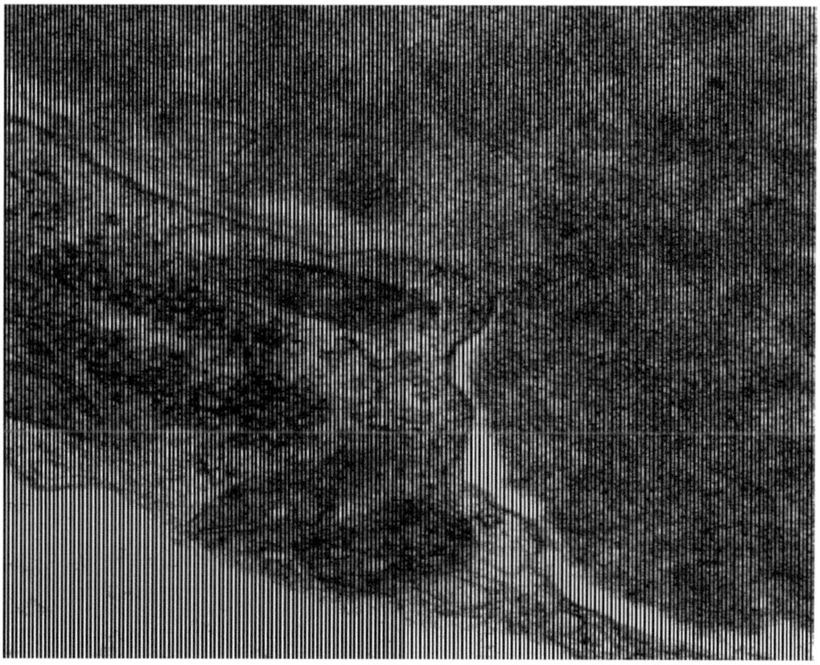

Fig. 11. Subendothelial concentric lamellae forming "finger prints", in a case of lupus nephritis. OM: x12000.

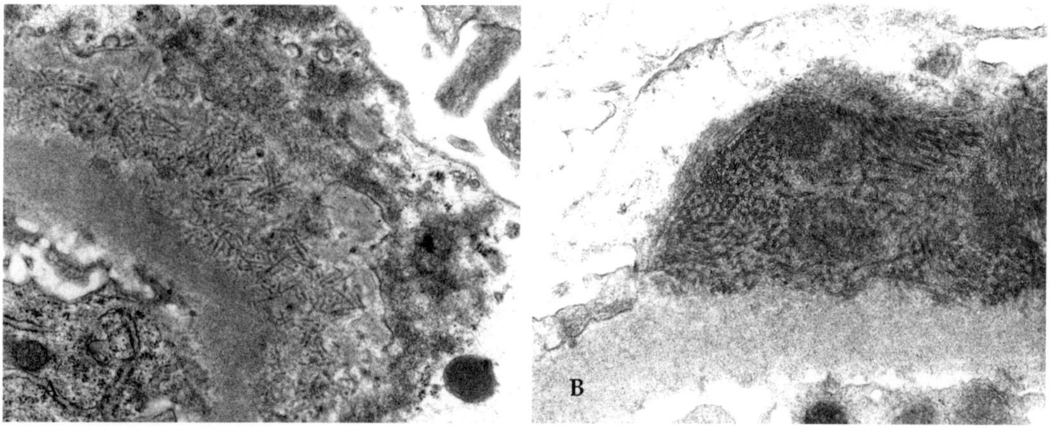

Fig. 12. A-B. Glomerular fibrillarry (A, OM: x12000; Nebuloni, 2009) and immunotactoid (B, OM: x12000) immunedeposits in subepithelial position. Fibrillarry deposits are composed by fibrils with a diameter less wide than 30nm, and they present a less ordered array than immunotactoid. The latter consist of microtubules, showing an hollow centre also at medium magnification.

Whereas most of structured deposits are easily distinguished from amyloid, fibrillar array in FGN may present various similarities with amyloid. FGN and ITG represent pathological entities characterized by the glomerular deposition of fibrillary/microtubular structures, whose identification is possible only by TEM. Rare cases of extraglomerular and extrarenal localization are also reported (Calls Ginestra et al., 1995; Adeyi et al., 2001; Sabatine et al., 2002). Pathologists generally maintain a conventional sub-structural distinction of FGN and ITG, based on diameters and random, or more ordered, arrangement of the fibrils. However, difference in clinicopathological correlation remain controversial (Alpers & Kowalewska, 2008; Schwartz et al., 2002). Clinical presentation in both varieties is nephrotic syndrome, with a tendency to early renal insufficiency. Because of the fact that cryoglobulins may present a similar morphology, definitive diagnosis generally include the exclusion of cryoglobulinemia by clinical analyses. In FGN, fibrils are Congo red negative, but present sub-structural similarities with amyloid fibrils. These include: a random arrangement, and, in rare cases, a wide range diameter, overlapping those of amyloid fibrils. Moreover, Yang et al. reported a case of Congo-red negative FGN with amyloid P associated to the fibrils, demonstrated by ITEM (Yang et al., 1992). However, in the majority of the cases of FGN, fibrils show a wider diameter than amyloid (range: 15-30). Amyloid fibrils have a more defined profile and generally a diameter smaller than 12nm. Amyloid ultrastructural appearance is sufficiently characteristic, so that the diagnosis of amyloidosis should continue to be considered even when Congo red staining is negative (Dember, 2006).

4.3 Glomerular immunecomplex diseases

The IF pattern of renal amyloidosis frequently shows glomerular deposition, including IgG, C3, IgA and IgM., the latter mainly in secondary AA. In fact, most cases of AA are associated to rheumatoid arthritis, which frequently presents an IgA and IgM glomerular deposition. In about one third of patient with AA, electron-dense IgA deposition in paramesangial areas may suggest a diagnosis of IgA nephropathy. TEM can easily prove the presence of unspecific immunecomplex in a context of amyloid deposition (Nishi et al., 2008; Yang & Gallo, 1990).

5. Ultrastructural detection of amyloid fibrils in non-conventional tissue preparations

In diagnostic practice, it happens that the need for ultrastructural analyses emerges after the results of histological examination on paraffin embedded tissue sections. In these cases, if there is no specific sample prepared for TEM, the residual formalin-fixed paraffin-embedded tissue can be recovered for ultrastruttural analysis. Briefly, the retrieving of tissues from paraffin consists on various changes in paraffin solvent (i.e. xylene, or rather, its less toxic substitutes), followed by rehydratation, using descendent scale of ethanol, prior to the specific preparation procedures for TEM (i.e. fixation and resin embedding). Ultrastructural diagnoses on tissues retrieved from paraffin have been often used in various diagnostic fields (Tosoni et al., 2002). In our experience, in kidney diseases, it allows the identification of immunecomplex deposits with good maintenance of sensitivity. This latter depends mainly by a good primary fixation in buffered formalin. Small tissues fragments, prepared without mechanical stress, immediately immersed in fixative, have a good preservation of the sub-structural detail. It should be noted that, contrary to the setting of glutaraldehyde fixation, formalin fixation for morphological studies is best carried out at room temperature. Ultrastructural general morphology of amyloid deposits of tissues retrieved from paraffin is conserved (Fig. 13).

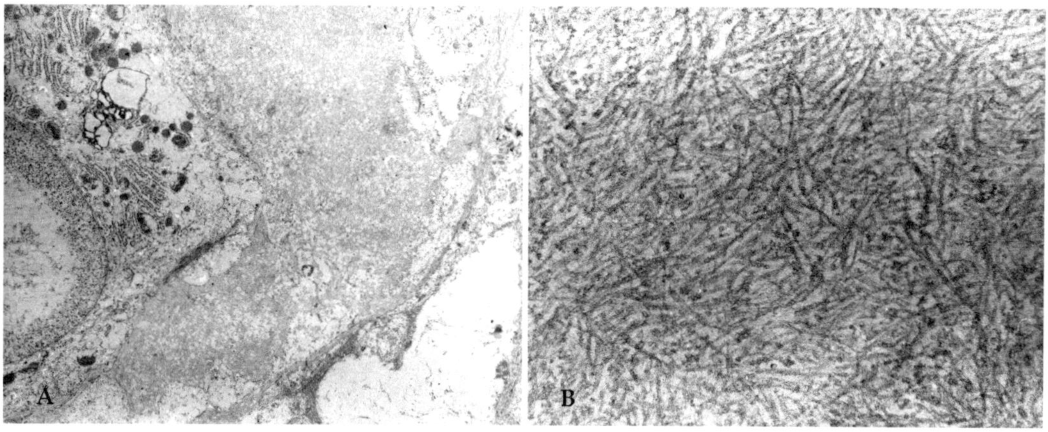

Fig. 13. A-B. Amyloid deposit in liver tissue retrieved from paraffin. Perisinusoidal space (A, OM x3000) is filled with a large amount of amyloid fibrils (B, x30000). The hepatocyte, on the left of panel A shows the relatively good sub-structural preservation after formalin fixation/paraffin embedding, and retrieving procedure.

Some authors report the possibility of change in fibrils diameter depending on formalin fixation (Sikorska et al., 2009), but fibrillar structure and aggregation patterns are maintained. Otherwise, sensitivity of TEM analysis may be reduced because of reduction in specificity. In fact, fibrillar ECM can appear more electrondense and can be difficult to distinguish from amyloid fibrils. Moreover, in the presence of poor preservation of cell's plasmalemma, intracytoplasmic intermediated filaments can mimic amyloid dense aggregates. Nevertheless, the presence of groups of randomly oriented non branched 10 nm fibrils is generally highly suspicious for amyloidosis. Our experience concerns mainly renal amyloidosis. TEM on renal biopsy retrieved from paraffin may be indicated in the following cases:

- Congo red positive / immunolabeling negative: TEM to confirm amyloidosis
- Clinical suspicion of renal amyloidosis, Congo red/immunolabeling with doubtful results: TEM to confirm amyloidosis
- Congo red positive, no glomeruli in frozen sections: TEM to evaluate concomitant immunecomplex glomerulopathy

Amyloid can also be detected in frozen tissues residues retrieved for TEM after immunofluorescence. However, frozen tissues should be preferably stored, to devote to any successive typing analyses, if necessary (Picken, 2010).

6. Conclusion

Amyloid is a characteristic conformational status of various proteins in specific conditions, frequently associated with disease. Morphology of amyloid fibrils is distinctive and useful in the diagnosis of amyloidosis, also in the early stage of disease. ITEM can provide a high sensitive typing approach, specially in unusual or new amyloid forms.

7. References

Adeyi, OA.; Sethi, S. & Rennke, HG. (2001). Fibrillary glomerulonephritis: a report of 2 cases with extensive glomerular and tubular deposits. Hum Pathol, Vol.32, No.6, (June 2001), pp. 660-663, ISSN 0046-8177

Allsop, D.; Kidd, M.; Landon, M. & Tomlinson, A. (1986). Isolated senile plaque cores in Alzheimer's disease and Down's syndrome show differences in morphology. *J Neurol Neurosurg Psychiatry*, Vol.49, No.8, (August 1986), pp. 886-892, ISSN 0022-3050

Alpers, CE. & Kowalewska, J. (2008). Fibrillary glomerulonephritis and immunotactoid glomerulopathy. *J Am Soc Neprol*, Vol.19, No.1, (January 2008), pp. 34-37, ISSN 1046-6673

Arbustini, E.; Verga, L.; Concardi, M.; Palladini, G.; Obici, L. & Merlini, G. (2002). Electron and immuno-electron microscopy of abdominal fat identifies and characterizes amyloid fibrils in suspected cardiac amyloidosis. *Amyloid*, Vol.9, No.2, (June 2002), pp. 108-14, ISSN 1350-6129

Bély, M.; Kapp, P.; Szabó, TS.; Lakatos, T. & Apáthy, A. (2005). Electron microscopic characteristics of beta2-microglobulin amyloid deposits in long-term haemodialysis. *Ultrastruct Pathol*, Vol.29, No.6, (November-December 2005), pp. 483-491, ISSN 0191-3123

Calls Ginesta, J.; Torras, A.; Ricart, MJ.; Ramirez, J.; Campo, E.; Darnell, A.; Andreu, J. & Revert, L. (1995). Fibrillary glomerulonephritis and pulmonary hemorrhage in a patient with renal transplantation. *Clin Nephrol*, Vol.43, No.3, (March 1995), pp. 180-183, ISSN 0301-0430

Caubet, C.; Bousset, L.; Clemmensen, O.; Sourigues, Y.; Bygum, A.; Chavanas, S.; Coudane, F.; Hsu, CY.; Betz, RC.; Melki, R.; Simon, M. & Serre, G. (2010). A new amyloidosis caused by fibrillar aggregates of mutated corneodesmosin. *FASEB J*, Vol.24, No.9, (September 2010), pp. 3416-3426, ISSN 0892-6638

Dember, LM. (2006). Amyloidosis-associated kidney disease. *J Am Soc Nephrol*, Vol.17, No.12, (December 2006), pp. 3458-3471, ISSN 1046-6673

Dikman, SH.; Churg, J. & Kahn, T. (1981). Morphologic and clinical correlates in renal amyloidosis. *Hum Pathol*, Vol.12, No.2, (February 1981), pp. 160-169, ISSN 0046-8177

Dzamba, BJ. & Peters, DM. (1991). Arrangement of cellular fibronectin in noncollagenous fibrils in human fibroblast cultures. *J Cell Sci.*, Vol.100, No.3, (November 1991), pp. 605-12, ISSN 0021-9533

Fändrich M. (2007). On the structural definition of amyloid fibrils and other polypeptide aggregates. *Cell Mol Life Sci*, Vol.64, No.16, (August 2007), pp. 2066-78, ISSN 1420-682X

Fändrich M, Meinhardt J, Grigorieff N. (2009). Structural polymorphism of Alzheimer Abeta and other amyloid fibrils. *Prion*, Vol.3, No.2, (April 2009), pp. 89-93, ISSN 1933-6896

Fournier, JG.; Escaig-Haye, F. & Grigoriev, V. (2000). Ultrastructural localization of prion proteins: physiological and pathological implications. *Microsc Res Tech*, Vol.50, No.1, (July 2000), pp.76-88, ISSN 1059-910X

Friedrich RP, Tepper K, Rönicke R, Soom M, Westermann M, Reymann K, Kaether C, Fändrich M. (2010). Mechanism of amyloid plaque formation suggests an intracellular basis of Abeta pathogenicity. *Proc Natl Acad Sci U S A*, Vol.107, No.5, (February 2010), pp. 1942-1947, ISSN 0027-8424

Gellermann, GP.; Appel, TR.; Tannert, A.; Radestock, A.; Hortschansky, P.; Schroeckh, V.; Leisner, C.; Lütkepohl, T.; Shtrasburg, S.; Röcken, C.; Pras, M.; Linke, RP.; Diekmann, S. & Fändrich, M. (2005). Raft lipids as common components of human extracellular amyloid fibrils. *Proc Natl Acad Sci U S A*, Vol.102, No.18, (May 2005), pp. 6297-6302, ISSN 0027-8424

Greenwald, J. & Riek, R. (2010). Biology of amyloid: structure, function, and regulation. *Structure*, Vol.18, No.10, (October 2010), pp. 1244-1260, ISSN 0969-2127

Inoue, S.; Kuroiwa, M.; Ohashi, K.; Hara, M. & Kisilevsky, R. (1997). Ultrastructural organization of hemodialysis-associated beta 2-microglobulin amyloid fibrils. *Kidney Int*, Vol.52, No.6, (December 1997), pp. 1543-1549, ISSN 0085-2538

Inoue, S.; Kuroiwa, M.; Saraiva, MJ.; Guimarães, A. & Kisilevsky, R. (1998). Ultrastructure of familial amyloid polyneuropathy amyloid fibrils: examination with high-resolution electron microscopy. *J Struct Biol*, Vol.124, No.1, (December 1998), pp. 1-12, ISSN 1047-8477

Inoue, S.; Kuroiwa, M. & Kisilevsky, R. (1999). Basement membranes, microfibrils and beta amyloid fibrillogenesis in Alzheimer's disease: high resolution ultrastructural findings. *Brain Res Rev*, Vol.29, No.2-3, (April 1999), pp. 218-31, ISSN 006-8993

Jadoul M, Garbar C, van Ypersele de Strihou C. (2001). Pathological aspects of beta(2)-microglobulin amyloidosis. *Semin Dial*, Vol.14, No.2, (March-April 2001), pp. 86-89, ISSN 0894-0959

Jiménez, JL.; Tennent, G.; Pepys, M. & Saibil, HR. (2001). Structural diversity of ex vivo amyloid fibrils studied by cryo-electron microscopy. *J Mol Biol*, Vol.311, No.2, (August 2001), pp. 241-247, ISSN 0022-2836

Joh, K. Pathology of glomerular deposition disease. (2007). *Pathol Int*, Vol.57, No.9, (September 2007), pp. 551-565, ISSN 1320-5463

Kaye, GC.; Butler, MG.; D'Ardenne, AJ.; Edmondson, SJ.; Camm, AJ. & Slavin, G. (1986). Identification of immunoreactive atrial natriuretic peptide in atrial amyloid. *J Clin Pathol*, Vol.39, No.5, (May 1986), pp. 581-582, ISSN 00219746

Keeling, J.; Teng, J. & Herrera, G. (2004). AL-amyloidosis and light-chain deposition disease light chains induce divergent phenotypic transformations of human mesangial cells. *Laboratory Investigation*, Vol.84, (August 2004), pp. 1322–1338, ISSN 0023-6837

King, JA.; Culpepper, RM.; Corey, GR.; Tucker, JA.; Lajoie, G. & Howell, DN. (2000). Glomerulopathies with fibrillary deposits. *Ultrastruct Pathol*, Vol.24, No.1, (January-February 2000), pp. 15-21, ISSN 0191-3123

Kluve-Beckerman, B.; Liepnieks, JJ.; Wang, L. & Benson, MD. (1999). A cell culture system for the study of amyloid pathogenesis. Amyloid formation by peritoneal macrophages cultured with recombinant serum amyloid A. *Am J Pathol*, Vol.155, No.1, (July 1999), pp. 123-133, ISSN 0002-9440

Korbet SM, Schwartz MM, Lewis EJ. (1994). The fibrillary glomerulopathies. *Am J Kidney Dis*, Vol.23, No.5, (May 1004), pp. 751-765, ISSN 0272-6386

Kronz, JD.; Neu, AM. & Nadasdy, T. (1998). When noncongophilic glomerular fibrils do not represent fibrillary glomerulonephritis: nonspecific mesangial fibrils in sclerosing glomeruli. *Clin Nephrol*, Vol.50, No.4, (October 1998), pp. 218-223, ISSN 0301-0430

Leonhardt, RM.; Vigneron, N.; Rahner, C.; Van den Eynde, BJ. & Cresswell, P. (2010). Endoplasmic reticulum export, subcellular distribution, and fibril formation by Pmel17 require an intact N-terminal domain junction. *J Biol Chem*, Vol.285, No.21, (May 2010), pp. 16166-16183, ISSN 0021-9258

Makin, OS. & Serpell, LC. (2005). Structures for amyloid fibrils. *FEBS J*, Vol.272, No.23, (December 2005), pp. 5950-61, ISSN 1742-464X

Merlini, G. & Bellotti, V. (2003). Molecular mechanisms of amyloidosis. *N Engl J Med*, Vol.349, No.6, (August 2003), pp. 583-96, ISSN 0028-4793

Morten, IJ.; Gosal, WS.; Radford, SE. & Hewitt, EW. (2007). Investigation into the role of macrophages in the formation and degradation of beta2-microglobulin amyloid fibrils. *J Biol Chem*, Vol.282, No.40, (October 2007), pp. 29691-29700, ISSN 0021-9258

Nebuloni, M.; Genderini, A.; Tosoni, A.; Caruso, S. & Barbiano di Belgiojoso, G. (2009). Fibrillary glomerulonephritis with prevalent IgA deposition associated with undifferentiated connective tissue disease: a case report. *NDT Plus*, Vol.3, pp. 57-59, ISSN 0931-0509

Nishi S, Alchi B, Imai N, Gejyo F. (2008). New advances in renal amyloidosis. *Clin Exp Nephrol*, Vol.12, No.2, (April 2008), pp. 93-101

Pan, KM.; Baldwin, M.; Nguyen, J.; Gasset, M.; Serban, A.; Groth, D.; Mehlhorn, I.; Huang, Z.; Fletterick, RJ. & Cohen, FE. (1993) Conversion of alpha-helices into beta-sheets features in the formation of the scrapie prion proteins. *Proc Natl Acad Sci U S A*, Vol.90, No.23, (December 1993), pp. 10962-10966, ISSN 0027-8424

Pedersen, JS.; Andersen, CB. & Otzen, DE. (2010). Amyloid structure--one but not the same:the many levels of fibrillar polymorphism. *FEBS J*, Vol.277, No.22, (November 2010), pp. 4591-4601, ISSN 1742-464X

Pettersson, T. & Konttinen, YT. (2010). Amyloidosis-recent developments. *Semin Arthritis Rheum*, Vol.39, No.5, (April 2010), pp. 356-68, ISSN 0049-0172

Picken, MM. & Linke, RP. (2009). Nephrotic syndrome due to an amyloidogenic mutation in fibrinogen A alpha chain. *J Am Soc Nephrol*, Vol.20, No.8, (August 2009), pp. 1681-1685, ISSN 1046-6673

Picken, MM. (2010). Amyloidosis-where are we now and where are we heading?. *Arch Pathol Lab Med*, Vol.134, No.4, (April 2010), pp. 545-551, ISSN 0003-9985

Prusiner, SB. (1998). The prion diseases. *Brain Pathol*, Vol.8, No.3, (July 1998), pp. 499-513, ISSN 1015-6305

Rozemuller, AJ.; Roos, RA.; Bots, GT; Kamphorst, W.; Eikelenboom, P. & Van Nostrand, WE. (1993). Distribution of beta/A4 protein and amyloid precursor protein in hereditary cerebral hemorrhage with amyloidosis-Dutch type and Alzheimer's disease. *Am J Pathol*, Vol.142, No. 5, (May 1993), pp. 1449-1457, ISSN 0002-9440

Sabatine, MS.; Aretz, HT.; Fang, LS. & Dec, GW. Images in cardiovascular medicine. Fibrillary/immunotactoid glomerulopathy with cardiac involvement. *Circulation*, Vol.105, No.15, (April 2002), e120-1, ISSN 0009-7322

Sachse C, Xu C, Wieligmann K, Diekmann S, Grigorieff N, Fändrich M. (2006). Quaternary structure of a mature amyloid fibril from Alzheimer's Abeta(1-40) peptide. *J Mol Biol*, Vol.362, No.2, (September 2006), pp. 347-354, ISSN 0022-2836

Santostefano, M.; Zanchelli, F.; Zaccaria, A.; Poletti, G. & Fusaroli, M. (2005). The ultrastructural basis of renal pathology in monoclonal gammopathies. *J Nephrol*, Vol.18, No.6, (November-December 2005), pp. 659-675, ISSN 1121-8428

Schreml, S.; Szeimies, RM.; Vogt, T.; Landthaler, M.; Schroeder, J. & Babilas, P. (2010). Cutaneous amyloidoses and systemic amyloidoses with cutaneous involvement. *Eur J Dermatol*, Vol.20, No.2, (March-April 2010), pp. 152-160, ISSN 1167-1122

Schwartz, MM.; Korbet, SM.& Lewis, EJ. (2002). Immunotactoid glomerulopathy. *J Am Soc Nephrol*, Vol.13, No.5, (May 2002), pp. 1390-1397, ISSN 1046-6673

Sen, S. & Sarsik, B. (2010). A proposed histopathologic classification, scoring, and grading system for renal amyloidosis: standardization of renal amyloid biopsy report. *Arch Pathol Lab Med*, Vol.134, No.4, (April 2010), pp. 532-544, ISSN 0003-9985

Serpell, LC. (2000). Alzheimer's amyloid fibrils: structure and assembly. *Biochim Biophys Acta*,Vol.1502, No.1 (July 26), pp. 16-30, ISSN 0304-4165

Sherratt, MJ.; Wess, TJ.; Baldock, C.; Ashworth, J.; Purslow, PP.; Shuttleworth, CA. & Kielty, CM. (2001). Fibrillin-rich microfibrils of the extracellular matrix: ultrastructure and assembly. *Micron*, Vol.32, No.2, (February 2001), pp. 185-200, ISSN 0968-4328

Sikorska, B.; Liberski, PP.; Sobów, T.; Budka, H. & Ironside, JW. (2009). Ultrastructural study of florid plaques in variant Creutzfeldt-Jakob disease: a comparison with amyloid plaques in kuru, sporadic Creutzfeldt-Jakob disease and Gerstmann-Sträussler-Scheinker disease. *Neuropathol Appl Neurobiol*, Vol.35, No.1, (February 2009), pp. 46-59, ISSN 0305-1846

Sipe, JD.; Benson, MD.; Buxbaum, JN.; Ikeda, S.; Merlini, G.; Saraiva, MJ. & Westermark, P. (2010). Amyloid fibril protein nomenclature: 2010 recommendations from the nomenclature committee of the International Society of Amyloidosis. *Amyloid*, Vol.17, No.3-4, (September 2010), pp. 101-4, ISSN 1350-6129

Sipe, JD. & Cohen, AS. (2000). Review: history of the amyloid fibril. *J Struct Biol*, Vol.130, No.2-3, (June 2000), pp. 88-98, ISSN 1047-8477

Stromer, T. & Serpell, LC. (2005). Structure and morphology of the Alzheimer's amyloid fibril. *Microsc Res Tech*, Vol.67, No.3-4, (July 2005), pp. 210-217, ISSN 1059-910X

Teng, J.; Russell, WJ.; Gu, X.; Cardelli, J.; Jones, ML. & Herrera, GA. (2004). Different types of glomerulopathic light chains interact with mesangial cells using a common receptor but exhibit different intracellular trafficking patterns. *Lab Invest*, Vol.84, No.4, (April 2004), pp. 440-451, ISSN 0023-6837

Tosoni, A.; Nebuloni, M.; Ferri, A.; Bonetto, S.; Antinori, S.; Scaglia, M.; Xiao, L.; Moura, H.; Visvesvara, GS.; Vago, L. & Costanzi, G. (2002). Disseminated microsporidiosis caused by Encephalitozoon cuniculi III (dog type) in an Italian AIDS patient: a retrospective study. *Mod Pathol*, Vol.15, No.5, (May 2002), pp. 577-583, ISSN 0893-3952

Vallat, JM.; Magy, L.; Richard, L.; Sturtz, F. & Couratier, P. (2008). Contribution of electron microscopy to the study of neuropathies associated with an IgG monoclonal paraproteinemia. *Micron*, Vol.39, No.2, (January 2007), pp. 61-70, ISSN 0968-4328

Weber, E.; Rossi, A.; Solito, R.; Sacchi, G.; Agliano', M. & Gerli, R. (2002). Focal adhesion molecules expression and fibrillin deposition by lymphatic and blood vessel endothelial cells in culture. *Microvasc Res*, Vol.64, No.1, (July 2002), pp. 47-55, ISSN 0026-2862

Westermark, P.; Davey, E.; Lindbom, K. & Enqvist, S. (2006). Subcutaneous fat tissue for diagnosis and studies of systemic amyloidosis. *Acta Histochem*, Vol.108, No.3, (May 2006), pp. 209-213, ISSN 0065-1281

Yazawa H, Yu ZX, Takeda, Le Y, Gong W, Ferrans VJ, Oppenheim JJ, Li CC, Wang JM. (2001). Beta amyloid peptide (Abeta42) is internalized via the G-protein-coupled receptor FPRL1 and forms fibrillar aggregates in macrophages. *FASEB* J, Vol.15, No.13, (November 2001), pp. 2454-2462, ISSN 0892-6638

Yamaguchi, H; Nakazato, Y.; Hirai, S.; Shoji, M. & Harigava, Y. (1989). Electron micrograph of diffuse plaques. Initial stage of senile plaque formation in the Alzheimer brain. *Am J Pathol*, Vol.135, No.4, (October 1989), pp.593-597, ISSN 0002-9440

Yang, GC. & Gallo, GR. (1990). Protein A-gold immunoelectron microscopic study of amyloid fibrils, granular deposits, and fibrillar luminal aggregates in renal amyloidosis. *Am J Pathol*, Vol.137, No.5, (November 1990), pp. 1223-1231, ISSN 0002-9440

Yang GC, Nieto R, Stachura I, Gallo G. (1992). Ultrastructural immunohistochemical localization of polyclonal IgG, C3, and amyloid P component on the Congo red-negative amyloid-like fibrils of fibrillary glomerulopathy. *Am J Pathol*, Vol.141, No.2, (August 1002), pp. 409-419, ISSN 0002-9440

8

Amyloidosis in Domestic Animals: Pathology, Pathogenesis, Gross and Microscopic Lesions and Clinical Findings

Moges Woldemeskel
University of Georgia, College of Veterinary Medicine, Department of Pathology, Tifton Veterinary Diagnostic and Investigational Laboratory, USA

1. Introduction

Amyloidosis refers to a group of protein misfolding diseases characterized by deposition of a particular amyloid protein in various organs and tissues of animals and humans. Although there are other components present in the deposit, the amyloid protein fibril is the main component of the amyloid substance. The amyloid substance differs in protein composition depending upon the types of amyloidosis (AA amyloidosis or AL amyloidosis) and the different clinical forms. Each clinical entity or form of amyloidosis may be manifested by a distinct clinical form with chemically specific amyloid fibril protein. This indicates that amyloid is a biochemically heterogeneous substance, although there are similarities in properties and staining characteristics.

Amyloidosis involving several tissues and organs throughout the body is referred to as systemic amyloidosis. This may be AA amyloidosis (including familial amyloidosis) or AL amyloidosis. Systemic amyloidosis can be deposited in several vital organs and tissues and may entail severe damage. Amyloid substance may be confined at a given area in the body in the form of localized amyloidosis.

The pathogenesis, pathology and clinical presentations of amyloidosis are protean consequent to the diverse underlying causes of its various forms, species of animals affected and the severity of functional disruption in different tissues and organs involved. The diagnosis of amyloidosis requires histopathologic identification of amyloid deposits in the affected tissues. This is confirmed by Congo red staining and green birefringence under polarized light.

In this chapter, the pathology, pathogenesis, lesions, and clinical syndromes encompassing various forms of amyloidosis in animals will be covered. Current knowledge available on amyloidosis in animals, which would be of importance as a reference for veterinary professionals and practitioners, and veterinary students will be elucidated in the chapter.

2. Pathology and pathogenesis

The pathology and pathogenesis of amyloidosis is a captivating enigma consequent to the diverse underlying causes of its various forms in different species affected. About 20-25

different types of proteins with the ability to aggregate, insolubilize, and deposit in tissue as amyloid have been identified (Murphy et al., 2001, Gruys, 2004). In animals, at least eight different amyloid precursors have been described (Ménsua et al., 2003). The precursor proteins in amyloid fibrils may be amyloidogenic mutants as in some familial amyloidosis, whereas other precursors are normal wild-type proteins (Westermark, 1998; Gruys, 2004). The exact mechanisms through which the proteins are converted into amyloid fibrils in vivo are not well known (Westermark, 1998). There are a number of divers conditions that can be associated with the formation of amyloid and each of these conditions are characterized by excessive production of amyloidogenic proteins that are prone to misfolding. Under normal conditions, the misfolded proteins are enzymatically degraded intracellularly within proteasomes or extracellularly by macrophages. In amyloidosis, these degradative processes are inadequate and may be responsible for the accumulation of misfolded protein extracellularly. The overproduction of precursor protein, although necessary, is not sufficient to result in the formation of amyloid by itself (Snyder, 2007). A single amyloidogenic protein may result in multiple forms of amyloid fibrils depending on their induction conditions. Multiple mechanisms for amyloidogenesis are expected to operate as witnessed with their fibrillar polymorphism (Bhak et al., 2009). Although there are divers proteins associated with the formation of amyloid, they are all characterized by misfolded proteins leading to the formation of fibrils that are unstable and self associated (Snyder, 2007). The protein fibril is the main component of the amyloid substance, however, there are other components present, the importance of which is yet not well established in the pathogenesis of amyloidosis. All forms of amyloid contain the pentraxin glycoprotein amyloid P-component (AP) that most probably is bound to the protein fibrils directly. The unique β-sheet fibril of amyloid is very resistant to physical agents and also gives the amyloid substance many of its characteristic properties, including affinity to the dye Congo red and green birefringence under polarized light after such staining (Westermark, 1998).
According to the WHO-IUIS Nomenclature Sub-Committee (1993) on the nomenclature of amyloid and amyloidosis, amyloid and amyloidosis are classified based on the amyloid fibril protein, followed by a designation of the fibril protein precursor. The capital letter A for amyloid is followed by the protein designation in abbreviated form. For example AL-amyloid refers to the amyloid derived from immunoglobulin light chain, whereas AA-amyloid refers to the amyloid derived from serum A-amyloid protein. Amyloid fibrils may be deposited locally in a given tissue (local amyloidosis) or it may be a systemic deposit (systemic amyloidosis) involving various tissues and organs in the body. Systemic deposits of amyloid are recognized as AL-amyloidosis (primary amyloidosis), AA-amyloidosis (secondary or reactive amyloidosis) or familial amyloidosis.

2.1 AA – Amyloidosis

AA-amyloidosis is described in literature as reactive or secondary amyloidosis. It is the most common form of amyloidosis in domestic animals. AA amyloidosis is associated with chronic inflammatory or neoplastic diseases (non-immunocyte dyscrasia) or it may be idiopathic, where no underlying disease is found (Kim et al., 2005; Snyder, 2007). In this form of amyloidosis, the deposited amyloid protein is derived from serum amyloid-A synthesized in the liver (Kim et al., 2005). Amyloid A is derived from the acute phase reactant, serum amyloid A (SAA) (Kisilevsky, 1990; Gruys, 2004), which is an apolipoprotein of high-density lipoproteins (HDL), classes 2 and 3. It is formed mainly in the liver upon stimulation by pro-inflammatory cytokines (Gruys, 2004) and normally plays a role in cholesterol transport (Kisilevsky, 1990) and as a chemoattractant (Badolato et al., 1994) in the inflammatory processes. When the concentration of this molecule is increased, typically as a result of chronic inflammation, certain isoforms of SAA are partially cleaved into fragments that have an increased propensity to form fibrillar aggregates of amyloid that are deposited systemically, mainly in the kidney, liver, and spleen (Johnson et al., 1996). In systemic AA amyloidosis (reactive systemic amyloidosis), macrophages are known to be activated and elaborate endogenous pyrogens IL-1 and IL-6, which stimulate hepatocytes to synthesize and secrete SAA. During an inflammatory reaction, the quantity of SAA in the serum may increase several 100 times normal concentrations. However, not all systemic inflammatory reactions lead to the formation of AA amyloid; but only some of the inflammatory reactions lead to amyloidosis. Either an enzyme defect in the system that normally degrades SAA protein or the synthesis of abnormal SAA protein that is resistant to the enzymatic degradation is suggested to underlie production of insoluble AA molecules that form the amyloid fibrils (Snyder, 2007). Some species of animals appear to have genetic predisposition to the deposition of AA amyloidosis. Analysis of SAA cDNA sequences from several animals identified a distinct genetic dimorphism that may be relevant to the susceptibility to secondary amyloid disease. The duck genome contained a single copy of the SAA gene that was expressed in the liver and lung tissues of ducklings, even in the absence of induction of acute phase response (Guo et al., 1996). Siamese and Abyssinian cats and Shar Pei dogs appear to have familial predisposition of AA proteins with different primary sequence and pattern of deposition in the body (Boyce et al., 1984; DiBartola et al., 1986 & 1990). Amyloid resistant mouse strains were found to have a non-amyloidogenic acute phase SAA (Gonnerman et al., 1995; Liang et al., 1998). Rats were shown not to form acute phase SAA and AA-amyloid at all (Ren et al., 1999; Yu et al., 2000).

AA amyloidosis is the most common type of amyloid in mammals and birds (**Fig. 1**) and often results in hepatic or renal failure due to physical disruption of normal cellular and organ processes (Terio et al., 2008). It is a common disease of water fowl and is characterized by the deposition of extracellular fibrils of amyloid A (AA) protein in the liver and certain other organs in this species (Guo et al., 1996). AA amyloidosis is also reported in a wide variety of domestic animal species including canines, equines, bovines, avian species, porcines, felines, sheep and goats (Jakob, 1971; Johnson & Jamison, 1984; Hayden et al., 1988; Zschiesche & Jakob, 1989; DiBartola, et al., 1990; Blunden & Smith, 1992; Seifi et al., 1997; Landman, 1998; Ménsua et al., 2003). It is described in association with different chronic diseases, in captive cheetah (*Acinonyx jubatus*), Siberian tigers (*Panthera tigris altaica*), mink (*Mustela vison*), black-footed cats (*Felis nigripes*), black-footed ferrets (*Mustela nigripes*), Dorcas gazelle (*Gazella dorcas*), mountain gazelle (*Gazella gazella*), bighorn and Dall's sheep, free living lioness and in swans and other anatidae (*Panthera leo*) (Hadlow & Jellison, 1962; Sato et al., 1981; Kingston et al., 1982; Linke et al., 1986; Rideout et al., 1989; Munson, 1993; Nieto et al., 1995; Papendick et al., 1997; Schulze et al., 1998; Williams et al., 2005; Garner et al., 2007; Terio et al., 2008). It is reported in association with chronic lymphoplasmacytic gastritis in the cheetahs and as idiopathic in the Siberian tigers. In the cheetahs and the Siberian tigers, the deposits were primarily in the medullary interstitium, with minimal glomerular involvement (Papendick et al., 1997; Schulze at al., 1998). Deposition of the amyloid in renal amyloidosis reported in the Dorcas gazelle was also mainly in the renal medulla, sparing the glomeruli (Rideout et al., 1989).

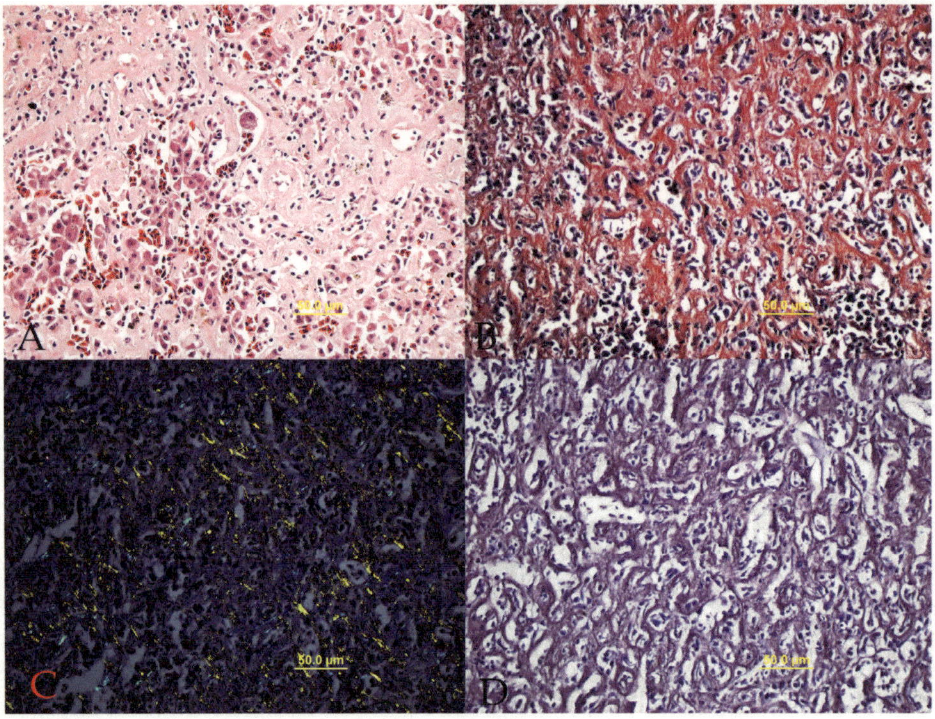

Fig. 1. A section of liver with hepatic amyloidosis in an American Coot with severe parasitism. (**A**) Light eosinophilic amorphous deposits disrupted the hepatic parenchyma (H&E stain). The deposit stained light red with Congo red stain (**B**) and exhibited green birefringens under polarized light (**C**). The amyloid deposit failed to stain with Congo red (**D**) after pretreatment with Potassium Permanganate solution, characteristic of AA-amyloid.

2.1.1 Familial forms of AA amyloidosis

Familial amyloidosis refers to the deposition of amyloid in tissues of animals in a given genetically associated family known to be prone to the deposition of amyloid fibrils. In veterinary medicine, it is reported in Siamese and Abyssinian cats (Boyce et al., 1984; DiBartola et al., 1986 & 1990) with the AA proteins differing in primary sequence and pattern of deposition in these cats (DiBartola et al., 1986 & 1990). Familial amyloidosis is also reported in Shar Pei dogs (DiBartola et al., 1990). The kidney is the main target organ for the deposition of amyloid in the Abyssinian cat, and Shar Pei dogs, while the amyloid protein is mainly deposited in the liver in Siamese cats (DiBartola et al., 1986 & 1990; Niewold et al., 1999). Furthermore, there are other animal species that appear to be prone to amyloid deposition. The high prevalence of amyloidosis in captive cheetahs is suggested to indicate some level of familial predisposition similar to the Abyssinian cats (Papendick et al., 1997). Amyloid arthropathy frequently occurred in brown layer chickens, but never in white layers. The suspected higher susceptibility of brown layers was confirmed experimentally by inducing amyloidosis with an arthropathic and amyloidogenic strain of *E. faecalis* (Ovelgönne et al., 2001). In the systemic amyloidosis reported in the black-footed cats, there was no association with concurrent chronic inflammatory conditions, indicating that the amyloid deposit was not secondary to inflammation. Heritability estimation suggested that amyloidosis might be familial in this species. Additionally, tissues from a single free-ranging black-footed cat had small amounts of amyloid deposition, suggesting that there could be a predilection for amyloidosis in this species too (Terio et al., 2008). Therefore, in addition to Siamese and Abyssinian cats and Shar Pei dogs, in which familial amyloidosis is well-recognized in veterinary medicine, certain species such as cheetahs (*Acinonyx jubatus*), Dorcas gazelles (*Gazella dorcas*), black-footed cat and brown layer chickens appear to be genetically predisposed to amyloidosis.

2.2 AL – Amyloidosis

The AL amyloid type derived from immunoglobulin light chains is the most common form of systemic amyloidosis in humans (Picken, 2001). Small-sized bone marrow plasma cell clones are reported to produce toxic light chains that cause fibrillar deposits in multiple organs (Merlini & Stone, 2006). The amyloid fibrils are formed by the N-terminal fragment of a monoclonal immunoglobulin light chain comprising the variable region and a portion of the constant region. Only a small proportion of free monoclonal light chains form amyloid fibrils in vivo. Thus, the ability to form amyloid is probably related to individual structural characteristics of the light chain variable region. Unlike most other plasma cell dyscrasias, the λ light chain isotype is prevalent in AL (κ/λ ratio, 1:3), suggesting the existence of amyloid-associated $V\lambda$ germ line genes (Merlini & Stone, 2006).

AL amyloidosis is very rare in domestic animals (Kim et al., 2005), unlike in humans, in which it is a common form of systemic amyloidosis. Report on systemic AL amyloidosis in domestic animals is very rare. It is reported in a horse gelding with multiple myeloma (Kim et al., 2005), a mare (Hawthorne et al., 1990) and in a cow with bovine leukocyte adhesion deficiency (Taniyama et al., 2000). Recently, non-AA amyloid is reported in two felines with thymomas (Burrough et al., 2011). In animals, the deposition of AL amyloid protein is generated following overproduction of monoclonal light chains associated with immunocyte dyscrasia. In this form of amyloidosis, plasma cells produce excessive quantities of immunoglobulin light chains that are resistant to complete enzymatic degradation and are susceptible to forming insoluble fibrils (Snyder, 2007). The most common immunocyte dyscrasia associated with AL amyloidosis in domestic animals is a neoplasm of plasma cell. The AL form of amyloid can contain complete immunoglobulin light chains, the NH_2-terminus portion of immunoglobulin light chains or both. Immunoglobulin secreting cells, B lymphocytes, and plasma cells are associated with the deposition of AL amyloid. In contrast to amyloidosis in humans, in which the majority of patients with AL do not have any overt B lymphocyte or plasma cell neoplasm, but do have monoclonal antibodies or light chains in their serum or urine, domestic species rarely have AL-type amyloid without evidence of an immune dyscrasia (Snyder , 2007).

2.3 Localized and other forms of amyloidosis

Localized amyloidosis refers to the deposition of amyloid fibrillar protein as a grossly visible mass or a microscopic deposit at a given site in an organ or tissue. Localized AL is an intriguing condition characterized by limited growth of monoclonal plasma cells and restriction of amyloid deposits to sites adjacent to those of the synthesis of the precursor (Merlini & Stone, 2006). In animals, localized amyloidosis is present in calcifying epithelial odontogenic tumors (amyloid producing odontogenic tumors) of the cat and dog and pancreatic islets in cats (Gruys, 2004; Snyder, 2007). Aβ-amyloid and APrPsc-amyloid can be encountered in the brains of old dogs and sheep with scrapie, respectively (Prusiner et al., 1983; Gruys, 2004). Some forms of naturally occurring transmissible spongiform encephalopathies such as chronic wasting diseases (CWD), are characterized by amyloid plaques in the brain in addition to the intraneural vacuolation (Snyder, 2007). In horses, localized cutaneous amyloidosis is described in association with lymphoma (Gliatto & Alroy, 1995), extramedullary plasmacytoma (Linke et al., 1991) and liver amyloidosis in serum-producing horses (Abdelkadir, et al., 1991). Local amyloidosis associated with plasma cell dyscrasia or focal extramedullary plasmacytoma occurs on the skin and along intestinal tracts in dogs (**Fig. 2**).

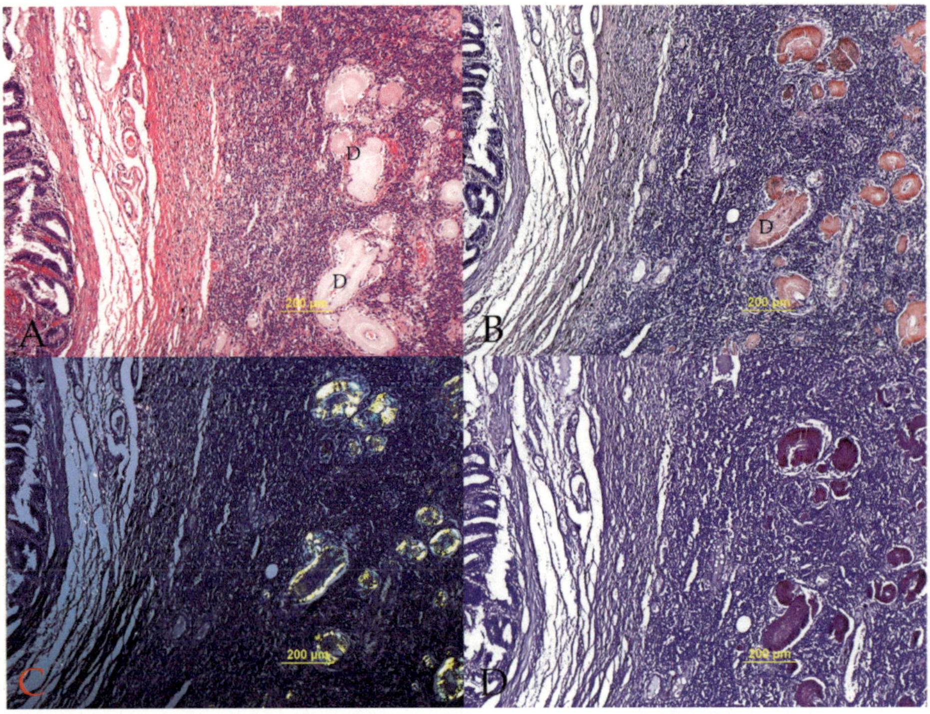

Fig. 2. A section of colon with amyloidosis in a dog with focal intestinal extramedullary plasma cell tumor. (**A**) Light eosinophilic amorphous deposits (D) surrounded by abundant plasmacytoid cells (H&E stain). The deposit stained light red with Congo red stain (**B**) and exhibited green birefringence under polarized light (**C**). The amyloid deposit stained with Congo red (**D**) after pretreatment with Potassium Permanganate solution, indicating that the amyloid is AL-amyloid.

Deposition of amyloid derived from islet amyloid polypeptide (IAPP), a normal protein secreted by the β cell of the pancreas, is reported in the pancreas of cats, and macaques. The mechanisms by which IAPP, a normal product of pancreatic islet beta cells, undergoes assembly and transformation into deposits of amyloid fibrils are not fully understood (O'Brien et al., 1996; Hoenig et al., 2000). However, the islet amyloid deposits in humans and feline and macaque animal models of type 2 diabetes mellitus are associated with significant loss of islet β cells (Hoenig et al., 2000). It is not known if the deposition of amyloid and the

development of clinical diabetes mellitus is the result of progressive loss of β cells from the amyloid deposit or if the deposition of the amyloid occurs as a result of prolonged stimulation of the β cells as a consequence of insulin resistance (Snyder, 2007).
Similar to human senile amyloidosis, old dogs develop neurodegenerative brain changes including cerebrovascular amyloidosis and senile plaques with amyloid deposition. The amyloid protein in the canine cerebrovascular amyloidosis is deposited in the medium- and small-caliber arterioles and capillaries of the leptomeninges and the brain parenchyma. Vascular or perivascular degeneration or cellular reactions were not detected in affected vessels (Borra's et al., 1999). Such amyloid deposits in the brain consist of a number of extracellular proteins, but most commonly contain Aβ type amyloid, which consists of a proteolytic fragment of the APP (Amyloid Precursor Protein). The Aβ form of amyloid is associated with the cerebral amyloid angiopathy of Alzheimer's disease in humans and with neurodegeneration in the canine brain (Snyder, 2007). In the brain tissue of aged dogs, Alzheimer-like pathology with lipofuscin being present in neurons and macrophages, Aβ-precursor protein in neurons, Aβ-positive plaques, 4-hydroxynonenal in neurons and macrophages, and limited intraneuronal accumulation of tau and advanced glycation end products increasing with longevity has been encountered (Gruys, 1995; Papaioannou et al., 2001; Rofina et al., 2001 & 2003). The amyloidosis which causes neurodegenerative disorders is almost always related to the intracerebral production of the pathogenic protein since most proteins, like immunoglobulins, do not cross the blood brain barrier. One exception may be the case of systemic amyloidosis related to transtiretin mutations, which produce peripheral neuropathy and cerebral changes in the white matter in some cases (Mena, 2009). Aβ-amyloid in the brain tissue of aged dogs showing signs of dementia forms a canine counterpart of senile dementia of the Alzheimer type (ccSDAT) in man. Other organ systems containing amyloid in the aged dog are the heart, gastrointestinal tract, and lungs. The deposition of amyloid in the pulmonary vasculature of the aged dogs was reported to be derived from apolipoprotein AI (Apo AI) (Snyder, 2007).

3. Clinical findings

Amyloidosis is a feature of several different pathologic mechanisms and as such should not be considered a single disease, but rather a group of diseases having in common the deposition of similar appearing proteins (Snyder, 2007). The animals affected with amyloidosis may show variable clinical signs due to the main underlying disease as commonly seen in AA amyloidosis (secondary amyloidosis) or those solely attributable to the deposition of amyloid in a given tissue or both. Some local amyloid depositions may be clinically non-significant incidental findings in certain tissues. In most cases, small local cutaneous amyloid masses pose no clinical problems. Therefore, the clinical finding of amyloidosis in affected animals is protean and reflects the extent of perturbed function of the predominantly affected organs and tissues due to the deposition of amyloid or may show variable clinical signs that may be associated to the underlying chronic disease and the concurrent amyloid deposit. For example, kidney is the main target organ for the deposition of amyloid in familial amyloidosis of the Abyssinian cat (glomerular deposit), and Shar Pei dogs (medullary deposit), while the amyloid is mainly deposited in the liver in Siamese cats (DiBartola et al., 1990; Niewold et al., 1999). Because amyloid deposit in the amyloidosis of the Abyssinian cat and Shar Pei dog is primarily a renal deposit, clinical signs associated with disrupted renal function will be seen in the affected

Abyssinian cats, and Shar Pei dogs, whereas clinical signs associated with derailed hepatic function may be manifested in Siamese cats. Deposition of amyloid in the pancreas of cats, non-human primates (macaques and baboons) and humans can lead to the development of type 2 diabetes mellitus (Hoenig et al., 2000; Snyder, 2007). Amyloid deposition can also occur in the cortex of the adrenal gland; however, it is not associated with any functional deficiencies (Snyder, 2007).

Reactive systemic amyloidosis secondary to chronic inflammatory conditions is often the most severe of the systemic forms. Liver, kidneys, spleen, lymph nodes, and adrenal glands are most commonly affected. Animals with renal amyloidosis frequently die from renal failure (Snyder, 2007). The clinical sign usually reflects the functional disruption and severity of the particular site of the kidney affected in renal amyloidosis. Progressive renal failure was the cause of death in Dorcas gazelles with renal medullary amyloidosis (Rideout et al., 1989). In contrast, renal medullary amyloidosis in cattle frequently occurs in conjunction with glomerular amyloidosis, and if the glomerular component is mild, it is usually a subclinical disease (Gruys, 1980, as cited by Rideout et al., 1989.) In Dorcas gazelle impairment of the renal function involved obstruction of the medullary tubules and collecting ducts, leading to atrophy and eventual loss of nephrons, with progressive interstitial fibrosis in the medulla and cortex (Rideout et al., 1989). Interstitial amyloidosis may also contribute to loss of concentrating ability and renal failure by interfering directly with maintenance of the medullary interstitial concentration gradient necessary for reabsorptive function in the renal tubules (Papendick et al., 1997). In 74% of the cheetahs with systemic amyloidosis associated with chronic gastritis, renal failure was determined to be the sole or partial cause of death (Papendick et al., 1997). Clinical signs including rapid weight loss, muscle atrophy, soft unformed stool, and ventral edema were noted in a horse gelding with multiple myeloma (Kim et al., 2005).

4. Gross and microscopic lesions

Several different pathologic mechanisms and conditions underlie various forms and types of amyloidosis, although abnormal proteins with similar staining characteristics are deposited in various organs and tissues of the affected animals. The gross feature of amyloidosis due to the deposited amyloid in these tissues and organs is not specific for amyloid. Grossly, the affected organs are often enlarged, moderately firm and abnormally discolored (Snyder, 2007). In AA-amyloidosis, the most frequently encountered amyloid type in veterinary medicine, the characteristic deposition pattern in most species is in the central organs such as spleen, liver, enteric mucosa and the arterial walls (Gruys, 1988 as cited by Gruys, 2004). Depending on the extent of the deposition, there may be splenomegaly, hepatomegaly and renomegaly as these organs are most commonly affected in systemic AA amyloidosis. Amyloid deposition was most severe in the renal medullary interstitium and glomeruli in systemic amyloidosis in black-footed cats (Terio et al., 2008). Renal lesions in AA amyloidosis in sheep and goats were characterized grossly by pale cortical surfaces with scattered, miliary, whitish-yellow foci and by straight, whitish-yellow striations on cut cortical surfaces (Ménsua et al., 2003). However, experimentally induced AA Amyloidosis in sheep principally affected the gastrointestinal tract. Amyloid was present from the tongue to the rectum, but was most prominent in the duodenum where the deposits disrupted the normal mucosal architecture. Other body organs had only mild amyloid deposition (Biescas et al., 2009).

Diffuse gastrointestinal hemorrhage, markedly thickened jejunal mucosa, and splenomegaly were present in a horse with AL amyloidosis associated with multiple myeloma (Kim et al., 2005). In Gallinae, it may also be deposited in the joints. In felines, pancreatic insular amyloid (AIAPP) is rather common (Gruys, 1988, as cited by Gruys, 2004). Amyloid deposits are occasionally limited to a single organ or tissue and may be visible grossly as masses (Snyder, 2007). Local amyloid deposits associated with plasma cell dyscrasia may be seen as variably sized grossly visible skin granulomas in cutaneous nodular amyloidosis in various animals. Rowland et al., (1991) reported local cutaneous amyloidosis associated with plasmacytoma involving the digits, forelimbs, lips, and ears in dogs (**Fig. 3**).

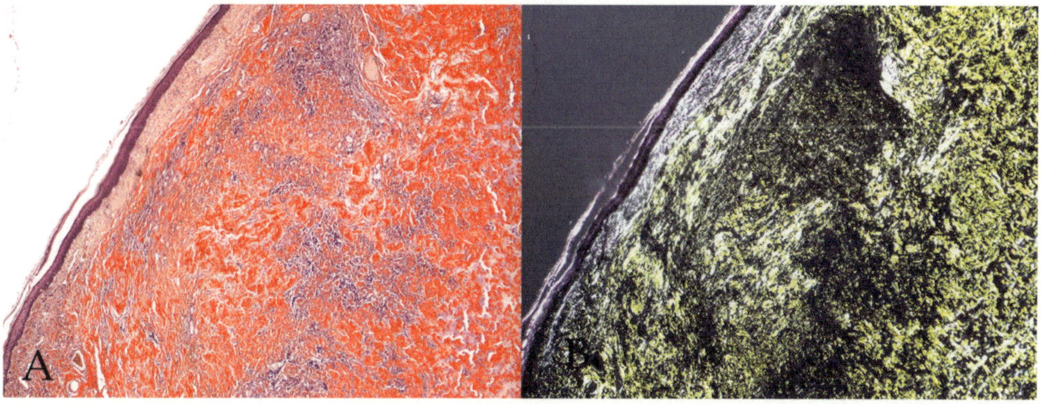

Fig. 3. Histological features of skin of a dog with nodular cutaneous amyloidosis, stained red with Congo red stain (left) and showed yellow-green birefringence (right) illuminated with polarized light, characteristic of amyloid deposits.

Microscopic findings of the deposition of amyloid protein may correspond to the grossly visible lesions, or it may be seen only after microscopic examination without distinct grossly discernible lesions. Amyloid should be differentiated from other similar-appearing extracellular deposits such as collagen and fibrin (Snyder, 2007). For a fibrillary protein to be considered amyloidogenic it should produce extracellular deposits with affinity for the red Congo dye and a green birefringence under polarized light. Congo red stain, which does not have chemical specificity for amyloid, but is dependent on the conformational property of being arranged in beta-pleated sheets, is the most commonly used stain for the identification of amyloid. Amyloid stains orange to red under light microscopy, which is seen under polarized light as an apple-green birefringent material (Ménsua et al., 2003; Snyder, 2007). Immunohistochemistry can also be used not only to identify amyloid deposits but also to identify the specific constituents composing the deposits such as the anti-β-light chain antibodies (Snyder, 2007). AA and AL amyloid deposits stain similar with Congo red stain. The identification of AA is usually based on its reactivity with specific anti-AA antibodies and sensitivity to permanganate pretreatment (Wright et al., 1977; Shtrasburg et al., 2005) (**Fig. 4**). The common ultra structure of amyloid proteins is made of some nonbranching, rigid fibrils, 7.5 to 10 nm wide and of variable length, which arrange themselves in anti-parallel sheets with β structure (Mena, 2009).

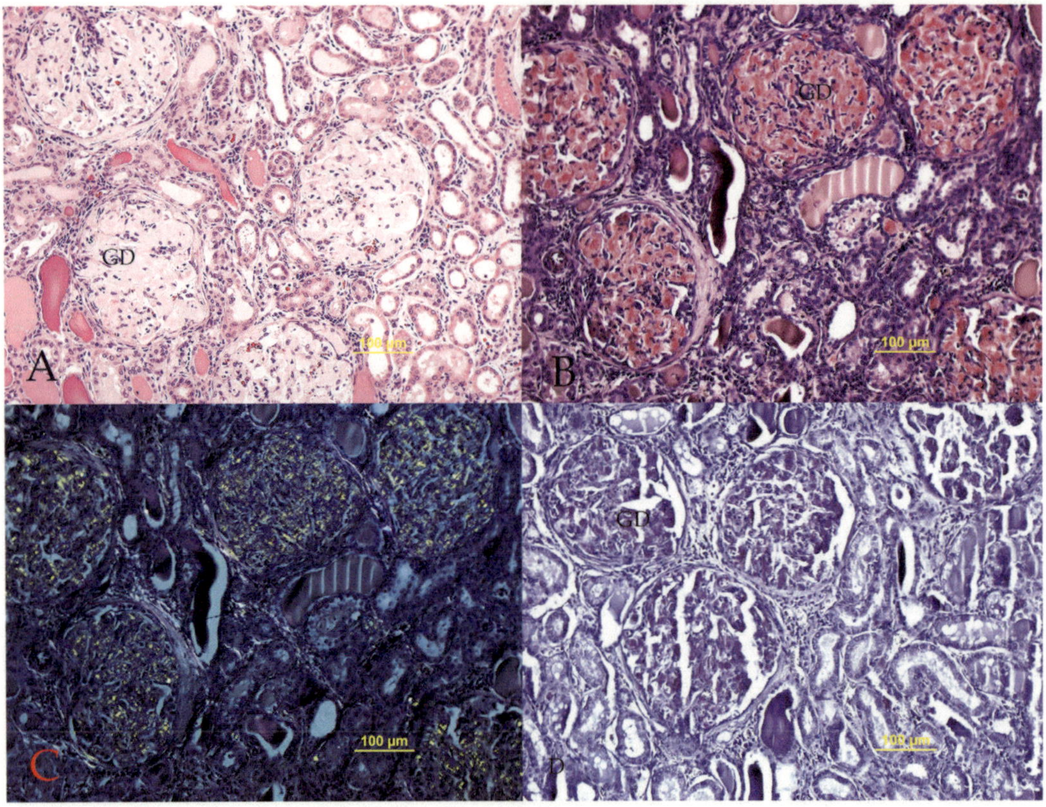

Fig. 4. A section of renal glomerular amyloidosis in a dog. (A) Light eosinophilic amorphous deposits partly effaced the glomerular architecture (H&E stain). The deposit stained light red with Congo red stain (**B**) and exhibited green birefringence under polarized light (**C**). The amyloid deposit failed to stain with Congo red (**D**) after pretreatment with Potassium Permanganate solution, indicating that the amyloid is AA-amyloid.

Microscopically, amyloid is deposited extracellularily in various affected tissues. Amyloid deposition was seen in the kidneys, blood vessels, spleen, liver, lymph nodes, gastrointestinal tract, and adrenal glands of sheep and goats with AA amyloidosis (Ménsua et al., 2003). There was widening of the medullary interstitium by eosinophilic homogeneous material, which encroached upon medullary tubules and collecting ducts with occasional renal papillary necrosis in Dorcas gazelle with medullary amyloidosis. The amyloid deposition significantly correlated with interstitial fibrosis, and tubular dilation and atrophy (Rideout, 1989).

In a horse with AL amyloidosis associated with multiple myeloma, diffuse severe extracellular amyloid deposits were present in the lamina propria of glandular stomach, duodenum, and jejunum. Much of the spleen and sternal bone marrow were replaced by neoplastic round cells, and multiple foci of amyloid were also present in the spleen and bone marrow. No significant microscopic changes were noted in the kidneys, liver, and lungs (Kim et al., 2005).

In a cow with systemic AL amyloidosis associated with bovine leukocyte adhesion deficiency, amyloid deposits immunohistochemically related to immunoglobulin kappa-light chains of precursor protein were present in the perivascular and intercellular spaces of the visceral organs, such as the liver, kidneys, pancreas, adrenal glands, and upper alimentary tract (Taniyama et al., 2000).

5. Conclusion

In summary, the pathology and pathogenesis of amyloidosis in animals is diverse depending upon the underlying causes and species affected. Similarly, the clinical findings are quite variable consequent to the variation of the tissues and organs involved and the extent of functional disruption of the affected organs in various animal species. The affected organs may be enlarged and exhibit variable pallor or the amyloid deposit may not be grossly visible and may be discernible only after microscopic examination of the affected tissues. Amyloid appears as a pale eosinophilic homogenous extracellular deposit in tissues. However, microscopic examination and Congo red staining with green birefringence under polarized light are needed to confirm amyloid and differentiated it from other similar extracellular deposits such as collagen and fibrin. Pretreatment of the affected tissues using potassium permanganate solution before staining with Congo red helps to differentiate AA-amyloid from AL-amyloid deposit.

6. References

Abdelkader, SV., Gudding, R. & Nordstoga, K. (1991). Clinical chemical constituents in relation to liver amyloidosis in serum-producing horses. *Journal of Comparative Pathology,* 105 (2):203-11

Badolato, R., Ming Wang, J., Murphy, WJ., Lloyd, AR., Michiel, DF., Bausserman, LL., Kelvin, DJ. & Oppenheim, JJ. (1994). Serum amyloid A is a chemoattractant: induction of migration, adhesion, and tissue infiltration of monocytes and polymorphonuclear leukocytes. *Journal of Experimental* Medicine, 180:203–209

Bhak, G., Choe, Y-J. & Paik, SR. (2009). Mechanism of amyloidogenesis: nucleation-dependent fibrillation versus double-concerted fibrillation. *BMB reports,* 541-551

Biescas, E., Jirón, W., Climent, S., Fernández, A., Pérez, M., Weiss, D.T., Solomon, A. & Luján. L. (2009). AA Amyloidosis induced in sheep principally affects the gastrointestinal tract. *Journal of Comparative Pathology,* 140 (4):238-246 doi:10.1016/j.jcpa.2008.12.004

Blunden, AS. & Smith, KC. (1992). Generalised amyloidosis and acute liver haemorrhage in four cats. *Journal of Small Animal Practice,* 33:566–570

Borra's, D., Ferrer, I. & Pumarola, M. (1999). Age-related Changes in the Brain of the Dog. *Veterinary Pathology,* 36:202–211

Boyce, JT., DiBartola, SP., Chew, DJ. & Gasper, PW. (1984). Familial renal amyloidosis in Abyssinian cats. *Veterinary Pathology,* 21(1):33-8

Burrough, ER ., Myers, RK., Hostetter, SJ., Fox, LE., Bayer, BJ., Felz, C L., Waller, K R. & Whitley, E. M. (2011). Amyloid deposition in 2 feline thymomas. *Veterinary Pathology,* 10.1177/0300985811400442

DiBartola, SP., Tarr, MJ., & Benson, MD. (1986). Tissue distribution of amyloid deposits in Abyssinian cats with familial amyloidosis. *Joural of Comparative Pathology,* 96(4):387-98

DiBartola, SP., Tarr, MJ., Webb, DM., & Giger, U. (1990). Familial renal amyloidosis in Chinese Shar Pei dogs. Journal of the American Veterinary Medical Association, 197(4):483-7

Garner, MM., Raymond, JT., O'Brien, TD., Nordhausen, RW. & Russell, WC. (2007). Amyloidosis in the black-footed ferret (*Mustela nigripes*). *Journal of* Zoo *and* Wildlife Medicine, 38(1):32-41

Gliatto, JM., & Alroy, J. (1995). Cutaneous amyloidosis in a horse with lymphoma. *The Veterinary Record,* 137(3):68-69

Gonnerman, WA., Elliott-Bryant, R., Carreras, I., Sipe, JD., & Cathcart, ES., (1995). Linkage of protection against amyloid fibril formation in the mouse to a single, autosomal dominant gene. *Journal of Experimental* Medicine, 181:2249-2252

Gruys E. (2004): Protein folding pathology in domestic animals: A review. *Journal of Zhejiang University Science,* 5(10):1226-1238

Gruys, E. (1995). First workshop and clinic on neuropathology in geriatric dogs and cats. Wiesbaden, Germany, May 4-5, 1995. *Amyloid, International Journal of Experimental and Clinical Investigation,* 2:280-283

Guo Ju-Tao, Aldrich, C E., Mason, WS. & Pugh, JC. (1996): Characterization of serum amyloid A protein mRNA expression and secondary amyloidosis in the domestic duck. Cell Biology, *Proceedings of the National Academy of Science,* December 1996, *USA,* Vol. 93, pp. 14548–14553

Hadlow, WJ. & Jellison WL. (1962). Amyloidosis in rocky mountain bighorn sheep. Journal of the American Veterinary Medical Association, 141:243–247

Hawthorne, TB., Bolon, B. & Meyer, DJ. (1990). Systemic amyloidosis in a mare. Journal of the American Veterinary Medical Association, 196:323–325

Hayden, DW., Johnson, KH., Wolf, CB. & Westermark, P. (1988). AA Amyloid-associated gastroenteropathy in a horse. *Journal of Comparative Pathology,* 98:195–204

Hoenig, M ., Hall, G., Ferguson, D., Jordan, K., Henson, M., Johnson, K. & O'Brien, T. (2000). A Feline Model of Experimentally induced islet amyloidosis. *American Journal of Pathology, Vol. 157 (6)* 2143–2150

Jakob, W. (1971). Spontaneous amyloidosis of mammals. *Veterinary Pathology,* 8:292–306

Johnson, KH., Westermark, P., Sletten, K. & O'Brien, TD. (1996). Amyloid proteins and amyloidosis in domestic animals. *Amyloid, International Journal of Experimental and Clinical Investigation,* 3:270–289

Johnson, R. & Jamison, K. (1984). Amyloidosis in six dairy cows. Journal of the American Veterinary Medical Association, 185:1538–1543

Kim, DY., Taylor, HW., Eades, SC. & Cho, D.-Y. (2005): Systemic AL amyloidosis associated with Multiple Myeloma in a horse. *Veterinary Pathology,* 42:81–84

Kisilevsky, R. (1990). Heparan sulfate proteoglycans in amyloidogenesis: an epiphenomenon, a unique factor, or the tip of a more fundamental process? Laboratory Investigation, 63:589–591

Kingston, RS., Shih, M. & Snyder, SP. (1982). Secondary amyloidosis in Dall's sheep. *Journal of* Wildlife *Diseases,* 18:381–383

Landman WJM. (1998). Amyloid arthropathy in chickens. *Veterinary Quarterly,* 21:78–82

Liang, J., Elliott-Bryant, R., Hajri, T., Sipe, JD. & Cathcart, ES. (1998). A unique amyloidogenic apolipoprotein serum amyloid A (apoSAA) isoform expressed by the amyloid resistant CE/J mouse strain exhibits higher affinity for macrophages than apoSAA1 and apoSAA2 expressed by amyloid susceptible CBA/J mice. *Biochimica et Biophysica Acta,* 1394:121-126

Linke, RP., Geisel, O. & Mann, K. (1991). Equine cutaneous amyloidosis derived from an immunoglobulin lambda-light chain. Immunohistochemical, immunochemical and chemical results. *Biological* Chemistry Hoppe-Seyler, 372(9):835-43

Linke, RP., Hol, PR. & Geisel, O. (1986). Immunohistochemical identification of generalized AA-amyloidosis in a mountain gazelle (*Gazella gazella*). *Veterinary Pathology,* 23:63–67

Mena, MA., Rodríguez-Navarro, JA. & García de Yébenes, J. (2009): The multiple mechanisms of amyloid deposition. The role of parkin. Commentary & View. *Prion* 3:1, 5-11

Ménsua, C., Carrasco, L., Bautista, MJ., Biescas, E., Fernández, A., Murphy, CL., Weiss, DT., Solomon, A. & Luján, L. (2003). Pathology of AA Amyloidosis in Domestic Sheep and Goats. *Veterinary Pathology,* 40: 71-81

Merlini, G. &. Stone, MJ. (2006). Dangerous small B-cell clones. *Blood,* 108, (8):2520-2530

Munson, L. (1993). Diseases of captive cheetahs (*Acinonyx jubatus*): results of the Cheetah Research Council pathology survey, 1989–1992. *Zoo Biology,* 12:105–124

Murphy, CL., Eulitz, M., Hrncic, R., Sletten, K., Westermark, P., Williams, T., Macy, SD., Wooliver, C., Wall, J., Weiss. DT. & Solomon, A. (2001). Chemical typing of amyloid protein contained in formalin-fixed paraffin-embedded biopsy specimens. *American Journal of Clinical Pathology,*116:135–142

Nieto, JM., Va´zquez, S., Quiroga, MI., Lo´pez-Pen˜a, M., Guerrero, F. & Gruys ,E. (1995). Spontaneous AA-amyloidosis in mink (*Mustela vison*). Description of eight cases, one of which exhibited intracellular amyloid deposits in lymph node macrophages. *European Journal of Veterinary Pathology,* 1 : 99–103

Niewold ,TA., van der Linde-Sipman, JS., Murphy, C., Tooten, PC. & Gruys, E. (1999). Familial amyloidosis in cats: Siamese and Abyssinian AA proteins differ in primary sequence and pattern of deposition. *Amyloid,* 6 (3):205-9

O'Brien, TD., Wagner, JD., Litwak, KN., Carlson, CS., Cefalu, WT., Jordan, K., Johnson, KH. & Butler, PC. (1996). Islet amyloid and islet amyloid polypeptide in Cynomolgus Macaques *(Macaca fascicularis):* An animal model of human non-insulin-dependent Diabetes Mellitus. *Veterinary Pathology,* 33 : 479-485

Ovelgönne, JH., Landman, WJ., Gruys, E., Gielkens , AL. & Peeters, BP. (2001). Identical amyloid precursor proteins in two breeds of chickens which differ in susceptibility to develop amyloid arthropathy. *Amyloid,* 8(1) : 41-51

Papaioannou, N., Tooten, PCJ., Van Ederen, AM., Bohl, JRE., Rofina, J., Tsangaris, T. & Gruys, E. (2001). Immunohistochemical investigation of the brain of aged dogs. I. Detection of neurofibrillary tangles and of 4-hydroxynonenal protein, an oxidative damage product, in senile plaques. *Amyloid Journal of Protein Folding Disorders,* 8:11-21

Papendick, RE., Munson, L., O'Brien, TD. & Johnson, KH. (1997). Systemic AA amyloidosis in captive cheetah (*Acinonyx jubatus*). *Veterinary Pathology,* 34:549-556

Picken MM. (2001). The changing concepts of amyloid. *Archives of* Pathology *& Laboratory* Medicine, 125:38–43

Prusiner, SB., McKinley, MP., Bowman, KA., Bolton, DC., Bendheim, PE., Groth, DF., & Glenner, GG. (1983). Scrapie prions aggregate to form amyloid-like birefringent rods. *Cell,* 35:349-358

Ren, Y., Reddy, SA. & Liao, WS. (1999). Purification and identification of a tissue-specific repressor involved in serum amyloid A1 gene expression. *Journal of Biological Chemistry,* 274:37154-37160

Rideout,BA., Montali, RJ., Wallace, RS., Bush, M., Phillips, LG., Antonovych, TT. & Sabnis, SG. (1989). Renal medullary amyloidosis in Dorcas Gazelles. *Veterinary Pathology,* 26:129–135

Rofina, JE., Papaioannou, N., Van Andel, I., Van Ederen, AM., Gossens, M., Secreve, M., Van der Meer, I., Toussaint, MJM., Terlou, M. & Gruys, E. (2001). Cerebrovascular amyloidosis may cause a decrease of blood supply leading to oxidative damage and formation of amyloid plaques in the aged canine brain. *In*: Bely, M., Apathy, A. (Eds.), *Amyloid and Amyloidosis* IX. Apathy, Budapest, Hungary, p.445-447

Rofina, JE., Van Andel, I., Van Ederen, AM., Papaioannou, N., Yamaguchi, H. & Gruys, E. (2003). Canine counterpart of senile plaques near capillaries but lack of spatial relationship with activated microglia and macrophages. *Amyloid Journal of Protein Folding Disorders,Dis* 10:86-96

Rowland, PH., Valentine, BA., Stebbins, KE. & Smith, CA. (1991). Cutaneous plasmacytomas with amyloid in six dogs. *Veterinary Pathology,* 28 (2): 125-130

Sato, A., Koga, T., Inoue, M. & Goto, N. (1981). Pathological observations of amyloidosis in swans and other anatidae. Japanese journal *of veterinary* science, 43:509–519

Seifi, HA., Karimi, K. & Movasseghi, R. (1997). Renal amyloidosis in cattle: a case report in Iran. *Journal of Veterinary Medicine,* 44:631–633

Shtrasburg, S., Gal, R., Gruys, E., Perl, S., Martin, BM., Artin, B., Kaplan, R., Koren, A., Nyska, A.,Pras, M. & Livneh, A. (2005). An ancillary tool for the diagnosis of amyloid A amyloidosis in a variety of domestic and wild animals. *Veterinary Pathology,* 42:132–139

Schulze, C., Brügmann, M., Bo¨er, M., Brandt, HP., Pohlenz, J. & Linke, RP. (1998). Generalized AA-amyloidosis in Siberian tigers (*Panthera tigris altaica*) with predominant renal medullary amyloid deposition. *Veterinary Pathology,* 35:70–74

Snyder, P.W. (2007). Diseases of Immunity: Amyloidosis . *In Pathologic basis of veterinary diseases, 4th edition. Editors,* McGavin, M.D, & Zachary, JF. Pp 246-251. Mosby Elsevier, ISBN-13:978-0-323-02870-7. St Lois Missouri

Taniyama, H., Yamamoto, S., Sako, T., Hirayama, K., Higuchi, H. & Nagahata H. (2000). Systemic κAL amyloidosis associated with bovine leukocyte adhesion deficiency. *Veterinary Pathology,* 37:98–100

Terio, KA., O'brien, T., Lamberski, N., Famula, TR. & Munson L. (2008). Amyloidosis in Black-footed Cats (*Felis nigripes*). *Veterinary Pathology,* 45:393–400

Westermark, P. (1998). The pathogenesis of amyloidosis. Understanding general principles. *American Journal of Pathology,* 152(5):1125-1127

WHO-IUIS, Nomenclature Sub-Committee. (1993). Nomenclature of amyloid and amyloidosis. *Bulletin of the World Health Organization,* 71(1): 105–112

Williams, JH., Van Wilpe, E. & Momberg, M. (2005). Renal medullary AA amyloidosis, hepatocyte dissociation and multinucleated hepatocytes in a 14-year-old free-ranging lioness (*Panthera leo*). *Journal of South African Veterinary Association,* 76(2):90-98

Wright, JR., Calkins, E. & Humphrey, RL. (1977). Potassium permanganate reaction in amyloidosis. *Laboratory Investigation,* 36:274-281

Yu, J., Guo, JT., Zhu, H. & Kindy, MS. (2000). Amyloid formation in the rat: adenoviral expression of mouse serum amyloid A proteins. *Amyloid International Journal of Experimental and Clinical Investigation,* 7:32-40

Zschiesche, W. & Jakob, W. (1989). Pathology of animal amyloidoses. *Pharmacology and Therapeutics,* 41:49–93

9

Mouse Models to Study Systemic Amyloidoses: Is Prion-Like Transmission a Common Pathogenic Mechanism?

Keiichi Higuchi et al.*
Department of Aging Biology, Institute on Aging and Adaptation, Shinshu University Graduate School of Medicine, Japan

1. Introduction

The amyloidoses are a group of protein-misfolding disorders characterized by the accumulation of amyloid fibrils formed from a variety of proteins. Currently, twenty- eight different kinds of human and animal proteins, in intact or fragmented forms, have been found to be associated with pathological disorders such as Alzheimer's disease, type II diabetes, prion diseases, dialysis-related amyloidosis, and various familial, senile and sporadic amyloidosis (Sipe et al., 2010; Benson et al 2008). Amyloidoses have been divided into two major classes: 1) systemic and 2) localized amyloidoses. In systemic amyloidoses, precursor proteins circulating in the blood associate to form amyloid fibrils that are then deposited throughout the body. For example, immunoglobulin light chains form deposits in patients with myeloma in AL amyloidosis. In reactive AA amyloidosis, serum amyloid A (SAA) protein forms deposits in patients with chronic inflammation, and transthyretin (TTR) forms deposits in patients with familial amyloid polyneuropathy (FAP) and senile systemic amyloidosis (SSA). Patients on long-term hemodialysis develop dialysis-related amyloidosis (DRA) due to the deposition of amyloid fibrils (A$ß_2$M) of $ß_2$-microglobulin ($ß_2$m). In contrast to systemic amyloidosis, precursor proteins produced in local organs deposit in one particular area of the body in various localized amyloidoses.

In mice, apolipoprotein A-II (apoA-II) in serum high density lipoproteins (HDL) forms amyloid fibrils (AApoAII) in age-associated systemic amyloidosis (senile AApoAII amyloidosis). AA amyloidosis, known as reactive or secondary amyloidosis associated with inflammation, is generally recognized as the predominant form of systemic amyloidosis that occurs in humans, mice, domestic animals and many species in the animal kingdom. These amyloidoses are characterized by the systemic deposition of extracellular fibrils composed of apoA-II in AApoAII amyloidosis or SAA (serum AA) in AA amyloidosis, primarily in the spleen, liver, heart, kidney, vessels walls, and to a lesser extent in other organs. In most

*Xiaoying Fu, Pengyao Zhang, Jinko Sawashita, Beiru Zhang, Jinze Qian, Wang Yaoyong and Masayuki Mori
Department of Aging Biology, Institute on Aging and Adaptation, Shinshu University Graduate School of Medicine, Japan

species, AApoAII and AA amyloidosis occurs sporadically and is associated with aging (AApoAII amyloidosis) and chronic inflammation (AA amyloidosis). However, intriguing recent data suggest that both AApoAII and AA amyloidoses could be transmitted by a prion-like infectious process through a seeding-nucleation mechanism (Qian et al., 2010; B. Zhang et al., 2008). In these amyloidoses, AApoAII and AA amyloid fibrils, abnormal forms of the host serum proteins (apoA-II and SAA), induce conformational changes in apoA-II and SAA to form AApoAII and AA fibrils, and this causes detectable phenotypes or diseases in affected individuals. Recently, Aß amyloid fibrils in Alzheimer's disease and intracellular amyloid fibril-like aggregated proteins were postulated to work as seeds for propagation of mis-folded and pathologic protein structures in various neurodegenerative disorders, including Huntington's disease, Parkinson's disease and tauopathies (Aguzzi et al., 2009; Brundin et al., 2010).

The prion-like transmission of amyloid fibrils or fibril-like materials, which could play an important role in the propagation of pathological events in systemic amyloidosis, will be discussed here.

2. Transmission of mouse senile AApoAII amyloidosis

Several senescence-prone inbred strains of mice (SAMP strains) have been developed with accelerated senescence, a shorter life span and various age-associated disorders and pathologic changes. These SAMP strains include SAMP1, SAMP6, SAMP8 and SAMP10. An accelerated senescence-resistant strain (SAMR1) has also been generated to serve as a control for the SAMP strains (Takeda et al., 1981; Higuchi et al., 1999). Severe senile amyloidosis is a characteristic age-associated disorder in the SAMP1 and SAMP10 strains, making them a valuable model to investigate amyloidosis pathogenesis and to assist in the development of effective therapeutic modalities. We identified apoA-II, a normal constituent of serum HDL, as the amyloid protein responsible for mouse senile amyloidosis in the SAMP1 strain, and the amyloid fibril was named AApoAII (Higuchi et al., 1983; Yonezu et al 1986; Higuchi et al. 1986). Recently we found that there was prion-like transmission in mouse AApoAII amyloidosis (Higuchi et al., 1998; Xing et al., 2001). Here, a brief history and the pathobiology of mouse AApoAII amyloidosis in SAMP1 and its related strains is described, followed by a discussion of AApoAII amyloidosis transmission.

2.1 Pathology of mouse AApoAII amyloidosis

Amyloid fibril deposition in aged SAMP1 mice is systemic and all organs except brain parenchyma are involved (Takeshita et al., 1982). The earliest AApoAII deposits are seen in the primary and secondary papillae of the tongue, the lamina propria and submucosa of the small intestine, the alveolar septa of the lungs and the squamous-glandular junction of the stomach. With advancing age, AApoAII deposits extend into the collecting tubules in the papillae of the kidneys, the perimedullary zone of the adrenal cortex, heart and skeletal muscle interstitium, thyroid gland interstitium, the papillary layer of the dermis, the testis interstitium, the corpora lutea, the atretic follicle and the ovarian interstitium, around the portal veins and in the spaces of Disse in the periportal sinusoid of the liver, the marginal zone around the lymphoid follicles of the spleen, and blood vessels throughout the body. In the final stage, the liver and spleen are enlarged and the kidneys are contracted with severe amyloid deposition (Higuchi et al. 1983) (Fig. 1).

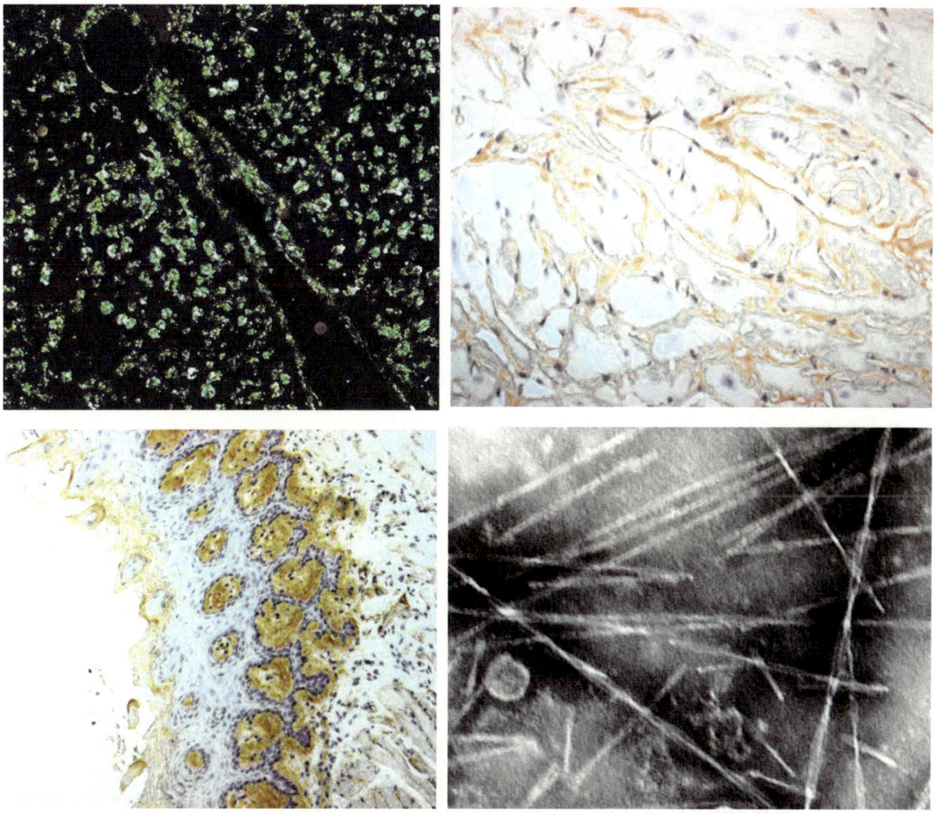

Fig. 1. **Mouse systemic senile amyloidosis in SAMP1 mice.** AApoAII amyloid fibrils were deposited in the whole body except for the brain parenchyma. **Upper-left**: heavy amyloid deposition in a liver section strained with Congo red was detected as green birefringence under the polarizing microscope (X100). **Upper-right** and **Lower-left**: AApoAII amyloid depositions were determined immunohistochemically in the heart and tongue, respectively (X400). **Lower-right**; Electron microscopic observation of AApoAII amyloid fibrils isolated from the liver (X50,000).

Although senile AApoAII amyloidosis is common in most mouse strains, severe senile amyloidosis has been reported in only a few strains, i.e. SAMP1, SAMP10, SJL/J, LLC, and PS strains. The complete nucleotide sequence of the apoA-II (gene is *Apoa2*) cDNA was determined in 41 inbred strains of mice (Kunisada et al., 1986; Kitagawa et al., 2003). Among these strains, six alleles containing amino acid substitutions (*Apoa2^a*, *Apoa2^b*, *Apoa2^c*, *Apoa2^d*, *Apoa2^e* and *Apoa2^f*) were identified. Severe amyloid deposition was observed in the strains with the *Apoa2^c* allele (Higuchi et al., 1991). Several genetic analyses indicated that the presence of the *Apoa2^c* allele markedly accelerates age-associated deposition of AApoAII and reduces the lifespan (Naiki et al., 1993; Higuchi et al., 1995; 1996). These results show that type C apoA-II protein in mice is highly amyloidogenic, while SAMR1 and strains with type B apoA-II protein are resistant to the development of amyloidosis. The mice expressing type A apoA-II protein, such as C57BL/6, are moderately amyloidogenic. *In vitro* amyloid fibril formation (fibril extension) has been reported with the type C apoA-II protein, but not with the type B apoA-II (Naiki et al., 1992; Fu et al., 2001). Recently we demonstrated that the combination of N- and C-terminal sequences of mouse apoA-II and a conformational change in their secondary structure are essential for polymerization into AApoAII amyloid fibrils (Sawashita et al., 2009). However, the mechanism behind the high amyloidogenicity of type C apoA-II protein *in vivo* is not yet known.

Congenic R1.P1-*Apoa2*^{c} mice have the amyloidogenic *Apoa2*^{c} SAMP1 gene on the genetic background of SAMR1 (Higuchi et al., 1993). Comparable to the donor SAMP1 strain, severe amyloid deposition is present in the R1.P1-*Apoa2*^{c} strain (Higuchi et al., 1995), and the R1.P1-*Apoa2*^{c} mice are more convenient for use in amyloidosis experiments. A transgenic mouse strain that over-expresses *Apoa2*^{c} mRNA has been established on the genetic background of R1.P1-*Apoa2*^{c}. This strain shows higher concentration of apoA-II and greater susceptibility to amyloidosis than the control R1.P1-*Apoa2*^{c} strain and should prove valuable in future studies of amyloidosis (Ge et al., 2007).

2.2 Transmission of mouse AApoAII amyloidosis

Nucleation-dependent polymerization is a postulated model consistent with the kinetics of *in vitro* amyloid protein fibrillization in amyloidoses such as prion diseases, Alzheimer disease and mouse AApoAII amyloidosis (Jarrett et al., 1993; Harper et al., 1997; Naki et al., 1991). This model is comprised of two phases: 1) nucleation and 2) extension. 1) Nucleus formation requires a series of thermodynamically unfavorable monomer association steps. Thus, the nucleation phase is the rate-limiting step in the development of amyloidosis. 2) Once the nucleus has formed, further addition of monomers becomes thermodynamically favorable, resulting in rapid extension of amyloid fibrils. The dramatically hastened *in vitro* fibril formation fueled by the addition of amyloid fibrils (nucleus) to a solution of amyloid protein monomers is an example of nucleation-dependent polymerization.

Prion diseases are associated with the accumulation of a pathologic conformational isomer (PrP^{Sc}) by a host-derived prion protein (PrP^c). Prion transmission or propagation involves the conversion of cellular PrP^c into PrP^{Sc} via an increase in its ß-sheet secondary structure content. According to the protein-only hypothesis, introduction of the abnormal conformer PrP^{Sc} into an organism would accelerate the conversion of PrP^c into its pathological conformation (Prusiner et al., 1998; 2006). Thus, the nucleation-dependent polymerization model provides a feasible mechanism for the *in vivo* conformational conversion of PrP^c to PrP^{Sc} via transmission of prions (Weissmann et al, 1999).

As predicted by the nucleation-dependent polymerization model, *in vitro* fibril formation experiments in which apoA-II monomers are converted to AApoAII fibrils indicate that the addition of AApoAII amyloid fibrils can facilitate the formation of amyloid fibrils from apoA-II monomers (seeding reaction)(Fig. 2A). Amyloid deposition was notably accelerated after a very small quantity of AApoAII fibrils was administered to R1.P1-*Apoa2*^{c} mice by peripheral injection (intravenous, intraperitoneal or intragastric) or in the diet (Fig. 2B) (Higuchi et al., 1998; Xing et al., 2001). Thus, fibril formation is greatly accelerated in mice through seeding with pre-formed fibrils *in vivo* in mice (transmission of amyloidosis). The acceleration of amyloidosis fibrils (transmissibility) disappeared completely after treatment with protein denaturing reagents including 6 M guanidine hydrochloride, strong alkaline solution or formic acid. Acceleration was slowed by 6 M urea or by autoclaving, and it was not changed by formalin, DNAse or RNAse treatments. This finding revealed that transmissibility of AApoAII depends on fibril conformation (H. Zhang et al., 2006).

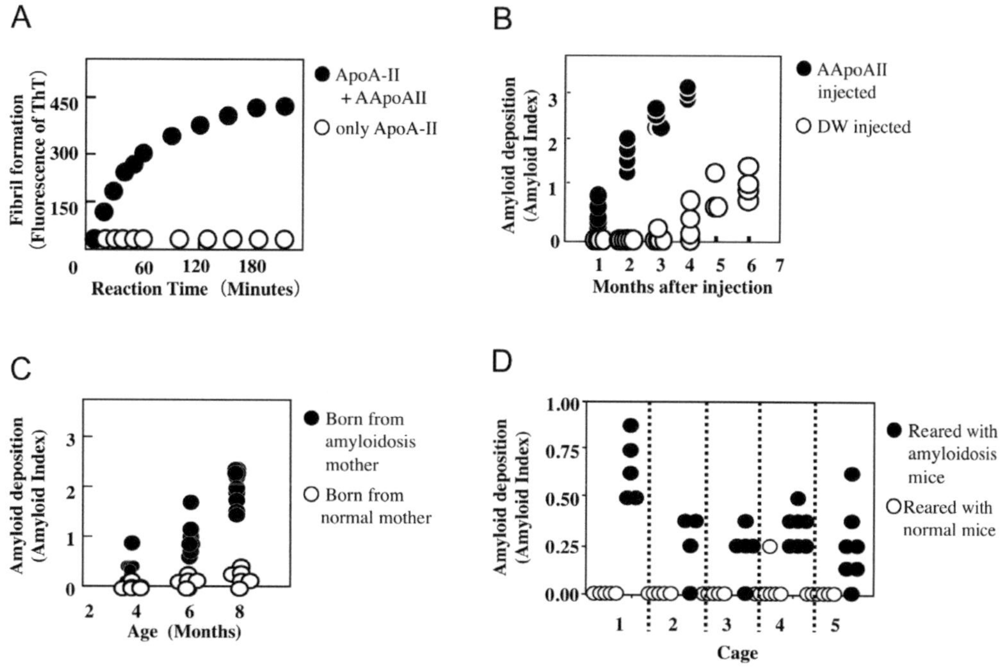

Fig. 2. **Transmission of mouse AApoAII amyloidosis in vitro and in vivo. A:** Addition of AApoAII amyloid fibrils to a solution of apoA-II monomers accelerates fibril formation in test tubes. **B:** Injection of AApoAII amyloid fibrils into R1.P1- *Apoa2^c^* mice accelerates amyloid deposition. **C:** Amyloid deposition is accelerated in offspring born to and nursed by mothers with amyloidosis. **D:** Young R1.P1- *Apoa2^c^* mice that were kept in the same cage with mice having amyloidosis for 3 months developed amyloidosis. The intensity of amyloid deposition in mice was determined semi-quantitatively using the amyloid index (AI) as a parameter. The AI parameter represents the average degree of deposition, graded 0 to 4, in Congo red - stained sections from the seven organs examined (liver, heart, spleen, tongue, stomach, intestine and skin).

Amyloidosis in the offspring of R1.P1- *Apoa2^c* mice was examined to further characterize this transmissibility. Acceleration of amyloidosis was observed in offspring born to, and nursed by, mothers with amyloidosis that was induced by injection of amyloid fibrils 3 months before pregnancy (Fig. 2C) compared with the offspring of control mothers that did not receive injections of amyloid fibrils (Korenaga et al., 2006). Acceleration of amyloidosis was also observed in offspring born to mothers that were not injected, but that were nursed by mothers injected with amyloid fibrils. However, this phenomenon was not observed in offspring born to amyloidosis mothers and nursed by control mothers. Injection of milk obtained from amyloid fibril-injected mothers induced AApoAII amyloidosis in young mice, and amyloid fibrils were detected in the milk of amyloid fibril-injected mothers by electron microscopy. Young mice were reared for 3 months in cages with old R1.P1- *Apoa2^c* mice that had severe amyloid-depositions. All of the young mice developed amyloid deposits (Fig. 1D)(Xing et al., 2001). Amyloid fibrils were detected in feces of mice with amyloidosis. Injection of amyloid fibrils found in feces induced amyloidosis in mice, raising the possibility that the oral transmission of amyloid fibrils through feces leads to acceleration of amyloidosis in AApoAII amyloidosis. AApoAII amyloid fibril deposits were found in the skeletal muscles of amyloid-affected mice, primarily in the blood vessels and in the interstitial tissues (endomysium) surrounding muscle fibers (Qian et al., 2010). Amyloid fibril fractions isolated from the muscles could also induce amyloidosis in young mice.

2.3 Cross-seeding of amyloidosis

The induction of AApoAII amyloidosis was studied *in vivo* using various kinds of amyloid fibrils that were isolated from human and mouse tissues or were formed *in vitro* from synthetic peptides and recombinant proteins. The fibrils were injected intravenously into young R1.P1-*Apoa2*^{c} mice. At 3 and 6 months after injection, the most severe amyloid depositions were detected in mice injected with mouse AApoAII(C) amyloid fibrils composed of amyloidogenic C type apoA-II, (Fu et al 2004, Yan et al., 2007). Mild amyloid depositions were also detected in tissues of mice that had been injected with other types of fibrils, including synthetic peptides and recombinant proteins. However, no amyloid depositions were found in mice injected with non-amyloid fibril proteins such as serum albumin, transthyretin and mouse apoA-II. This cross-seeding model postulates that there is a direct interaction between newly forming and preexisting heterologous amyloid fibrils *in vivo*. Thus, induction by various amyloid fibrils supports the prospect of amyloidosis acceleration in animals and humans by heterogeneous amyloid and amyloid-like fibrils in foods or the environment.

AApoAII(C) fibrils were injected intravenously into 2-month-old SAMR1 mice, which carry the less amyloidogenic apoA-II allele (*Apoa2*^{b}) and develop few, if any, spontaneous amyloid deposits. Ten months after the amyloid injection, deposits were detected on the tongue, and the intensity of deposition increased thereafter, whereas no amyloid was detected in SAMR1 mice injected with distilled water, even after 20 months (Xing et al., 2002). The deposited amyloid fibrils were composed of endogenous type B apoA-II protein, with a different amyloid fibril conformation of the proto-fibril-like figure. Subsequent injection of these AApoAII(B) fibrils induced earlier and more severe amyloidosis in SAMR1 mice than did the first injection of AApoAII(C) fibrils. Thus, adaptation of amyloid fibril structure might happen during deposition in SAMR1 mice.

AApoAII(A) fibrils composed of mild amyloidogenic apoA-II allele (*Apoa2*^{a}) were isolated from the intestine and liver of C57BL/6 mice. Atomic force microscopy and transmission electron microscopy revealed that the majority of isolated AApoAII(A) fibrils have fine, proto-fibril-like shapes. The AApoAII(A) fibril has a much weaker affinity for thioflavin T than does the AApoAII(C) fibril. The injection of AApoAII(A) fibrils induced amyloid deposition in C57BL/6 mice (*Apoa2*^{a}) as well as in R1.P1-*Apoa2*^{c} mice (*Apoa2*^{c}). However, the AApoAII(A) fibrils induced more severe amyloidosis in *Apoa2*^{a} strains than in the *Apoa2*^{c} strain (Korenaga et al., 2003).

These findings indicate that AApoAII(A) fibrils isolated from mice having the mild-amyloidogenic type A apoA-II, and AApoAII(B) fibrils isolated from mice having the less-amyloidogenic type B apoA-II, have distinct morphological, pathological and structural characteristics that differ from those of the AApoAII(C) fibrils of amyloidogenic type C apoA-II. Consequently, cross-seeding with the amyloid fibrils induced amyloid deposition in mice that had amyloid protein monomers with different primary structures.

3. Transmission of mouse reactive AA amyloidosis

AA amyloidosis, also known as reactive or secondary amyloidosis, is generally recognized as the predominant form of systemic amyloidosis that occurs in the human and animal kingdoms (Sipe & Cohen, 2000). The disease is characterized by systemic deposition, primarily in the spleen, liver and, to a lesser extent, in other organs, of extracellular fibrils composed of amyloid A protein. In most species, AA amyloidosis typically occurs secondary to chronic inflammation, infection or neoplasia. SAA protein is an acute phase apolipoprotein reactant primarily produced by hepatocytes under the control of interleukin-1, interleukin-6, and tumor necrosis factor-α (Betts et al., 1993; Hagihara et al., 2005). The plasma concentration of SAA is normally very low, but it can increase to > 1,000 mg/liter following an inflammatory stimulus. This protein can be proteolytically processed to produce an N-terminal cleavage product of approximately 44 to 100 residues that is deposited as amyloid in vital organs including the spleen, liver, and kidneys (Kisilevsky et al., 1994). AA amyloidosis occurs in patients with rheumatoid arthritis and other chronic inflammatory diseases. AA can also be induced experimentally in mice by injecting them with silver nitrate, casein, or lipopolysaccharide (LPS), which greatly increases the concentration of circulating SAA (Hoffman & Benditt, 1982). Intriguing recent data have led to the suggestion that AA amyloidosis might also be transmitted by a prion-like infectious process that involves a seeding-nucleation mechanism, a model that is widely accepted (Lundmark, et al., 2002, 2005; Cui et al., 2002). The lag phase of AA amyloidogenesis can be dramatically shortened by co-injection of "amyloid enhancing factor (AEF)" with an acute inflammatory stimulus. There is evidence that AEF is actually AA fibrils, and that AA amyloidosis might be transmitted by a prion-like mechanism.

3.1 Transmission of AA amyloidosis in cheetah and cattle

The cheetah species (*Acinonyx jubatus*) is in danger of extinction and is included on The World Conservation Union list of vulnerable species. Although efforts have been made in wildlife sanctuary parks and zoos worldwide to prevent extinction, a steady increase in the size of the cheetah population is hampered by the high prevalence of systemic AA amyloidosis, which is regarded as an increasingly important cause of morbidity and mortality in captive cheetahs (Papendick et al 1997). Inflammatory diseases, especially chronic lymphoplasmacytic gastritis, were found in 100% of cheetahs with AA amyloidosis, and environmental epidemiological studies indicate that breeding conditions have a prominent effect on the incidence of AA amyloidosis. A high rearing density is always associated with early age of onset and with a high incidence and severity of AA amyloidosis. We hypothesize that the propagation of AA amyloidosis among captive cheetah populations may depend on a horizontal transmission pathway (B. Zhang et al., 2008).

Captive cheetahs with severe AA amyloidosis were studied. AA amyloid fibrils were isolated from several tissues and the biochemical and pathological future outcomes of the animals were recorded. In particular, we hypothesized that amyloid fibrils in feces, urine and saliva would be important for the conveyance of amyloid fibrils from the body into the environment and hence for horizontal transmission. We found that cheetah feces contained AA amyloid fibrils that were different from those in the liver, having a smaller molecular weight and a shorter and finer shape. However, we could not find amyloid fibrils in the urine, and unfortunately we could not collect saliva from cheetahs. We compared the transmissibility of fecal and liver AA amyloid fibrils using the mouse experimental AA amyloidosis system. Fecal amyloid fibrils had significantly greater transmissibility (Fig. 3A). The infectious activity of fecal AA amyloid fibrils was reduced or abolished by the protein denaturants 6 M guanidine HCl and formic acid or by AA immunodepletion. With regard to the liver fraction, formic acid treatment caused a nearly complete loss of amyloid-inducing activity, whereas the guanidine-HCl-treated fraction retained high amyloid-inducing activity (Fig. 3B). Thus, we unexpectedly found that the amyloid fibril fraction from feces had smaller amyloid fibrils and higher sensitivity to denaturation treatment than the liver amyloid fibril fraction. In yeast prions, it also has been indicated that [PSI+] with stronger infectivity typically have less stable fibrils *in vivo* than strains with weaker infectivity (Krishnan & Lindquist, 2005), and the prion strain with relatively smaller prion particles is always associated with greater fragility and increased sensitivity to denaturants (Tanaka et al., 2006). Thus, we propose that feces are a potential transmission vehicle that may accelerate AA amyloidosis in captive cheetah populations. These results provide a pathogenic mechanism for AA amyloidosis and suggest possible measures for rescuing cheetahs from extinction.

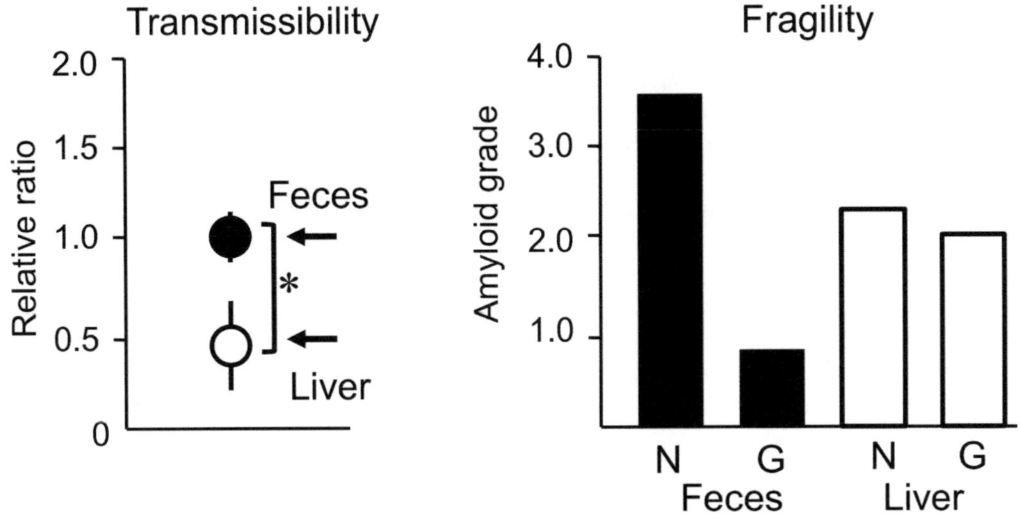

Fig. 3. **Transmissibility and fragility of fecal AA amyloid fibrils. A**: Quantification of transmissibility of AA amyloid fibrils from feces and liver. The degree of AA deposition in AA-induced mice was determined by isolation of AA amyloid fibril fractions from the spleens of mice in each group (filled circle is fecal; open circle is liver) followed by Western blot analysis and quantification using an image analyzer. The means and SE were determined by the relative ratios of AA amyloid protein levels versus the group receiving 10 μg of amyloid fibrils fraction from the feces (*, $P < 0.05$). **B**: Fecal and liver AA amyloid fibril fractions were untreated (N), or treated with guanidine-hydrochloride (G) or formic acid (F) and injected into mice to induce AA amyloidosis. Equal quantities of amyloid fractions (100 μg) were used in each experiment. The degree of amyloidosis was determined by the amyloid deposition observed in Congo red-stained sections of the spleen.

4. Analysis of transmission in mouse models of another systemic amyloidosis

Patients on long-term hemodialysis can develop dialysis-related amyloidosis (DRA) due to deposition of ß$_2$-microglobulin (ß$_2$m) into amyloid fibrils (Aß$_2$M) (Gejyo et al., 1985). Despite intensive biochemical studies, the pathogenesis of amyloid deposition in DRA patients remains poorly understood. Intact wild type ß$_2$m is unable to form amyloid fibrils under physiological conditions in test tubes. However, the addition of Aß$_2$M amyloid fibrils induces fibril formation following a nucleation dependent polymerisation model (Yamaguchi et al., 2001; Xue et al., 2008). To elucidate the mechanisms that underlie Aß$_2$M fibril formation in DRA, transgenic mice were generated that overexpress human ß$_2$m protein on a mouse ß2m gene knockout background (hB2MTg$^{+/+}$mB2m $^{-/-}$), and the possibility of transmission was examined using these model mice (P. Zhang et al., 2009).

Families with a variant transthyretins (TTR V30M)-associated familial amyloidotic polyneuropathy (FAP) exhibit genetic anticipation, with TTR V30M-amyloid depositing noted at an earlier age in successive generations (Yamamoto et al., 1998). The molecular basis of anticipation in FAP remains to be determined. The possibility that ATTR amyloid fibrils might be excreted in the milk of the FAP patients was suggested (Tokuda et al., 2007). We asked if administration of TTR-amyloid fibrils (ATTR) extracted from the heart of an FAP TTR V30M patient would accelerate ATTR deposition in transgenic mice expressing the human mutant TTR gene responsible for FAP TTR V30M (Wei et al., 2004).

4.1 Analysis of the transmission of Aß$_2$M amyloidosis in human ß$_2$m transgenic mice

Transgenic mice that overexpress human ß2m protein were generated on a mouse B2m gene knockout background (hB2MTg$^{+/+}$, mB2m$^{-/-}$). First, the pCAGGS-hB2M vector was created, and a human ß2m gene (hB2M) cDNA fragment was isolated by reverse transcription-PCR (RT-PCR) of messenger RNA extracted from human liver and cloned into pCAGGS. The hB2M cDNA was expressed under the control of the cytomegalovirus immediate early gene enhancer (CMV-IE)/chicken ß-actin promoter and rabbit ß-globin poly(A) signal (Fig. 4). The hB2M transgene copy number was determined by real-time PCR and calculated as 10 for homozygous hB2MTg$^{+/+}$. To exclude possible effects of endogenous mouse ß2m, transgenic mice were crossed with mouse ß2m (mB2m) knockout mice. The hB2MTg$^{+/+}$, mB2m$^{-/-}$ mice express a high level of human ß2m protein in many tissues and also have a high plasma ß2m concentration (192.8 mg/L). This concentration is >100 times higher than that observed in healthy humans and >4 times higher than that detected in patients on dialysis. These mice were checked for spontaneous amyloidosis, but amyloid deposition of ß2m protein was not observed in aged (~2 years) mice. Next we attempted to accelerate amyloidosis by injecting human Aß2M amyloid fibrils isolated from the amyloid-laden ligaments of the patient, and artificial amyloid fibrils were produced from recombinant human ß2m protein. Amyloid deposition of ß2m protein was not observed in animals injected with amyloid fibrils. However, mouse senile AApoAII amyloidosis was detected, particularly in the joints of mice that were injected with amyloid fibrils.

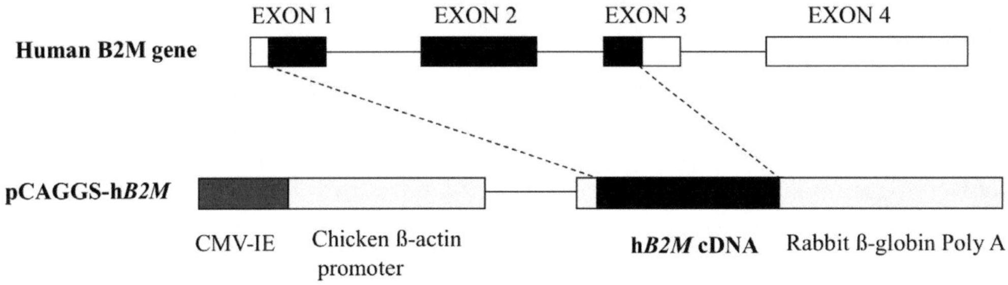

Fig. 4. **Establishment of hB2M transgenic mice.** The pCAGGS-hB2M targeting vector containing the human ß$_2$m cDNA inserted between the CMV-IE enhancer/chicken ß-actin promoter and the rabbit ß-globin poly(A) site.

This study demonstrates that this mouse model could be valuable in studying the components and conditions that promote DRA, and the results indicate that neither high plasma concentrations of hß$_2$m nor seeding with pre-existing amyloid fibrils may be sufficient to induce Aß$_2$M. We attempted to enhance amyloidosis by inducing arthritis through injection of the following substances: a monoclonal antibody against type II collagens, LPS (which induces inflammatory reactions), type I collagen and heparin solution, all of which are known to induce amyloid fibril formation in the test tube (Relini et al., 2006; Bellotti & Chiti, 2008). However, we have not been able to induce Aß$_2$M amyloid deposition in mice.

4.2 Analysis of the transmission of TTR amyloidosis in human variant TTR transgenic mice

Transgenic mice producing human variant TTR due to a mutant TTR (V30M) gene with its endogenous 6.0 kb upstream region were generated by Maeda et al (Kohno et al., 1997). The variant TTR transgene copy number was determined to be ~ 60 for homozygous h*TTR-V30M*Tg$^{+/+}$. To exclude possible effects of endogenous mouse *Ttr*, transgenic mice were crossed with *Ttr* knockout mice. The *Ttr*$^{-/-}$, h*TTR-V30M*Tg$^{+/?}$ mice expressing a high level of human variant TTR protein, which was produced mainly in the liver, were used (Fig. 5).

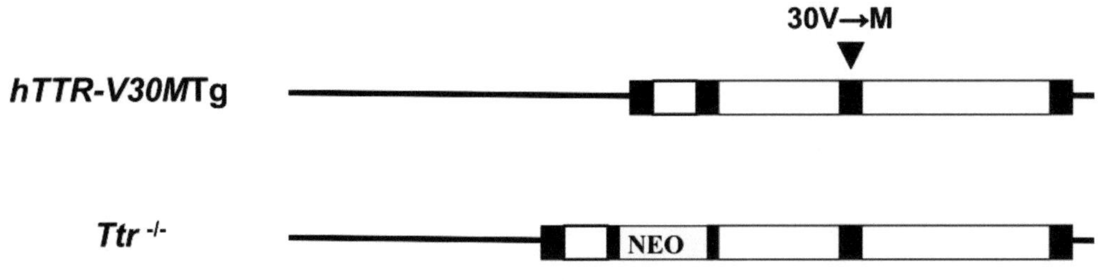

Fig. 5. **Establishment of Ttr$^{-/-}$, hTTR-V30MTg$^{+/?}$ mice.** Variant human *Ttr* transgenic mice were crossed with mouse *Ttr* knockout mice.

We asked if administration of TTR-amyloid fibrils (ATTR) extracted from the heart of an FAP TTR V30M patient would accelerate ATTR deposition in these transgenic mice. Although the administration of amyloid fibrils did accelerate deposition of AApoAII fibrils in several organs including intestine, esophagus, heart kidney, liver and so on by a cross-seeding effect, deposition of ATTR was not observed. Thus, these experiments present, for the first time, evidence that the degree of ATTR inducibility is low relative to that of AApoAII. This leads us to suggest that administration of ATTR may not explain the genetic anticipation that occurs in FAP.

5. Discussion and conclusion

The amyloidogenic SAMP1, congenic R1.P1-*ApoA2*^{c} and transgenic m*ApoA2*^{c}Tg strains did not experience spontaneous amyloid deposition when they were reared in specific pathogen free (SPF) and amyloidosis-free conditions. This finding suggested that environmental conditions affect amyloidosis and that pre-existing amyloid fibrils make a significant contribution to the transmission or induction of AApoAII amyloidosis *in vivo*. (Higuchi et al., unpublished data). Moreover, cross-seeding between heterogeneous amyloid fibrils or fibril-like structures and amyloidogenic proteins has been reported *in vitro* and *in vivo* in both mouse AApoAII and AA amyloidosis (Fu et al., 2004; P. Westermark et al., 2009). Thus, the possibility of acceleration and induction of amyloidosis in animals and humans by heterogeneous amyloid fibrils in foods or the environment should be considered (Fig.6).

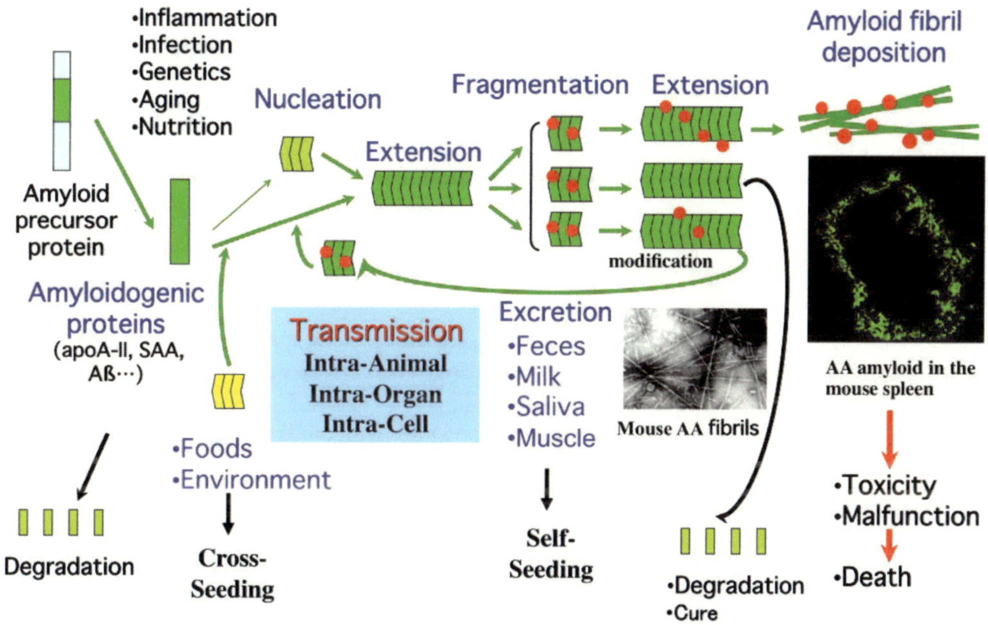

Fig. 6. **Transmission mechanism in systemic AApoAII and AA amyloidosis**. HDL-associated ApoA-II and SAA circulate in the blood. Spontaneous formation of the nucleus is slow and rare. Homologous or heterologous amyloid fibrils act as seeds and facilitate the formation of amyloid fibrils (self and cross-seeding). Extended amyloid fibrils were fragmented to make new seeds. ●: Fibril associated molecules that stabilize or modify the amyloid fibril structure. Amyloid fibrils are excreted from the body into feces, milk, saliva and muscle, and other animals may then take these into their bodies. Transmission should be observed at 3 levels; intra-animal, intra-organ and intra cells.

Recently, researchers have recognized that misfolded proteins play important roles in many neuro- degenerative diseases, including Alzheimer's disease (Eisele et al., 2010), Parkinson's disease (Hansen et al., 2011), Huntington's disease (Ren et al., 2009), tauopathies (Clavaguera et al 2009) and so on. These disorders resemble classic prion diseases, as the disease can be spread by imparting the pathological structure of the proteins to new and normal cellular counterparts, and these seeds can recruit endogenous proteins (Angot et al., 2010). Although none of these mis-folded proteins behave like typical infectious agents, the possible exception is systemic AApoAII and AA amyloidosis (Walker et al., 2006; G.T. Westermark & P. Westermark, 2010). Inter-individual infectivity of these two amyloidoses has been revealed experimentally and clinical outcomes are similar to those of the prion diseases. However, a paucity of epidemiological evidence argues against the role that transmission of amyloidosis may play in the human amyloidosis. How do the pathologic agents (amyloid fibrils) penetrate the recipient body? How do they spread throughout the body? Our studies have revealed that feces, milk, saliva and muscle are possible transporters through nasal and gastric pathways for inter-animal transmission. In particular, the amyloid fibrils in feces are noteworthy, since these fibrils showed higher fragility and transmissibility. Unstable species of infections prion (PrP^{Sc}) and yeast prion (Sup35) fibrils, which readily break and generate further free ends that can then act as seeds, have been reported to be important for transmission (Tanaka et al., 2006; Wille et al., 2009).

Analysis of amyloid fibril formation of ß$_2$m protein in test tubes revealed clearly the acceleration of fibril extension in the presence of pre-existing amyloid fibrils. However, injection of Aß$_2$M fibrils did not induce amyloidosis in transgenic mice having a high blood concentration of human ß$_2$m. Thus, transmission seems to not contribute to the development of systemic Aß$_2$M amyloidosis associated with long-term dialysis. However, the connections between *in vitro* studies performed in extreme and simplified conditions and *in vivo* observations in more complex organisms are important, and we need to improve and extend future experiments using model systems in order to understand the pathogenesis of human diseases.

The concept of transmission via self-propagating structures of proteins or by seeding is unique, and it is important to understand the pathogenesis of protein mis-folding diseases. The animal models of systemic amyloidosis described here should prove valuable in further studies of the pathogenesis, genetics, therapeutics and transmission of amyloidosis.

6. Acknowledgments

We thank Drs. Matsumoto K and Tomozawa H, Ms. Nishio A and Suzuki K, Mr. Kamatani K. (Research Support Center for Human and Environmental Sciences, Shinshu University) for animal care and technical assistance. This work was supported by the Ministry of Education, Culture, Sports, Science and Technology of Japan, Grants-in-Aid for Scientific Research (B) 20300144 and Science Research on Priority Areas 22020015, and by grants from the Intractable Disease Division, the Ministry of Health, Labor and Welfare to Research Committees for Amyloidosis.

7. References

Aguzzi, A. (2009) Beyond the prion principle. *Nature,* Vol. 459(7249): 924-925.

Bellotti, V. & Chiti F. (2008) Amyloidogenesis in its biological environment: challenging a fundamental issue in protein misfolding diseases. *Curr Opin Struct Biol,* Vol. 18 (6): 771–779.

Benson, MD., James, S., Scott, K., Liepnieks, JJ. & Kluve-Beckerman, B. (2008). Leukocyte chemotactic factor 2: A novel renal amyloid protein. *Kidney Int,* Vol.74(2): 218-222.

Betts, JC., Cheshire, JK, Akira, S., Kishimoto, T. & Woo, P. (1993) The role of NF-kappa B and NF-IL6 transactivating factors in the synergistic activation of human serum amyloid A gene expression by interleukin-1 and interleukin-6. *J. Biol. Chem,* Vol. 268 (34): 25624-25631.

Brundin, P., Melki, R., & Kopito, R. (2010) Prion-like transmission of protein aggregates in neurodegenerative diseases. *Nat Rev Mol Cell Biol.* Vol 11(4): 301-307.

Clavaguera, F., Bolmont, T., Crowther, RA., Abramowski, D., Frank, S., Probst, A., Fraser, G., Stalder, AK., Beibel, M., Staufenbiel, M., Jucker, M., Goedert, M. & Tolnay, M. (2009) Transmission and spreading of tauopathy in transgenic mouse brain. *Nat Cell Biol.* Vol. 11(7): 909-913.

Cui, D., Kawano, H., Takahashi, M., Hoshii, Y., Setoguchi, M., Gondo. T. & Ishihara, T. (2002) Acceleration of murine AA amyloidosis by oral administration of amyloid fibrils extracted from different species. *Pathol. Int,* Vol. 52(4): 264-270.

Eisele, YS., Obermüller, U., Heilbronner, G., Baumann, F., Kaeser, SA., Wolburg, H., Walker, LC., Staufenbiel, M., Heikenwalder, M. & Jucker, M. (2010) Peripherally applied Abeta-containing inoculates induce cerebral beta-amyloidosis. *Science,* Vol. 330(6006): 980-982.

Fu, L., Matsuyama, I., Chiba, T., Xing, Y., Korenaga T, Guo Z, Fu X, Nakayama J, Mori M, & Higuchi K. (2001) Extrahepatic expression of apolipoprotein A-II in mouse tissues: possible contribution to mouse senile amyloidosis. *J Histochem Cytochem,* Vol. 49(6): 739-748.

Fu, X., Korenaga, T., Fu, L., Xing, Y., Guo, Z., Matsushita, T., Hosokawa, M., Naiki, H., Baba S., Kawata, Y., Ikeda, S., Ishihara, T., Mori, M. & Higuchi K. (2004) Induction of AApoAII amyloidosis by various heterogeneous amyloid fibrils. *FEBS Lett,* Vol. 563(1-3): 179-184.

Ge, F., Yao, J., Fu, X., Guo, Z., Yan, J., Zhang, B., Zhang, H., Tomozawa, H., Miyazaki, J., Sawashita, J., Mori, M. & Higuchi, K. (2007) Amyloidosis in transgenic mice expressing murine amyloidogenic apolipoprotein A-II (*Apoa2^{c}*). *Lab Invest,* Vol. 87(7): 633-643.

Gejyo, F., Yamada, T., Odani, S., Nakagawa, Y., Arakawa, M., Kunitomo, T., Kataoka, H., Suzuki, M., Hirasawa, Y., Shirahama, T., et al. (1985) A new form of amyloid protein associated with chronic hemodialysis was identified as b2-microglobulin. *Biochem Biophys Res Commun,* Vol. 129(3): 701–706.

Hagihara, K., Nishikawa, T., Sugamata, Y., Song, J., Isobe, T., Taga, T. & Yoshizaki, K. (2005) Essential role of STAT3 in cytokine-driven NF-kappaB-mediated serum amyloid A gene expression. *Genes Cells.* Vol.10 (11): 1051-1063.

Hansen, C., Angot, E., Bergström, AL., Steiner, JA., Pieri, L., Paul, G., Outeiro, TF., Melki, R., Kallunki, P., Fog, K., Li, JY. & Brundin, P. (2011) α-Synuclein propagates from mouse brain to grafted dopaminergic neurons and seeds aggregation in cultured human cells. *J Clin Invest.* Vol. 121(2): 715-725.

Harper, JD., & Lansbury, PT Jr. (1997) Models of amyloid seeding in Alzheimer's disease and scrapie: mechanistic truths and physiological consequences of the time-dependent solubility of amyloid proteins. *Annu Rev Biochem,* Vol. 66: 385-407.

Higuchi, K., Matsumura, A., Hashimoto, K., Honma, A., Takeshita, S., Hosokawa, M., Yasuhira, K. & Takeda, T. (1983) Isolation and characterization of senile amyloid--related antigenic substance (SASSAM) from mouse serum. Apo SASSAM is a low molecular weight apoprotein of high density lipoprotein. *J Exp Med,* Vol. 158((5): 1600-1614.

Higuchi, K., Matsumura, A., Honma, A., Takeshita, S., Hashimoto, K., Hosokawa, M., Yasuhira., K. & Takeda, T. (1983) Systemic senile amyloid in senescence-accelerated mice. A unique fibril protein demonstrated in tissues from various organs by the unlabeled immunoperoxidase method. *Lab Invest,* Vol. 48(2): 231-240.

Higuchi, K,. Yonezu, T., Kogishi, K., Matsumura, A., Takeshita, S., Higuchi, K., Kohno, A., Matsushita, M., Hosokawa, M. & Takeda, T. (1986) Purification and characterization of a senile amyloid-related antigenic substance (apoSASSAM) from mouse serum. apoSAS$_{SAM}$ is an apoA-II apolipoprotein of mouse high density lipoprotein *J Biol Chem,* Vol. 261(27): 12834-12840.

Higuchi, K., Kitagawa, K., Naiki, H., Hanada, K., Hosokawa, M. & Takeda T. (1991) Polymorphism of apolipoprotein A-II (apoA-II) among inbred strains of mice. Relationship between the molecular type of apoA-II and mouse senile amyloidosis. Biochem J, 279 (2): 427-433.

Higuchi, K., Kitado, H., Kitagawa, K., Kogishi, K., Naiki, H. & Takeda T. (1993) Development of congenic strains of mice carrying amyloidogenic apolipoprotein A-II (*Apoa2^c*). *Apoa2^c* reduces the plasma level and the size of high density lipoprotein. *FEBS Lett,* Vol. 317(3): 207-210.

Higuchi, K., Naiki, H., Kitagawa, K., Kitado H, Kogishi K, Matsushita T. & Takeda T. (1995) Apolipoprotein A-II gene and development of amyloidosis and senescence in a congenic strain of mice carrying amyloidogenic ApoA-II. *Lab Invest,* Vol. 72(1): 75-82.

Higuchi, K., Wang, J., Kitagawa, K., Matsushita, T., Kogishi, K., Naiki, H., Kitado, H., & Hosokawa, M. (1996) Accelerated senile amyloidosis induced by amyloidogenic ApoA-II gene shortens the life span of mice but does not accelerate the rate of senescence. *J Gerontol A Biol Sci Med Sci,* Vol. 51(4): B295-B302.

Higuchi, K., Kogishi, K., Wang, J., Chen, X., Chiba, T., Matsushita, T., Hoshii, Y., Kawano, H., Ishihara, T., Yokota, T. & Hosokawa M. (1998) Fibrilization in mouse senile amyloidosis is fibril conformation-dependent. *Lab. Invest.* Vol.78(12): 1535-1542.

Higuchi, K., Hosokawa, M. & Takeda, T. (1999) Senescence-accelerated mouse. *Methods Enzymol.* Vol. 309: 674-686.

Hoffman, J.S, & Benditt, EP. (1982) Changes in high density lipoprotein content following endotoxin administration in the mouse. Formation of serum amyloid protein-rich subfractions. *J Biol Chem,* Vol. 257(17): 10510-10517.

Jarrett, JT. & Lansbury, PT Jr. (1993) Seeding "one-dimensional crystallization" of amyloid: a pathogenic mechanism in Alzheimer's disease and scrapie? *Cell.* Vol. 73(6): 1055-1058.

Kisilevsky, R., Narindrasorasak, S., Tape, C., Tan, R., & Boudreau, L. (1994) During AA amyloidogenesis is proteolytic attack on serum amyloid A a pre- or post-fibrillogenic event? *Amyloid,* Vol. 1(3), 174-183.

Kitagawa, K., Wang, J., Mastushita, T., Kogishi, K., Hosokawa, M., Fu, X., Guo, Z., Mori, M. & Higuchi K. (2003) Polymorphisms of mouse apolipoprotein A-II: seven alleles found among 41 inbred strains of mice. *Amyloid,* Vol. 10(4): 207-214.

Kohno, K., Palha, JA., Miyakawa, K., Saraiva, MJ., Ito, S., Mabuchi, T., Blaner, WS., Iijima, H., Tsukahara, S., Episkopou, V., Gottesman, ME., Shimada, K., Takahashi, K., Yamamura, K. & Maeda S. (1997) Analysis of amyloid deposition in a transgenic mouse model of homozygous familial amyloidotic polyneuropathy. *Am J Pathol.* Vol. 150(4): 1497-508.

Korenaga, T., Fu, X., Xing, Y., Matsusita, T., Kuramoto, K., Syumiya, S., Hasegawa, Z., Naiki, H., Ueno, M., Ishihara, T., Hosokawa, M., Mori, M. & Higuchi K. (2004) Tissue distribution, biochemical properties, and transmission of mouse type A AApoAII amyloid fibrils. *Am. J. Pathol,* Vol. 164(5): 1597-19606.

Korenaga, T., Yan, J., Sawashita, J., Matsushita, T., Naiki, H., Hosokawa, M., Mori, M., Higuchi, K. & Fu X. (2006) Transmission of amyloidosis in offspring of mice with AApoAII amyloidosis. *Am J Pathol,* Vol. 168(3): 898-906.

Krishnan, R. & Lindquist, SL (2005) Structural insights into a yeast prion illuminate nucleation and strain diversity. *Nature* Vol. 435 435(7043): 765-772

Kunisada, T., Higuchi, K., Aota, S., Takeda, T. & Yamagishi, H. (1986) Molecular cloning and nucleotide sequence of cDNA for murine senile amyloid protein: nucleotide substitutions found in apolipoprotein A-II cDNA of senescence accelerated mouse (SAM). *Nucleic Acids Res,* Vol. 14(14): 5729-5740.

Lundmark, K., Westermark, GT., Nystrom, S., Murphy, CL., Solomon, A. & Westermark P. (2002) Transmissibility of systemic amyloidosis by a prion-like mechanism.*Proc. Natl. Acad. Sci. U S A.*, Vol. 99(10): 6979-6984. Erratum. 2003, *Proc. Natl. Acad. Sci. U S A.* Vol. 100(6), 3543.

Lundmark, K., Westermark, GT, Olsén A. & Westermark, P. (2005) Protein fibrils in nature can enhance amyloid protein A amyloidosis in mice: Cross-seeding as a disease mechanism. *Proc Natl Acad Sci U S A.* Vol. 102(17): 6098-6102.

Naiki, H., Higuchi, K., Nakakuki, K. & Takeda, T. (1991) Kinetic analysis of amyloid fibril polymerization in vitro. *Lab Invest,* Vol. 65(1): 104-110. Erratum in: *Lab Invest,* 67(5): 652.

Naiki, H., Higuchi, K., Shimada, A., Takeda, T. & Nakakuki, K. (1993) Genetic analysis of murine senile amyloidosis. *Lab Invest,* Vol. 68(3): 332-337.

Papendick, RE., Munson, L., O'Brien, TD. & Johnson, KH (1997) Systemic AA amyloidosis in captive cheetahs (Acinonyx jubatus). *Vet Pathol,* Vol. 34(6): 549–556.

Prusiner, SB., Scott, MR., DeArmond, SJ. & Cohen, FE. (1998) Prion protein biology. *Cell,* Vol. 93(3): 337-348.

Prusiner, SB. & McCarty, M. (2006) Discovering DNA encodes heredity and prions are infectious proteins. *Annu Rev Genet*, Vol. 40: 25-45.

Qian, J., Yan, J., Ge, F., Zhang, B., Fu, X., Tomozawa, H., Sawashita, J., Mori, M. & Higuchi, K. (2010) Mouse senile amyloid fibrils deposited in skeletal muscle exhibit amyloidosis-enhancing activity. *PLoS Pathog*. Vol. 6(5): e1000914.

Ren, PH., Lauckner, JE., Kachirskaia, I., Heuser, JE., Melki, R. & Kopito, RR. (2009) Cytoplasmic penetration and persistent infection of mammalian cells by polyglutamine aggregates. *Nat Cell Biol*, Vol. 11(2): 219-225.

Sawashita, J., Kametani, F., Hasegawa, K., Tsutsumi-Yasuhara S, Zhang B, Yan J, Mori M, Naiki H. & Higuchi K. (2009). Amyloid fibrils formed by selective N-, C-terminal sequences of mouse apolipoprotein A-II. *Biochim Biophys Acta*; Vol. 1794(10): 1517-1529.

Sipe, JD. & Cohen, AS. (2000) Review: history of the amyloid fibril.*J Struct Biol*. Vol. 130(2-3): 88-89.

Sipe, JD.; Benson, MD., Buxbaum, JN., Ikeda, S., Merlini, G., Saraiva, MJ. & Westermark, P. (2010). Amyloid fibril protein nomenclature: 2010 recommendations from the nomenclature committee of the International Society of Amyloidosis. *Amyloid.* Vol.17 (3-4), 101-104.

Takeda, T., Hosokawa, M., Takeshita, S., Irino, M., Higuchi, K., Matsushita, T., Tomita, Y., Yasuhira, K., Hamamoto, H., Shimizu, K., Ishii, M. & Yamamuro, T. (1981) A new murine model of accelerated senescence. *Mech. Ageing Dev.*, Vol 17(2): 183-194.

Takeshita, S., Hosokawa, M., Irino, M., Higuchi, K., Shimizu, K., Yasuhira, K. & Takeda, T. (1982) Spontaneous age-associated amyloidosis in senescence-accelerated mouse (SAM). *Mech Ageing Dev,* Vol. 20(1): 13-23.

Tanaka, M., Collins, SR., Toyama, BH. & Weissman, JS. (2006) The physical basis of how prion conformations determine strain phenotypes. *Nature* Vol. 442 (7102): 585–589.

Tojo, K., Tokuda, T., Hoshii, Y., Fu, X., Higuchi, K., Matsui, T., Kametani, F., & Ikeda S. Unexpectedly high incidence of visceral AA-amyloidosis in slaughtered cattle in Japan. *Amyloid.* 12(2): 103-108.

Tokuda, T., Takei, Y., Takayama, B., Hoshii, Y. & Ikeda S. (2007) Severe amyloid deposition in mammary glands of familial amyloid polyneuropathy patients. *Amyloid.* Vol. 14(3): 249-253.

Walker, LC., Levine, H3rd., Mattson, MP. & Jucker, M. (2006) Inducible proteopathies. *Trends Neurosci,* Vol. 29(8): 438-443.

Wei, L., Kawano, H., Fu, X., Cui, D., Ito, S., Yamamura, K., Ishihara, T., Tokuda, T., Higuchi, K. & Maeda S. (2004) Deposition of transthyretin amyloid is not accelerated by the same amyloid *in vivo*. *Amyloid.* Vol. 11(2): 113-120.

Weissmann, C. (1999) Molecular genetics of transmissible spongiform encephalopathies. *J Biol Chem,* Vol. 274(1): 3-6.

Westermark, GT. & Westermark P. (2010) Prion-like aggregates: infectious agents in human disease. *Trends Mol Med.* Vol. 16(11): 501-507.

Westermark, P., Lundmark, K. & Westermark GT. (2009) Fibrils from designed non-amyloid-related synthetic peptides induce AA-amyloidosis during inflammation in an animal model. *PLoS One*. Vol. 4(6): e6041.

Wille, H., Bian, W., McDonald, M., Kendall, A., Colby, DW., Bloch, L., Ollesch, J., Borovinskiy, AL., Cohen, FE., Prusiner, SB. & Stubbs, G. (2009) Natural and synthetic prion structure from X-ray fiber diffraction. *Proc Natl Acad Sci U S A*. Vol. 106(40): 16990-16995.

Xing, Y., Nakamura, A., Chiba, T., Kogishi, K., Matsushita, T., Li, F., Guo, Z., Hosokawa, M., Mori, M. & Higuchi K. (2001) Transmission of mouse senile amyloidosis. *Lab Invest*. Vol. 81(4): 493-499.

Xing, Y., Nakamura, A., Korenaga, T., Guo, Z., Yao, J., Fu, X., Matsushita, T., Kogishi, K., Hosokawa, M., Kametani, F., Mori, M. & Higuchi, K. (2002), Induction of protein conformational change in mouse senile amyloidosis. *J Biol Chem*, 277(36): 33164-33169.

Xue, WF., Homans, SW. & Radford, SE. (2008) Systematic analysis of nucleation-dependent polymerization reveals new insights into the mechanism of amyloid self-assembly. *Proc Natl Acad Sci U S A*, Vol. 105(26): 8926–8931

Yamada, M., Kotani, Y., Nakamura, K., Kobayashi, Y., Horiuchi, N., Doi, T., Suzuki, S., Sato, N., Kanno, T. & Matsui T. (2006) Immunohistochemical distribution of amyloid deposits in 25 cows diagnosed with systemic AA amyloidosis. *J Vet Med Sci*. 68(7): 725-729.

Yamaguchi, I., Hasegawa, K., Naiki, H., Mitsu, T., Matuo, Y. & Gejyo, F. (2001) Extension of Aß$_2$M amyloid fibrils with recombinant human ß$_2$-microglobulin. *Amyloid* Vol. 8(1): 30–40.

Yamamoto, K., Ikeda, S., Hanyu, N., Takeda, S. & Yanagisawa, N. (1998) A pedigree analysis with minimised ascertainment bias shows anticipation in Met30-transthyretin related familial amyloid polyneuropathy. *J Med Genet*. Vol.35(1): 23-30.

Yan, J., Fu, X., Ge F., Zhang, B, Yao, J., Zhang, H., Qian, J., Tomozawa, H., Naiki, H., Sawashita, J., Mori, M. & Higuchi K. (2007) Cross-seeding and cross-competition in mouse apolipoprotein A-II amyloid fibrils and protein A amyloid fibrils. *Am J Pathol*. 171(1): 172-1780.

Yonezu, T., Higuchi, K., Tsunasawa, S., Takagi, S., Sakiyama, F. & Takeda, T. (1986) High homology is present in the primary structures between murine senile amyloid protein (ASSAM) and human apolipoprotein A-II. *FEBS Lett*, Vol. 203(2): 149-152.

Yoshida, T., Zhang, P., Fu, X., Higuchi, K. & Ikeda S. (2009) Slaughtered aged cattle might be one dietary source exhibiting amyloid enhancing factor activity. *Amyloid*. 16(1): 25-31.

Zhang, B., Une, Y., Fu, X., Yan, J., Ge, F., Yao, J., Sawashita, J., Mori, M., Tomozawa, H., Kametani, F. & Higuchi, K. (2008) Fecal transmission of AA amyloidosis in the cheetah contributes to high incidence of disease. *Proc Natl Acad Sci U S A*. Vol. 105(20): 7263-7268.

Zhang, H., Sawashita, J., Fu, X., Korenaga, T., Yan, J., Mori, M., & Higuchi. K. (2006) Transmissibility of mouse AApoAII amyloid fibrils: inactivation by physical and chemical methods. *FASEB J* Vol. 20(7): 1012–1014.

Zhang, P., Fu, X., Sawashita, J., Yao, J., Zhang, B., Qian, J., Tomozawa, H., Mori, M., Ando, Y., Naiki, H. & Higuchi K. (2010) Mouse model to study human Aß2M amyloidosis: generation of a transgenic mouse with excessive expression of human ß2-microglobulin. *Amyloid*. Vol. 17(2): 50-62.

10

Transthyretin Amyloidosis in Aged Vervet Monkeys, as a Candidate for the Spontaneous Animal Model of Senile Systemic Amyloidosis

Shinichiro Nakamura[1], Mitsuharu Ueda[2], Naohide Ageyama[3], Yukio Ando[2] and Ryuzo Torii[1]

[1]*Research Center for Animal Life Science, Shiga University of Medical Science,*
[2]*Department of Diagnostic Medicine, Graduate School of Medical Sciences, Kumamoto University,*
[3]*Tsukuba Primate Research Center, National Institute of Biomedical Innovation, Japan*

1. Introduction

Transthyretin (TTR) amyloidosis is classified into systemic senile amyloidosis (SSA), due to senescent events caused by the wild type TTR gene, and familial amyloidotic cardiomyopathy (FAC) and familial amyloidotic polyneuropathy (FAP), which are inherited diseases caused by mutant TTR genes (Ando et al., 2005; Buxbaum, 2009; Rapezzi et al., 2010). TTR is biochemically stable as a tetramer; however unstable as a monomer when the amyloid fibrillogenesis is higher (Damas et al., 2005). Non-fibrillar TTR deposits can be first detected immunohistochemically in the heart of humans with SSA, and finally in the peripheral nerves of those with FAP. After the non-fibrillar TTR deposits, congophilic and/or fibrillar amyloids consisting of TTR can be detected and are consistent with immunopositive lesions for TTR (Damas et al., 2005; Sousa et al., 2002).

Although animal models of SSA and FAP are strong tools to develop therapeutic agents and diagnostic materials, as well as to understand the pathomechanism (Buxbaum, 2009), spontaneous TTR amyloidosis has not yet been reported in animals. Therefore, a model has been developed using transgenic (Tg) techniques, such as Tg mice and rats with human mutant TTR genes (Buxbaum, 2009; Ueda et al., 2007). However, these model rodents do not show enough phenotypes resembling the clinical signs and histopathological features of SSA and FAP. In histopathological examinations, some Tg rodents tended to be hardly detected with fibrillar amyloid deposits, even if they reveal abundant non-fibrillar TTR immunoreactivity.

Nakamura et al. (2008) observed SSA in an aged vervet monkey that showed typical clinical symptoms and histopathological features, as well as the human form of SSA. Furthermore, another group followed up on our findings (Chambers et al., 2010). Both cases revealed not only non-fibrillar TTR immunoreactivity but also fibrillar amyloid deposits. Thus, since the vervet monkey shows more mature TTR amyloid formation than Tg rodents, it could be a novel animal model for TTR amyloidosis.

2. Animal models for TTR amyloidosis

2.1 Rodent models

The main strategy used to develop an animal model for TTR amyloidosis is to transfect mutant human TTR genes to mice because spontaneous TTR amyloidosis has not been reported in mammalian species before 2008 other than in humans. Because TTR is synthesized from hepatocytes, most Tg rodent lines are produced using the hepatocyte-specific metallothionein promoter (Karin et al., 1987). The first Tg mice, transfected with human V30M TTR (valine substituted for methionine at the human TTR 30 residue), expressed mutant TTR in the fetal liver and yolk sac (Yamamura et al., 1987) and showed significant increase in serum concentrations of a TTR variant (Sasaki et al., 1986) but failed to show TTR immunoreactivity or amyloid deposits. Yi et al. (1991) improved the next Tg mouse line, which they attempted to create by transfecting mice with an increased number of TTR V30M gene copies. This Tg line showed slight TTR amyloid deposition in the gastrointestinal and cardiovascular organs in 6-month-old mice, which revealed SSA-like systemic amyloid deposits at 24 months. Takaoka et al. (1997) inserted 0.6 kb or 6 kb fragments upstream of the V30M TTR gene. Tg mice with the 6-kb upstream insert showed a high enough concentration of human TTR in serum, corresponding with that in normal humans, but 10-fold greater than that in wild type-mice. An increasing TTR concentration was seen in 1-month-old animals with the 6-kb upstream insert, whereas TTR amyloid deposits appeared in the gastrointestinal tract of mice at 9 months and in their systemic organs at 21 months. In Tg mice with the 0.6-kb upstream insert, some amyloid deposits appeared at 15 months, particularly in the gastrointestinal tract. The density of the amyloid deposits in mice with the 6-kb upstream insert was more severe than in mice with the 0.6-kb insert. However, no TTR immunoreactivity or amyloid deposits were found in peripheral nerves of either mouse types.

Additional TTR Tg mice transfected with the human wild type TTR gene and an L55P mutant TTR gene (leucine substituted for proline at the human TTR 55 residue) were developed by Sousa and Teng et al. (Sousa et al., 2001; Teng et al., 2001). Mice with the L55P TTR mutant did not reveal amyloid deposition at 2.5 years because they had only one copy of the inserted gene. In contrast, mice with wild type TTR gene, which had 100 copies inserted, revealed amyloid deposits consisting of TTR in the heart, gastrointestinal tract, and kidneys at 18 months. Amyloid-affected male mice were more abundant than amyloid-affected female mice. Thus, the incidence and histopathological features mimicked human SSA. Furthermore, TTR immunoreactivity was observed in both females and males before the appearance of congophilic amyloid deposits formed, as the early stage of FAP (Sousa et al., 2002).

However, amyloid deposits in Tg mice are less frequently observed than in human SSA or FAP cases. Indeed, amyloid formation is inhibited by the human/mouse hybrid hetero-tetramer TTR in all Tg mice lines, which is extremely stable biochemically (Reixach et al., 2008; Tagoe et al., 2007). Human TTR immunoreactivity of amyloid deposits increased in interstitial tissues of a crossbreed between L55P TTR Tg and TTR null-mice due to decreased formation of the hybrid hetero-tetramer TTR (Tagoe et al., 2007).

An association between co-factors and TTR-amyloid formation in Tg mice is easy to confirm. Another line of crossbred mice (KO) was developed between L55P TTR Tg and heat shock factor protein 1 (HSF1), a TTR molecular chaperone protein in KO mice (Santos et al., 2010). These mice showed 2–3-fold more frequent amyloid deposits than in wild type TTR Tg mice and revealed TTR immunoreactivity not only in the cutaneous tissues and gastrointestinal system but also in the peripheral nerves at 3 months of age. The extra-neural tissue lesions developed further into congophilic amyloid deposits, whereas those in peripheral nerves did not. TTR immunoreactivity in peripheral nerves is thought to be an early change prior to congophilic amyloid formation (Sousa et al., 2001).

A retinol-biding site occurs at residue 84 in the TTR amino acid sequence. TTR Tg mice with I84S (isoleucine substituted for serine at human TTR residue 84) failed to show any amyloid deposits (Waits et al., 1995).

According to the findings from these crossbred mice, strong overexpression of the mutant TTR gene is insufficient for TTR amyloid fibrogenesis. Amyloid formation increase in V30M TTR Tg mice were maintained under standard conditions but not under specific pathogen-free conditions (Inoue et al., 2008; Noguchi et al., 2002), suggesting that microbiological conditions and consequent immunological events are closely associated with amyloid formation. Amyloid formation is required not only for misfolding of the precursor proteins but also other factors including microbiological exposure to the immune system (Muchowski, 2002; Noguchi et al., 2002). Moreover, possible associations with chaperone proteins, such as amyloid P component, apolipoprotein E, and HSF1 should also be considered (Nakamura et al., 2008; Santos et al., 2010; Wood et al., 2005).

Other than Tg rodents, amyloid deposits consisting of mouse endogenous TTR have been found in senescence-accelerated mice, but this is supported by only one spontaneous report of TTR amyloidosis in rodents (Higuchi et al., 1991), although the strain in this report possessed a unique genetic background. Ueda et al. (2007) reported a TTR Tg rat transfected with V30M TTR that was TTR immunoreactive but did not have congophilic amyloid deposition in the gastrointestinal tract.

2.2 Nonhuman primate models

TTR amyloidosis has been reported in two male vervet monkeys (Table 1, cases 3 and 5) (Chambers et al., 2010, Nakamura et al., 2008), and we obtained one additional aged male case (Table 1, case 4) that revealed TTR amyloid deposits (data not shown). The remaining four monkeys (Table 1, cases 1, 2, 6, and 7) were examined histopathologically but did not contain amyloid deposits. Although all positive cases were males (similar to human SSA findings), understanding the epidemiological aspects of the disease is expected with additional cases. A characteristic symptom in case 5, mimicking human SSA, was an arrhythmia detected by electrocardiography (Fig. 1), whereas the SSA characteristics were confirmed by gross and histopathological findings in case 3. In both cases, the hearts revealed dilatation of both ventricles at necropsy, but the dilatation in case 3 was more severe than in case 5. In contrast, the histopathological density of amyloid deposits was more severe in case 5 than in case 3. The most severe amyloid deposits were observed in the heart of case 5. Myocardium and stroma were multifocally replaced by hyaline deposits as amyloid. The amyloid deposits were further found in the thyroid gland, tonsils, salivary glands, trachea, esophagus, thymus, lungs, gastrointestinal organs, kidneys, prostate gland, urinary bladder, lymph nodes, and skeletal muscle. In case 3, amyloid deposits were observed not only in the heart, gastrointestinal tract, liver, spleen, and kidneys, but also in the tenosynovium tissues, which were grossly hemorrhaged. These amyloid deposits are resistant to potassium permanganate, show apple green birefringence under a polarizing microscope (Fig. 2), and are TTR immunopositive (Fig. 3). Although most amyloid deposits in vervet monkeys are consistent with TTR immunoreactivity, TTR immunopositivity without congophilic amyloids was observed only in the testes of case 5. These were thought to be non-fibrillar precursor amyloid deposits that occur prior to congophilic amyloid deposits (Sousa et al., 2001, Teng et al., 2001).

Case No.	Age (Year)	Sex *	Facility **	Cause of death ***	TTR-amyloid deposits
1	17	F	E	Uterine myoma	-
2	25	M	E	Cardiac failure	-
3	26	M	Z	Cardiac failure	+
4	27	M	E	Thoracic tumor	+
5	29	M	E	Cardiac failure	+
6	>30	F	E	ND	-
7	>30	F	Z	ND	-

*: F; Female, M; Male

**: E; Experimental Animal Facility, Z; Zoo

***: ND; Not determined

+: Positive

-: Negative

Table 1. Profiles of postmortem specimen of aged vervet monkey.

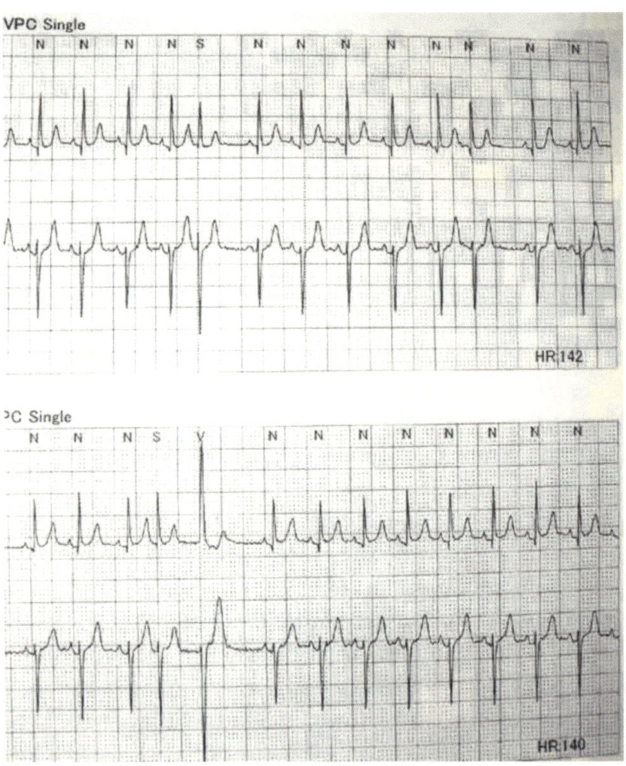

Fig. 1. Arrhythmia detected by electrocardiography in case 5.

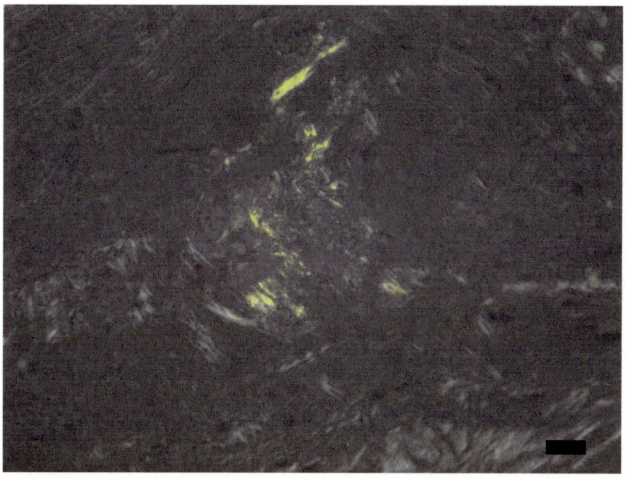

Fig. 2. Apple green birefringence was observed under a polarizing microscope in the heart of case 5; Congo red staining; bar, 25 μm.

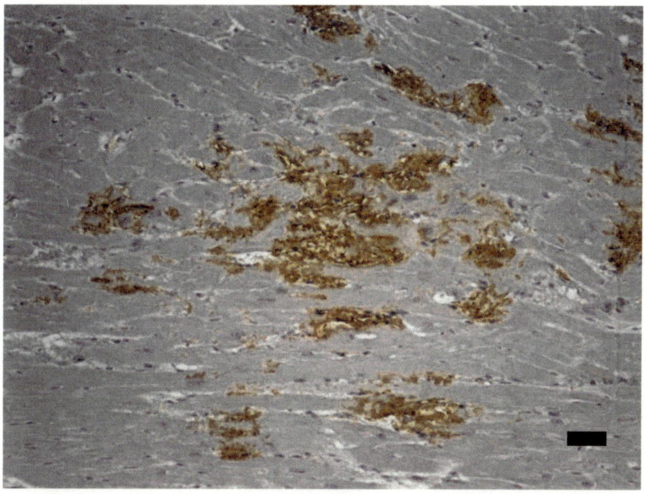

Fig. 3. Transthyretin (TTR) immunoreactivity in the heart of case 5; TTR immunostain; bar, 50 μm.

We observed seven vervet monkey cases (Table 1; average age, 26.3 ± 1.71 years; range, 17–30 years). Three of the four males were positive for amyloid deposits, whereas all three females were negative. The incidence of TTR in aged male monkeys seems to be very high and reflects the features of human SSA (Rapezzi et al., 2010). In contrast, 42 cynomolgus monkeys (*Macaca fascicularis*; average age, 18.5 ± 1.33 years; range, 4–36 years) failed to show any TTR immunoreactivity or amyloid deposits in heart specimens (data not shown).

Both vervet and cynomolgus monkeys belong to Cercopithecoidea, and they have a close evolutionary relationship. However, the onset of TTR amyloidosis differs, which may be due to differences in amino acid sequences. The TTR amino acid sequence in nonhuman primates has been clarified in the chimpanzee (*Pan troglodytes*, AAV41026; Nadezhdin et al., 2001), orangutan (*Pongo abelii*, CAI29591), cynomolgus monkey (BAC20609), rhesus monkey (*Macaca mulatta*, XP_001099005), common marmoset (*Callithrix jacchus*, XP_002757195), and Bolivian squirrel monkey (*Saimiri boliviensis*, AAV74285) (Fig. 4). Homologies between human and nonhuman primate TTRs (including the signal peptide) are 97.3% with chimpanzee, 95.2% with orangutan, 93.9% with cynomolgus monkey, 93.2% with rhesus monkey, and 78.9% with the common marmoset and Bolivian squirrel monkey. The lower homology with New world monkeys (marmoset and squirrel monkey) is due to a deletion of four to six residues and some TTR N-terminal substitutions. The homology of human and mouse TTRs is 81.0%. Although human FAP is induced by an amino acid substitution, major residues with substitution in FAP (residues at 30, 33, 45, 53, 55, 60, 69, 77, 84, 88, 111, and 122) (Rapezzi et al., 2010) are conserved as human wild type in nonhuman primate species. The TTR amino acid sequence in vervet monkeys is expected to be clarified and is predicted to be very similar to cynomolgus and rhesus monkeys because they are very closely related species, belonging to Cercopithecoidea. However, substitution at the mutated residue position in FAP is predicted in vervet monkeys.

Signal peptide

	-20	-19	-18	-17	-16	-15	-14	-13	-12	-11	-10	-9	-8	-7	-6	-5	-4	-3	-2	-1		1	2	3	4	5	6	7	8	9	10	11	12	13	14	15	16	17	18	19
Human	M	A	S	H	R	L	L	L	L	C	L	A	G	L	V	F	V	S	E	A		G	P	T	G	T	G	E	S	K	C	P	L	M	V	K	V	L	D	A
Chimpanzee	M	A	S	H	R	L	L	L	L	C	L	A	G	L	V	F	V	S	E	A		G	P	T	G	T	G	E	S	K	C	P	L	M	V	K	V	L	D	A
Orangutan	M	A	S	H	R	L	L	L	L	C	L	A	G	L	V	F	V	S	E	A		G	P	T	G	A	G	E	S	K	C	P	L	M	V	K	V	L	D	A
Cynomolgus monkey	M	A	S	H	R	L	L	L	L	C	L	A	G	L	V	F	V	S	E	A		G	P	T	G	V	D	E	S	K	C	P	L	M	V	K	V	L	D	A
Rhesus monkey	M	A	S	H	R	L	L	L	L	C	L	A	G	L	V	F	V	S	E	A		G	P	T	G	V	D	E	S	K	C	P	L	M	V	K	V	L	D	A
Marmoset	M	A	S	H	R	L	L	L	L	C	L	A	G	L	V	F	V	S	E	A		G	P	T	-	-	-	G	Y	S	C	P	L	M	V	K	V	L	D	A
Borivian squirrel monkey	M	A	S	H	H	L	L	L	L	C	L	A	G	L	V	F	V	S	E	A		G	H	T	-	-	-	G	Y	S	C	P	L	M	V	K	V	L	D	A
Mouse	M	A	S	L	R	L	F	L	L	C	L	A	G	L	V	F	V	S	E	A		G	P	A	G	A	G	E	S	K	C	P	L	M	V	K	V	L	D	A

	21	22	23	24	25	26	27	28	29	30	31	32	33	34	35	36	37	38	39	40	41	42	43	44	45	46	47	48	49	50	51	52	53	54	55	56	57	58	59	60
Human	R	G	S	P	A	I	N	V	A	V	H	V	F	R	K	A	A	D	D	T	W	E	P	F	A	S	G	K	T	S	E	S	G	E	L	H	G	L	T	T
Chimpanzee	R	G	S	P	A	I	N	V	A	V	H	V	F	K	K	A	A	D	E	T	W	E	P	F	A	S	G	K	T	S	E	S	G	E	L	H	G	L	T	T
Orangutan	R	G	S	P	A	V	N	V	A	V	N	V	F	K	R	A	A	D	E	T	W	E	P	F	A	S	G	K	T	S	E	S	G	E	L	H	G	L	T	T
Cynomolgus monkey	R	G	S	P	A	V	N	V	A	V	N	V	F	K	K	A	A	D	E	T	W	A	P	F	A	S	G	K	T	S	E	S	G	E	L	H	G	L	T	T
Rhesus monkey	R	G	S	P	A	V	N	V	A	V	N	V	F	K	K	A	A	D	E	T	W	A	P	F	A	S	G	K	T	S	E	S	G	E	L	H	G	L	T	T
Marmoset	Q	G	R	P	A	V	N	V	A	V	S	V	F	K	K	A	A	D	E	T	W	E	P	F	A	F	G	K	T	S	E	S	G	E	L	H	G	L	T	T
Borivian squirrel monkey	Q	G	R	P	A	I	N	V	A	V	S	V	F	K	K	A	A	D	E	T	W	E	P	F	A	L	G	K	T	S	E	S	G	E	L	H	G	L	T	T
Mouse	R	G	S	P	A	V	D	V	A	V	K	V	F	K	K	T	S	E	G	S	W	E	P	F	A	S	G	K	T	A	E	S	G	E	L	H	G	L	T	T

	61	62	63	64	65	66	67	68	69	70	71	72	73	74	75	76	77	78	79	80	81	82	83	84	85	86	87	88	89	90	91	92	93	94	95	96	97	98	99	100
Human	E	E	E	F	V	E	G	I	Y	K	V	E	I	D	T	K	S	Y	W	K	A	L	G	I	S	P	F	H	E	H	A	E	V	V	F	T	A	N	D	S
Chimpanzee	E	E	E	F	V	E	G	I	Y	K	V	E	I	D	T	K	S	Y	W	K	A	L	G	I	S	P	F	H	E	H	A	E	V	V	F	T	A	N	D	S
Orangutan	E	E	E	F	V	E	G	I	Y	K	V	E	I	D	T	K	S	Y	W	K	A	L	G	I	S	P	F	H	E	H	A	E	V	V	F	A	A	N	D	S
Cynomolgus monkey	E	E	E	F	V	E	G	I	Y	K	V	E	I	D	T	K	S	Y	W	K	S	L	G	I	S	P	F	H	E	H	A	E	V	V	F	T	A	N	D	S
Rhesus monkey	E	E	E	F	V	E	G	I	Y	K	V	E	I	D	T	K	S	Y	W	K	S	L	G	I	S	P	F	H	E	H	A	E	V	V	F	T	A	N	D	S
Marmoset	E	E	K	F	V	K	G	V	Y	K	V	E	I	N	S	K	S	Y	W	H	T	L	G	I	T	S	F	H	E	H	A	D	V	V	F	S	A	N	D	S
Borivian squirrel monkey	E	E	K	F	V	K	G	I	Y	K	V	E	I	D	S	K	S	Y	W	H	N	L	G	I	A	S	F	H	E	H	A	D	V	V	F	A	A	N	E	S
Mouse	D	E	K	F	V	E	G	V	Y	R	V	E	L	D	T	K	S	Y	W	K	T	L	G	I	S	P	F	H	E	F	A	D	V	V	F	T	A	N	D	S

	101	102	103	104	105	106	107	108	109	110	111	112	113	114	115	116	117	118	119	120	121	122	123	124	125	126	127		Homology (%)
Human	G	P	R	R	Y	T	I	A	A	L	L	S	P	Y	S	Y	S	T	T	A	V	V	T	N	P	K	E		**100.0**
Chimpanzee	G	P	R	R	Y	T	I	A	A	L	L	S	P	Y	S	Y	S	T	T	A	V	V	T	I	P	K	E		**97.3**
Orangutan	G	P	R	R	Y	T	I	A	A	L	L	S	P	Y	S	Y	S	T	T	A	V	V	T	N	P	K	E		**95.2**
Cynomolgus monkey	G	P	R	H	Y	T	I	A	A	L	L	S	P	Y	S	Y	S	T	T	A	V	V	T	N	P	K	E		**93.9**
Rhesus monkey	G	P	R	H	Y	T	I	A	A	L	L	S	P	Y	S	Y	S	T	T	A	V	V	T	N	P	K	E		**93.2**
Marmoset	G	P	R	H	Y	I	V	A	A	L	L	S	P	Y	S	Y	S	T	T	A	V	V	S	D	P	R	K		**78.9**
Borivian squirrel monkey	G	P	R	H	Y	I	V	A	A	L	L	S	P	Y	S	Y	S	T	T	A	V	V	S	D	P	K	N		**78.9**
Mouse	G	H	R	H	Y	T	I	A	A	L	L	S	P	Y	S	Y	S	T	T	A	V	V	S	N	P	Q	N		**81.0**

Fig. 4. Amino acid sequences of TTR in nonhuman primate species, as compared with that in human and mice.

3. Discussion and conclusion

At present, animal models for TTR amyloidosis are restricted to Tg rodents and vervet monkeys. The vervet monkey more obviously reflects the clinical symptoms and histopathological features of human SAA compared to those of TTR Tg mice (Nakamura et al., 2008), as some Tg mice lines do not reveal sufficient congophilic amyloid deposits. Because mice do not show spontaneous TTR amyloidosis but form extensive amyloid deposits following transfection with the human wild type or mutant TTR genes, the higher homology of TTR with humans may be important. Thus, the TTR amino acid sequence is key for primary amyloid formation. However, even if mutant TTR genes are strongly expressed in mice, amyloid formation has not been found in the peripheral nerves of any TTR Tg mice lines. Vervet monkeys also do not form TTR amyloid deposits in peripheral nerves, even if abundant TTR amyloid is deposited in extra-neural organs. Amyloid deposition of TTR in peripheral nerves is exclusively a human phenomenon, observed as terminal TTR amyloidosis lesions. Namely, other factors, such as molecular chaperones, immunological events, and time are required for development of TTR amyloidosis lesions prior to deposits in peripheral nerves.

For example, differences between human and animals are well known in animal models of Alzheimer's disease (AD). Senile plaques (SPs), consisting of amyloid protein (Aβ) and amyloid formation, are found in various mammalian species other than rodents (Selkoe et al., 1987), whereas neurofibrillary tangles (NFTs), consisting of phosphorylated tau, are found mostly in humans. In general, SPs appear first and NFTs appear consequently in the brain during the development of AD pathology. In mammalian species other than humans, the formation of NFTs is restricted to very old macaque monkeys (Oikawa et al., 2010). The Aβ amino acid sequence is completely homologous between humans and most mammalian species but not in rodents (Selkoe et al., 1987), and SPs can be found in various mammalian species. Furthermore, Tg mice transfected with mutant Aβ precursor protein (APP) show well developed SP formation but little or only slight formation of NFTs, whereas double Tg mice lines with APP and one of some other factors, such as presenilin-1, also form NFTs (Ashe et al., 2010). Thus, the formation of NFTs at the later stage of AD pathology is a phenomenon particular to humans, and not only Aβ amino acid sequence homology but also some other factors are required to develop NFTs in mammalian species.

When animals develop the pathological changes of TTR and Aβ amyloidosis, the lesions seem to stop developing at the middle period before reaching the terminal period, as in humans. Unfortunately, the factors participating as thresholds for the onset of these diseases are unknown. Absolute time, amino acid sequence, the presence of molecular chaperones, and other factors may lead to these differences between humans and animals. Of these factors, life span is easy to understand. The longest lived cynomolgus monkey was 36 years (Oikawa et al., 2010), which is less than one-third of the longest lived human. More importantly, how a long term event that occurs in humans is shortened by model animals may be very difficult to ascertain.

TTR Tg mice are useful for basic in vivo studies, whereas aged male vervet monkeys are useful for developing novel therapeutic chemicals and diagnostic materials in preclinical studies. Vervet monkeys have often been used to provide red blood cells for the measles hemagglutination inhibition test. However, the number of captive vervet monkeys is decreasing in Japan because of new diagnostic methods for measles (Fujino et al., 2007). Although there is a US primate center with a vervet monkey colony (http://www.ncrr.nih.gov/comparative_medicine/resource_directory/primates.asp#verv), funds are insufficient for maintaining such a huge facility in Japan. Shimozawa et al. (2010) developed embryonic stem cells from a vervet monkey, which may help reproduce them in the future. Now, captive vervet monkeys possess a novel raison d'etre under the field of biomedical science based on characteristics similar to human SSA. Here, we propose vervet monkeys as a novel biomedical science resource that will contribute to understanding TTR amyloidosis.

4. Acknowledgment

We thank Dr. Yumi Une and Dr. James Kenn Chambers for providing some of the vervet monkey cases.

5. References

Ashe, KH. & Zahs, KR. (2010). Probing the biology of Alzheimer's disease in mice. *Neuron*, Vol.66, No.5, pp. 631-645, ISSN 0896-6273

Ando, Y., Nakamura, M. & Araki, S., (2005). Transthyretin-related familial amyloidotic polyneuropathy. *Arch Neurol*, Vol.62, No.7, pp. 1057-1062, ISSN 0003-9942

Buxbaum, JN. (2009). Animal models of human amyloidoses: Are transgenic mice worth the time and trouble? *FEBS Lett*, Vol.583, No.16, pp. 2663-2673, ISSN 0014-5793

Chambers, JK., Kanda, T., Shirai, A., Higuchi, K., Ikeda, S. & Une, Y. (2010). Senile systemic amyloidosis in an aged savannah monkey (Cercopithecus aethiops) with tenosynovial degeneration. *J Vet Med Sci*, Vol.72, No.5, pp. 657-659, ISSN 0916-7250

Damas, AM. & Saraiva, MJ. (2005). *Transthyretin, In: Amyloid proteins*, Sipe JD. (Ed), pp. 571-588, WILEY-VCH, ISBN 3-527-31072-X, Weinheim, Germany

Fujino, M., Yoshida, N., Kimura, K., Zhou, J., Motegi, Y., Komase, K. & Nakayama, T. (2007). Development of a new neutralization test for measles virus. *J Virol Methods*, Vol.142, No.1-2, pp. 15-20, ISSN 0166-0934

Higuchi, K., Naiki, H., Kitagawa, K., Hosokawa, M. & Takeda, T. (1991). Mouse senile amyloidosis. ASSAM amyloidosis in mice presents universally as a systemic age-associated amyloidosis. *Virchows Arch B Cell Pathol Incl Mol Pathol*, Vol.60, No.4, pp. 231-238, ISSN 0340-6075

Inoue, S., Ohta, M., Li, Z., Zhao, G., Takaoka, Y., Sakashita, N., Miyakawa, K., Takada, K., Tei, H., Suzuki, M., Masuoka, M., Sakaki, Y., Takahashi, K. & Yamamura K. (2008). Specific pathogen free conditions prevent transthyretin amyloidosis in mouse models. *Transgenic Res*, Vol.17, No.5, pp. 817-826, ISSN 0962-8819

Karin, M., Haslinger, A., Heguy, A., Dietlin, T. & Imbra, R. (1987). Transcriptional control mechanisms which regulate the expression of human metallothionein genes. *Experientia Suppl*, Vol.52, pp. 401-405, ISSN 0071-335X

Muchowski, PJ. (2002). Protein Misfolding, Amyloid Formation, and Neurodegeneration: A Critical Role for Molecular Chaperones? *Neuron*, Vol.35, No.1, pp. 9-12, ISSN 0896-6273

Nadezhdin, EV., Vinogradova, TV. & Sverdlov, ED. (2001). Interspecies subtractive hybridization of cDNA from human and chimpanzee brains. *Dokl Biochem Biophys*, Vol.381, No.5, pp. 415-418, ISSN 1607-6729

Nakamura, S., Okabayashi, S., Ageyama, N., Koie, H., Sankai, T., Ono, F., Fujimoto, K. & Terao, K. (2008). Transthyretin amyloidosis and two other aging-related amyloidoses in an aged vervet monkey. *Vet Pathol*, Vol.45, No.1, pp. 67-72, ISSN 0300-9858

Noguchi, H., Ohta, M., Wakasugi, S., Noguchi, K., Nakamura, N., Nakamura, O., Miyakawa, K., Takeya, M., Suzuki, M., Nakagata, N., Urano, T., Ono, T. & Yamamura, K. (2002). Effect of the intestinal flora on amyloid deposition in a transgenic mouse model of familial amyloidotic polyneuropathy. *Exp Anim*, Vol.51, No.4, pp. 309-316, ISSN 1341-1357

Oikawa, N., Kimura, N. & Yanagisawa, K. (2010). Alzheimer-type tau pathology in advanced aged nonhuman primate brains harboring substantial amyloid deposition. *Brain Res*, Vol.1315, No.22, pp. 137-149, ISSN 0006-8993

Rapezzi, C., Quarta, CC., Riva, L., Longhi, S., Gallelli, I., Lorenzini, M., Ciliberti, P., Biagini, E., Salvi, F. & Branzi, A., (2010). Transthyretin-related amyloidoses and the heart: a clinical overview. *Nat Rev Cardiol*, Vol.7, No.7, pp. 398-408, ISSN 1759-5002

Reixach, N., Foss, TR., Santelli, E., Pascual, J., Kelly, JW. & Buxbaum, JN., (2008). Human-murine transthyretin heterotetramers are kinetically stable and non-amyloidogenic. A lesson in the generation of transgenic models of diseases involving oligomeric proteins. *J Biol Chem*, Vol.283, No.4, pp. 2098-2107, ISSN 0021-9258

Santos, SD., Fernandes, R. & Saraiva, MJ., (2010). The heat shock response modulates transthyretin deposition in the peripheral and autonomic nervous systems. *Neurobiol Aging*, Vol.31, No.2, pp. 280-289, ISSN 0197-4580

Sasaki, H., Tone, S., Nakazato, M., Yoshioka, K., Matsuo, H., Kato, Y. & Sakaki Y. (1986). Generation of transgenic mice producing a human transthyretin variant: a possible mouse model for familial amyloidotic polyneuropathy. *Biochem Biophys Res Commun*, Vol.139, No.2, pp. 794-799, ISSN 0006-291X

Selkoe, DJ., Bell, DS., Podlisny, MB., Price, DL. & Cork, LC. (1987). Conservation of brain amyloid proteins in aged mammals and humans with Alzheimer's disease. *Science*, Vol.235, No.4791, pp. 873-877, ISSN 1095-9203

Shimozawa, N., Nakamura, S., Takahashi I., Hatori, M. & Sankai, T. (2010). Characterization of a novel embryonic stem cell line from an ICSI-derived blastocyst in the African green monkey. *Reproduction*, Vol.139, No.3, pp. 565-573, ISSN 1470-1626

Sousa, MM., Cardoso, I., Fernandes, R., Guimarães, A. & Saraiva, MJ. (2001). Deposition of transthyretin in early stages of familial amyloidotic polyneuropathy: evidence for toxicity of nonfibrillar aggregates. *Am J Pathol*, Vol.159, No.6, pp. 1993-2000, ISSN 0002-9440

Sousa, MM., Fernandes, R., Palha, JA., Taboada, A., Vieira, P. & Saraiva, MJ. (2002). Evidence for early cytotoxic aggregates in transgenic mice for human transthyretin Leu55Pro. *Am J Pathol*, Vol.161, No.5, pp. 1935-1948, ISSN 0002-9440

Tagoe, CE., Reixach, N., Friske, L., Mustra, D., French, D., Gallo, G. & Buxbaum, JN. (2007). In vivo stabilization of mutant human transthyretin in transgenic mice. *Amyloid*, Vol.14, No.3, pp. 227-236, ISSN 1350-6129

Takaoka, Y., Tashiro, F., Yi, S., Maeda, S., Shimada, K., Takahashi, K., Sakaki, Y. & Yamamura K. (1997). Comparison of amyloid deposition in two lines of transgenic mouse that model familial amyloidotic polyneuropathy, type I. *Transgenic Res*, Vol.6, No.4, pp. 261-269, ISSN 0962-8819

Teng, MH., Yin, JY., Vidal, R., Ghiso, J., Kumar, A., Rabenou, R., Shah, A., Jacobson, DR., Tagoe, C., Gallo, G. & Buxbaum, J. (2001). Amyloid and nonfibrillar deposits in mice transgenic for wild-type human transthyretin: a possible model for senile systemic amyloidosis. *Lab Invest*, Vol.81, No.3, pp. 385-396, ISSN 0023-6837

Ueda, M., Ando, Y., Hakamata, Y., Nakamura, M., Yamashita, T., Obayashi, K., Himeno, S., Inoue, S., Sato, Y., Kaneko, T., Takamune, N., Misumi, S., Shoji, S., Uchino, M. & Kobayashi, E. (2007). A transgenic rat with the human ATTR V30M: a novel tool for analyses of ATTR metabolisms. *Biochem Biophys Res Commun*, Vol.352, No.2, pp. 299-304, ISSN 0006-291X

Waits, RP., Uemichi, T., Zeldenrust, SR., Hull, MT., Field, L. & Benson, MD., (1995). Development of lines of transgenic mice expressing the human transthyretin Ser 84 variant, In Proc III Int. Symp. FAP and other TTR Disorders, Vol.6, pp. S31

Wood, SP. & Coker, AR. (2005). Serum amyloid P component - structural fetures and amyloid recognition, In: Amyloid proteins, Sipe JD. (Ed). pp. 189-209, WILEY-VCH, ISBN 3-527-31072-X, Weinheim, Germany.

Yamamura, K., Wakasugi, S., Maeda, S., Inomoto, T., Iwanaga, T., Uehira, M., Araki, K., Miyazaki, J. & Shimada, K. (1987). Tissue-specific and developmental expression of human transthyretin gene in transgenic mice. *Dev Genet*, Vol.8, No.4, pp. 195-205, ISSN 0192-253X

Yi, S., Takahashi, K., Naito, M., Tashiro, F., Wakasugi, S., Maeda, S., Shimada, K., Yamamura, K. & Araki, S. (1991). Systemic amyloidosis in transgenic mice carrying the human mutant transthyretin (Met30) gene. Pathologic similarity to human familial amyloidotic polyneuropathy, type I. *Am J Pathol*, Vol.138, No.2, pp. 403-412, ISSN 0002-9440

11

Amyloidosis Associated to *Leishmania* Infection in Murine Model

Ana Lucia Abreu-Silva[1,2], Gabriel Xavier-Silva[1], Marlise Neves Milhomem[1], Mylena Andrea Oliveira Torres[1] and Kátia da Silva Calabrese[2]
[1]*Department of Pathology - Universidade Estadual do Maranhão, São Luís - Maranhão*
[2]*Laboratory of Imunomodulação and Protozoologia, Instituto Oswaldo Cruz, Rio de Janeiro*
Brazil

1. Introduction

Amyloidosis comprises a group of chronic disease characterized by the deposition in different organs of an insoluble and fibrilar protein known as amyloid. AA-amyloidosis is commonly found in mammalian, including mice, and has been associated with inflammatory chronic diseases, such as leprosy, tuberculosis and rheumatoid arthritis, due to persistent high plasma concentration of SAA, a conserved protein. Leishmanasis are chronic diseases; however, the amyloidosis associated to them is rarely reported in the human being. Nevertheless, the association of leishmaniasis and amyloidosis has been described in the animal model during the course of infection. Mice experimentally infected by *Leishmania amanozensis* may present, after six months of infection, amyloid deposition in the liver, the spleen and less frequently in the ovaries. Macroscopically, these organs presented a whitish yellow-coloration diffusely distributed in the organ parenchyma. Histologicaly, the amyloid deposition is observed mainly among hepatocytes, in marginal zone of the spleen or in the renal glomerular tufts.

Proteins are found in all cells and carry out a variety of important cellular functions. Folding and unfolding are crucial ways of regulating biological activity and targeting proteins to different cellular locations. Failure to fold correctly, or to remain correctly folded, will therefore give rise to the malfunctioning of living systems and hence to disease (Dobson, 2003).

The largest group of misfolding diseases, which include numerous neurodegenerative disorders and the amyloidosis, originates from the conversion of specific proteins from their soluble functional states into stable, highly ordered, filamentous protein aggregates, known as amyloid fibrils (Uversky, 2003)

In accordance to Xue et al. (2010), the time course of amyloidogenesis and the cellular responses to the presence of amyloid fibrils depends on the extent of fibril fragmentation and that length, width and surface area of amyloid fibrils may play important roles in the mechanism of amyloid deposition.

The term amyloid was coined by the pathologist Virchow, in 1854, to describe an extracellular material found in the liver during the necroscopic exam. This term was used because when this affected organ was treated with an iodine-sulfuric acid test, it turned blue, a positive test for starch .

It has been described 27 amyloid protein in human being and at least 9 in animal (Sipe et al., 2010). This protein in histological sections stained by hematoxylin has an amorphous hyaline appearance and when it stained by red Congo and viewed by conventional polarized light the amyloid protein present a green birefringence. The amyloid is not a unique protein presented in tissue deposition it comprises substance such as glicosaminoglycans, substance P and amyloid protein.

Based on the distribution of the amyloid, amyloidosis is classified in systemic and localized. The systemic amyloidosis are classified in four types: AA amyloidosis, AL amyloidosis, B2 microglobulin and ATR amyloidosis.

AA amyloidosis, in both animals and human, is associated with long-standing chronic infections or inflammatory reaction. In animals is more frequent in bovine suffering from mastitis, traumatic reticuloperintonitis, metritis and pododermatitis (Elitok et al., 2008). This type of amyloidosis is characterized by high concentration in the blood stream of SAA.

SAA is an acute phase protein serum amyloid A produced mainly hepatocytes, has a molecular weight of approximately 12-14 kD and plays a role in reparation of tissue damaged by the inflammatory response. Can be proteolytically processed into an N-terminal cleavage product of approximately 44 to 100 residues that is deposited as amyloid in vital organs, which under normal conditions, all of the SAA is completely degraded. The deposition of this substance lead to cellular dysfunction and the clinical signs depend on the affected organs (Elimova et al., 2009; Sandri et al., 2008).

2. Amyloidosis x Leishmaniasis

Leishmaniasis are infectious and parasitic diseases that affect animals and human beings, caused by protozoan parasites of the *Leishmania* species. The genus *Leishmania* comprises protozoa parasites with a digenetic life cycle, living alternately in vertebrates hosts and phebotomine sandflies. The insect is responsible for transmission of parasites of a mammalian to another (Asfhord, 2000). In vertebrate hosts, *Leishmania* survives as amastigotes form, primarily in macrophages, that are ingested when the female sandfly takes a blood meal from an infected host. Several clinical syndromes are subsumed under the term leishmaniasis: most notably visceral, cutaneous, and mucosal leishmaniasis, which result from replication of the parasite in macrophages in the mononuclear phagocyte system, dermis, and naso-oropharyngeal mucosa, respectively (Herwaldt, 1999).

AA amyloidosis is rarely described in naturally infection by *Leishmania* spp. However several author have been reported the occurrence of this disease in experimental infection (Carvalho et al., 2008; Barbosa-Santos et al., 1984).

Even in murine model it has been observed that AA amyloidosis occur only in some strains of mice. In different experiment where DBA/2, Swiss, BALB/c, C57BL/6 female were infected with promastigote and amastigote of L. amanozensis just Swiss and C57BL/6 presented amyloidosis in the course of the infection (Cupolillo et al., 1998 Carvalho et al., 2008). Several hypotheses have been postulated to explain why a minority of patients displayed AA amyloidosis during chronic inflammatory infection. In accordance to Westermark and Westermark al., 2009, the individuals probably have deficient degradation system for aggregated proteins or they had received one or several nucleation or seeding factors. Even C57BL/6 mice, an inbred strain, challenged with that same inoculum some animals did not display AA amyloidosis after the long term after the infection. Studies show that Swiss male mice were more prone to AA amyloid deposition than female. This may be one of explanation why not all C57BL/6 mice displayed amyloidosis. On the other hands, BALB/c mice did not present amyloid deposition probably due to high susceptibility to *L. amazonensis,* what lead to generalized disease at 60 or 90 days post infection. Thus, several factors such as sex, duration and type of infection and polymorphism can contribute to onset of AA amyloidosis (Shtrasburg et al., 2004; van der Hilst, 2011).

The pathogenesis of leishmaniasis is related to the genetic background of the host and the *Leishmania* species and the modulation of T-cell immune response can be influenced by the infective *Leishmania* species as described by Silveira et al. (2009), since the clinical manifestation of cutaneous depends on both the host immune response and the specie of *Leishmania* involved.

All mice that presented amyloid deposition develop palpable lesion in skin in the delayed phase of the infection, which allowed that this animals were maintained for long period after infection. When mice presented primary lesion they were euthanatized. The necropsy exam revealed that liver, spleen and kidney presented pale and enlargement. The other organs did not present macroscopic lesions.

The histological sections stained by haematoxylin and eosin showed the liver presented an inflammatory reaction in portal area and deposition of a hyaline and amorphous substance among the hepatocytes. The same substance was seen in renal corpuscle and in the splenic marginal zone. In additional, C57BL/6 mouse showed a diffuse amyloid deposition in the ovary. The Congo red staining revealed that the amorphous substance presented in the sampled organs had a yellow-green birefringence under polarized light, confirming the occurrence of amyloid protein deposition. This dye presents a linear molecule that permits that hydrogen bonding of its azo and amino radicals to hydroxyls radicals of amyloid protein, which explain the birefringence under polarized light.

Amyloid A fibril protein in secondary amyloidosis is designated as AA protein, which is derived from the precursor protein known as serum amyloid A, or SAA. SAA protein is an acute-phase reactant produced by liver cells in response to macrophage-derived inflammatory cytokines such as interleukin 1, interleukin 6 and tumor necrosis factor-alpha. A major factor responsible for the development of AA amyloidosis is the increased synthesis and subsequent degradation of the precursor protein SAA1 under chronic inflammatory conditions (Ray et al., 2006). Approximately 45% of systemic amyloidosis reported in the literature is AA amyloidosis.

Amyloidosis has been described in spleen and liver of dogs naturally infected with *L. infantum* (Bely and Apathy, 2000; Poli et al., 1991; George et al., 1976). In hamsters, this pathology has been reported in adrenal gland (Novoa et al., 1990) in mice amyloidosis is most common in liver (Figure 1), spleen and kidney (Figure 2) Here, inflammatory infiltrates were observed in both medullary and cortical regions, however amyloidosis depositions were not demonstrated, suggesting passage of parasitic antigen though these organs but without evidence of parasites. Previous studies showed that Swiss mice infected with *L. amazonensis* amastigotes had developed amyloidosis in spleen, liver , and kidney 10 months post-infection (Barbosa-Santos et al., 1984).

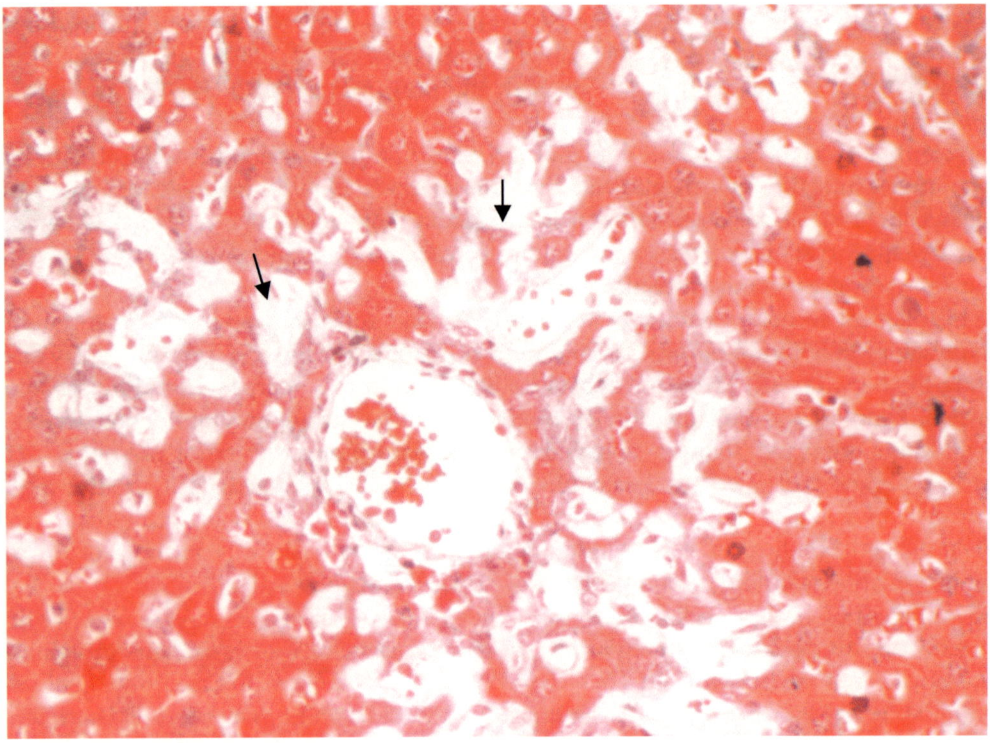

Fig. 1. Liver – Amyloidal deposits among hepatocytes cells (arrows) – Gomori Trichrome Stain. Scale bar 100 μm.

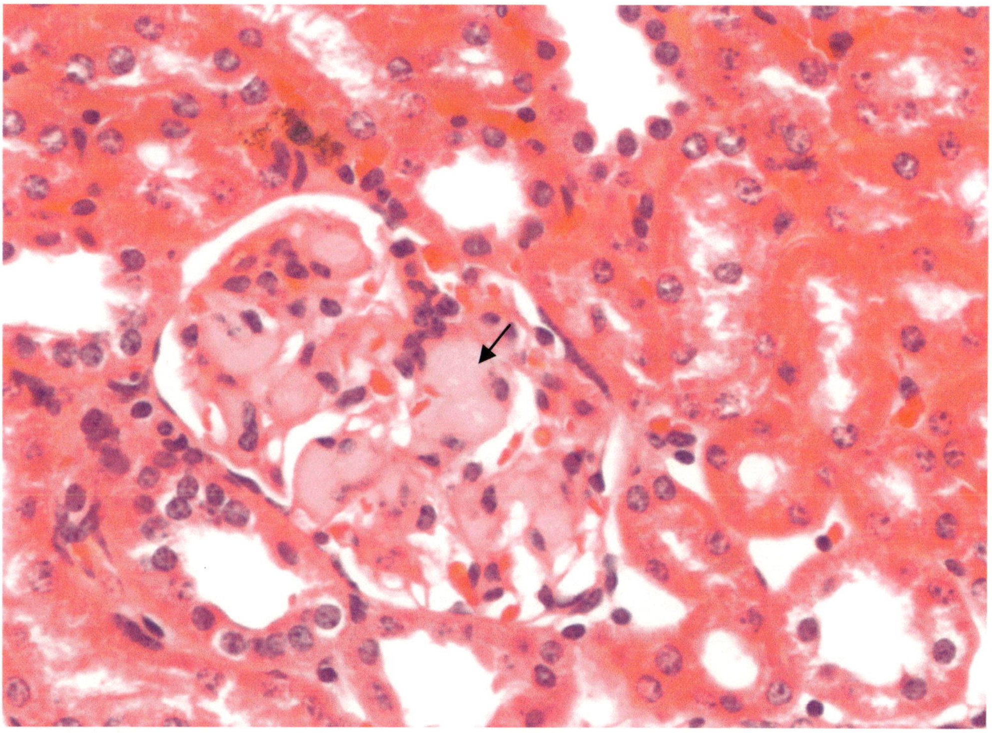

Fig. 2. Kidney - Amyloidal deposits in the glomerular tuft (arrows) - Hematoxylin-Eosin. Scale bar 100 μm

2.1 Conclusions remarks

In murine model, the persistence of the *Leishmania* infection lead to amyloid deposition, which may impair the function of several organs, including, liver, spleen, kidney and ovary. The tecidual damage is caused by several factor.

3. Acknowledgment

Dr. Abreu-Silva and Dr Calabrese hold a research fellowship from the Brazilian National Research Council (CNPq), Brazil.

4. References

Ashford, R. W.(2000). The leishmaniases as emerging and reemerging zoonoses. *International journal for parasitology*, Vol. 30, N. 12-13, (November 2000), pp. 1269-1281, ISSN 1879-0135

Barbosa-Santos E.G. , Gonçalves da Costa, S. C., and Alencar, A., Amyloidosis in experimental tegumentary leishmaniasis in mice, *The American Journal of Tropical Medicine and Hygiene* **33** (1984), pp. 1270–1271, ISSN 0002-9637

Bely, M. and Apathy, A., Histochemical and immunohistochemical differential diagnosis of amyloidosis—a brief illustrated essay and personal experience with Romhanyi's method, *Amyloid* **7** (2000), pp. 212–217, ISSN 1350-6129

Carvalho, L. O.; Calabrese, K. da S.; da Costa, S. C.; Mendes, V. G.; da Silva, A. P.; Barros, A. C.; Melo, S. de A. & Abreu-Silva, A. L.(2003). Leishmania (Leishmania) amazonensis: experimental cutaneous leishmaniasis associated with systemic amyloidosis in mice. *Experimental Parasitology*, Vol. 120, N. 1, (June 2008), pp. 123-125, ISSN 0014-4894

Cupolillo, E.; Momen H. & Grimaldi, G. Jr. (1998). Genetic diversity in natural populations of New World Leishmania. *Memórias do Instituto Oswaldo Cruz*, Vol. 93, N. 5, (September/October 1998), pp. 663-668, ISSN 0074-0276

Dobson C. M.(2003). Protein folding and misfolding. *Nature*, Vol 426, N. 6968, (December 2003), pp. 884-890, ISSN 0028-0836

Elimova, E.; Kisilevsky, R. & Ancsin, J. B.(2009). Heparan sulfate promotes the aggregation of HDL-associated serum amyloid A: evidence for a proamyloidogenic histidine molecular switch. *FASEB*, Vol. 23, N. 10, (June 2003), pp. 3436-3448, ISSN *0892-6638*

Elitok, O. M. & Unver, O.(2008). Renal amyloidosis in cattle with inflammatory diseases. *Journal of Veterinary Internal Medicine*, Vol. 22, N. 2,(February 2008), pp. 450-455, ISSN 1939-1676

George, J.W., Nielsen, S.W., Shiyeley, J.N., Hopek, S. and Mroz, S. , Canine leishmaniasis with amyloidosis, *Veterinary Pathology* **13** (1976), pp. 365–373, ISSN 0300-9858

Herwaldt, B. L.(1999). Leishmaniasis. *Lancet*, Vol. 354, N. 9185, (October 1999), pp. 1191-1199, ISSN 1040-6736

Hubng-Hsu, H; De-Feng, H.; Cheng-Hwai, T.; Cheng-Hsi, S.; Tung-Ping, S.; Hunf-Chieh, C.; Shyh-Haw, T.; Han-Chich, L.; Jaw-Ching, W.; Shou-Dong, L. & Chien-Wei, S.(2010). Systemic Amyloidosis Manifesting as a Rare Cause of Hepatic Failure. *Journal of the* Chinese Medical Association, *Vol.75, N.3, (Mach 2010), pp. 161-165, ISSN* 1726-4901

Kleiner, E. & Benson, M. D.(1980). Synthesis and secretion of serum amyloid protein A (SAA) by hepatocytes in mice treated with casein. *The Journal of Immunology*, Vol. 124, N. 2, pp. 495-499, ISSN 0022-1767

Lavatelli, F.; Perlman, D. H.; Spencer, B.; Prokeaeve, T.; McComb, M. E., Théberge, R.; Connors, L. H.; Bellotti, V.; Seldin, D. C.; Merlini, G.; Skinner, M. & Costello, C. E.(2008). *Molecular & Cellular Proteomics*, Vol. 7, N. 8,(May 2008), pp. 1570-15783, ISSN 1535-9484

Martins, R. G.; Roncon-Albuquerque, R. J.; Cabral, R.; Frazão, J. & Von Hafe, P.(2010). Primary Amyloidosis Associated With Kappa Light Chain Myeloma. *Acta Medica Portuguesa*, Vol. 23, N. 2,(March/April 2010), pp. 281-284, ISSN 1646-0758

Monsellier, E.; Ramazzoti, M.; Tadei, N. & Chiti, F. (2010). A Computational Approach for Identifyng the Chemical Factors Involved in Glycosaminoglycans-Mediated Acceleration of Amyloid Fibril Formation. *PLoS ONE*, Vol.5, No.11363, (June 2010), p. e11363, ISSN 1932-6203

Novoa, C., Garcia, P., Rollan, E. and Gonzalez, J.L., Amyloidosis in adrenal glands of hamsters experimentally infected with Leishmania infantum, *Histology and Histopathology* **5** (1990), pp. 225–229, ISSN 1699-5848

Poli, A., Abramo, F., Mancianti, F.,,Nigro, M.,Pieri, S. and Bionda, A., Renal involvement in canine leishmaniasis. A light-microscopic, immunohistochemical and electron-microscopic study, *Nephron* **57** (1991), pp. 444–452, ISSN 0028-2766

Ray,A., Shakya, A.,Kumar, D.,Benson M.D. and Ray, B. K., Inflammation-responsive transcription factor SAF-1 activity is linked to the development of amyloid A amyloidosis, *Journal of Immunology* 177 (2006), pp. 2601–2609, ISSN 0022-1767

Sandri, S.; Rodriguez, D.; Gomes, E.; Monteiro, H. P.; Russo, M. & Campa, A.(2008). Is serum amyloid A an endogenous TLR4 agonist?. *Journal of leukocyte biology*, Vol. 83, N. 5, (February 2008), pp. 1174-1180, ISSN 0741-5400

Shtrasburg, S.; Pras, M.; Dulitzky, M.; Pariente, C.; Gal, R.; Mor, A. & Livneh, A.(2004). Increased propensity for amyloidogenesis in male mice. *Clinical and Experimental Rheumatology*, Vol. 22, N. 4, (July-August 2004), pp. 241-246, ISSN 0392-856

Silveira, F. T.; Lainson, R; de Souza, A. A.;Campos, M.B.; Carneiro, L. A.; Lima, L. V.; Ramos, P. K.; de Castro Gomes, C. M.; Laurenti, M. D. & Corbett, C. E.(2009). Further evidences on a new diagnostic approach for monitoring human Leishmania (L.) infantum chagasi infection in Amazonian Brazil. *Parasitology research*, Vol.106, N. 2, (November 2009), pp. 367-386, ISSN 0932-0113

Sipe, J. D.; Benson, M. D.; Buxbaum, J. N.; Ikeda, S.; Merlini, G.; Saraiva, M.J. & Westermark, P.(2010). Amyloid fibril protein nomenclature: 2010 recommendations from the nomenclature committee of the International Society of Amyloidosis. *Amyloid*, Vol. 17, N. 3-4, (November 2010), pp. 101-104, ISSN 1744-2818

Snow, A. D.; Bramson, R.; Mar, H.; Wight, N. T. & Kisilevsky, R.(1991). A Temporal and Ultrastructural Relatonship Between Heparan Sulfate Prteogycans and AA Amyloid in Experimental Amyloidosis. Journal of Histochemistry *&* Cytochemistry, *Vol. 39, N. 10,(May 1991), pp. 1321-1330, ISSN* 0022-1554

Steel, D. M.; Rogers, J. T.; DeBeer, M. C.; DeBeer, F. C. & Whitehead, A. S.(1993). Biosynthesis of human acute-phase serum amyloid A protein (A-SAA) in vitro: the roles of mRNA accumulation, poly(A) tail shortening and translational efficiency. *Biochemical Journal*, Vol. 291, N. Pt 3, (May 1993), pp. 701-707, ISSN 0264-6021

Shtrasburg, S.; Pras, M.; Dulitzky, M.; Pariente, C.; Gal, R.; Mor, A. & Livneh, A.(2004). Increased propensity for amyloidogenesis in male mice. *Clinical and experimental rheumatology*, Vol. 22, N. 4, (July-August 2004), pp. 421-426, ISSN 0392-856X

Strokes, M. I. & Trickey, R. J.(1973). Screening for neurofibrillary tangles and argyrophilic plaques with Congo Red and polarized light. *Journal of Clinical* Pathology, *Vol.26, N.3, (March 1973), pp. 241-242, ISSN* 0021-9746

Uversky V. N.(2003). Protein folding revisited. A polypeptide chain at the folding-misfolding-nonfolding cross-roads: which way to go?. *Cellular and Molecular Life Sciences*, Vol. 60, N. 9, (September 2003), pp. 1852-1871, ISSN 1420-682 van der Hilst, J.(2011). Recent Insights into the Pathogenesis of Type AA Amyloidosis. *TheScientificWorld*, Vol. 11, (March 2011), pp. 641-650, ISSN 1537-744

Westermark G. T. & Westermark P.(2009). Serum amyloid A and protein AA: molecular mechanisms of a transmissible amyloidosis. *FEBS Letters*, Vol. 583, N. 16, (August 2009), pp. 2685-2690, ISSN 0014-5793

Xue, W. F.; Hellewell, A. L.; Hewitt, E. W. & Radford, S. E.(2010). Fibril fragmentation in amyloid assembly and cytotoxicity. When size matters. *Prion*, Vol. 4, N. 1, (January-March 2010), pp. 20-25, ISSN 1933-6896

12

Modeling Amyloid Diseases in Fruit Fly *Drosophila Melanogaster*

Svetlana Sarantseva[1] and Alexander Schwarzman[1,2]
[1]*Petersburg Nuclear Physics Institute, Russian Academy of Sciences*
[2]*Institute for Experimental Medicine, Russian Academy of Medical Sciences*
Russia

1. Introduction

Amyloidoses are a heterogeneous group of diverse etiology diseases. They are characterized by an endogenous production of abnormal proteins called amyloid proteins, which are not hydrosoluble, form depots in various organs and cause functional dysfunctions [Westermark et al., 2007]. Despite of their different structures, these proteins are probably generated by a common pathological pathway. Twenty-seven such proteins have been identified as amyloid precursors in humans [Sipe et al., 2010]. However, the question how and why these proteins form aggregates and cause disease is not still completely clear. A wide range of common neurodegenerative diseases is associated with amyloidosis such as Alzheimer's disease and Creutzfeldt-Jakob disease, as well as non-neuropathic diseases, such as senile systemic amyloidosis and type II diabetes. At present, there is not an effective treatment to prevent these amyloid diseases.

To understand the pathogenesis and to develop novel therapeutic strategies, it is crucial to generate animal models of amyloid diseases in genetically tractable organisms. During the last decades, the genetically amenable fruit fly *Drosophila melanogaster* was established as a valuable model system for the study of variety of human neurodegenerative disorders including Alzheimer's disease, Huntington's disease, amyotrophic lateral sclerosis and familial amyloidotic polyneuropathy [Bilen & Bonini., 2005; Lu & Vogel., 2009]. The advantages of using the *Drosophila* model are that flies have a short lifespan, small size, large number of individuals and simplicity in genetic manipulation [Hirth, 2010]. In addition, *Drosophila* represents a useful model for screening and testing chemical compounds. Moreover, *Drosophila* is an ideal model for screening genetic modifiers of pathogenic process due to their potential to prevent or ameliorate the disease [Marsh & Thompson., 2006].

In this review we will summarize recent progress in developing of fly models for amyloid disease. We address the following issues: (1) creating models of human amyloidosis in *Drosophila* (Alzheimer' disease, prion disease, senile systemic amyloidosis, familial amyloidotic polyneuropathy) and (2) screening of chemical and peptide compounds, as well as modifier genes of protein toxicity in the fly model.

2. Advantages in using *Drosophila melanogaster* to model amyloid diseases

One of the most interesting approaches to research of genetic forms of human diseases is their modeling on fruit fly *Drosophila melanogaster*. For these purposes two basic experimental approaches are used: an expression in *Drosophila* of human genes playing the role in development of diseases, and studying of own genes of *Drosophila*, orthologs of human genes involved in development of diseases [Bier, 2005]. The recent sequencing of the human and *Drosophila* genome has shown that more than 50% of genes of *Drosophila melanogaster* have homologs in humans, and at the same time not less than 60%-70% of genes of human hereditary diseases have the *Drosophila* counteracts [Fortini, 2000; Reiter, 2001]. Therefore, when acting with various models of diseases on *Drosophila* direct research of mutant protein can characterize substantially its participation in a pathogenesis of human disease. Moreover, use of transgenic technology allows to create the strains carrying the human genes and to use them for modulation of concrete physiological mechanisms. On the other hand, genetic experiments with gene knockout can be a basis for definition of unknown cellular protein functions involved in the development of pathological process.

Well-established techniques on the *Drosophila* [Rubin & Spradling, 1982] allows receiving transgenic flies not only according to the certain gene, but also to define an expression of this gene in tissues at various stages of an ontogenesis of the *Drosophila*, due to binary system UAS-GAL4 [Brand & Perrimon, 1993]. The system imported from yeast consists of two independent strains one of which carries an investigated gene under promoter UAS control (Upstream Activating Sequence), and the second strain contains its transcription activator - transcription factor GAL4. For the induction of transgenic expression, UAS strain is crossed to the strain expressing GAL4 under control of the endogenous or specially designed promoter that leads to the expression of investigated gene in tissues where GAL4 expresses. Hundreds of different activator-expressing strains have been generated by the Drosophila community and are available to other investigators.

Temperature- sensitive character of transgenic expression in UAS-GAL4 system has been used for creation of temporal and regional gene expression targeting (TARGET) [McGuire, 2003]. TARGET system is based on ability of yeast protein GAL80 to suppress the GAL4 expression. Joint expression of UAS-GAL4 strain and temperature-sensitive allele $Gal80^{TS}$ [Matsumoto, 1978], under tubulin 1α promoter control leads to the greatest suppression of GAL4 expression at 19°C and synthesis depressions of this protein at 30°C.

The other approach for the direct temporary gene expression by using UAS-GAL4 system is based on creation of hormone-inducible chimeric GAL4 variants: Gal4-estrogen receptor [Han, 2000] and GAL4-progesterone receptor (Gene Switch) [Nicholson, 2008; Osterwalder, 2001; Roman, 2001]. The transgenic expression is controlled with addition of ligands in food of flies or larvae during certain time period that allows excluding deleterious effects of the early expression of transgene. However, it imposes restriction on the use of these approaches on embryonal and pupal development stages [Elliott & Brand, 2008].

The method of insertional mutagenesis has been developed on *Drosophila melanogaster* and became widely used, based on application of mobile genetic elements (ME). ME represent the DNA segments capable to independent transpositions inside the genome. The share of mobile elements in human and mammal genome can reach 40% of the nuclear DNA [Kazazian, 2004]. The quantity of copies of mobile elements from various families changes

from one to several hundreds. ME insertion can essentially change the character of gene expression, and it has become the cause for wide ME application in creation of regulated tissue specific expression vectors [Enerly et al., 2002; Rorth P.,1996; Staudt et al., 2005]. The largest extension in *Drosophila* researches belongs to vectors, framed on the basis of mobile P-element [Adams & Sekelsky, 2002; Bellen et al., 2004]; however property of the P-element to be built in only certain genome sites, limits the mutagenesis in the whole genome. Therefore now approaches with use of other mobile elements preferring insertion sites distinct from the P-element, in particular, *hobo* [Huet et al., 20002; Myrick et al., 2009; Smith et al, 1993] and *Minos* [Metaxakis et al., 2005], are developed.
It is necessary to notice that use of *Drosophila* models allows avoiding such restrictions arising in action with human material, as incomplete family pedigrees, genetic heterogeneity of population, duration of the sampling. At the same time, fundamental aspects of cellular biology, such as regulation of gene expression, membrane transport, cell signaling, synaptogenesis, cellular death, neurotransmitter systems are similar enough in humans and *Drosophila* [Sang & Jackson, 2005].

3. *Drosophila* models of Alzheimer's amyloidosis

Alzheimer's disease (AD) is the most frequent reason of a dementia in elderly and senile age [Davis and Samuels, 1998]. Clinically, AD manifests as a gradual decline of cognitive functions such as learning and memory, which significantly correlates with synaptic loss. The main neuropathological features of AD are well known and characterized by the accumulation of aggregated phosphorylated tau in neurofibrillary tangles (NFTs) and amyloid beta peptide (Aβ) in senile amyloid plaques. Aβ is the peptide with 39 - 42 *amino acid*, a product of the proteolytic processing of the big transmembrane protein which has received a name of **A**myloid **P**recursor **P**rotein (APP). Normally, Aβ in nanomolar quantities is found out in the blood flow and cerebrospinal fluid; however, according to modern representations, accumulation of toxic intermediates of amyloid fibril in AD brain is the central link in all neuropathological processes, including dysfunction of synapses, neurodegeneration, neuron loss and dementia development [De Strooper & Annaert, 2001; Hardy & Selkoe, 2002; Selkoe, 1998]. The appreciable part of works specifies that such intermediates may be soluble oligomers of Aβ [Walh & Selkoe, 2004].
Different membrane proteases known as alpha, beta (BACE) and gamma-secretases, are involved in proteolytic APP processing. The coordinated action of β– and γ-secretases results in the formation of Aβ. γ-secretase represents the protein complex, in which basic component are transmembrane proteins presenilin 1 (PSN1) or presenilin 2 (PSN2) [De Strooper & Annaert, 2000]. All known familial AD forms are caused by mutations in *APP, PSN1, PSN2* genes [Selkoe, 1999]. There are a fly homologue of presenilin genes (*Psn*) [Ye & Fortini, 1998] and homologue of *APP* gene (*Appl*) [Luo et al., 1990] in *Drosophila melanogaster* genome.
Appl is characterized by high degree of homology with APP, it is exposed to similar proteolytic processing, but it lacks the Aβ peptide region and its processing does not lead to neurotoxic effects [Luo et al., 1990; Rosen et al., 1989]. Appl knockout didn't lead to lethal effect, but caused change of behavioral reactions which were restored at APP expression. This indicates functional conservatism between *Drosophila* Appl and human APP[Luo et al., 1992]. Many researches specify the key role of Appl in formation and maintenance of synapses in *Drosophila* [Ashley et al., 2005; Torroja et al., 1996]. Experiments by definition of Appl localization have shown significant Appl enrichment in growing axons and synaptic

structures and participation of Appl in formation and differentiations of synapses in neuromuscular junctions of larvae [Torroja et al., 1996, 1999b]. The overexpression both Appl, and human APP caused disturbance of axon transport [Gunawardena and Goldstein, 2001; Torroja et al., 1999a]. At APP human overexpression in *Drosophila melanogaster* it also was transported in the presynaptic terminal of neurons and postsynaptic sites of neuromuscular junctions [Yagi et al., 2000].

Fly models of human Aβ peptide-induced amyloidosys have been generated employing direct expression Aβ40 and Aβ42, in nervous system in *Drosophila* strains [Iijima-Ando & Iijima, 2010; Moloney et al., 2010]. Interestingly, diffusive amyloid deposits and neuron loss have been detected only in flies carrying the sequence of more amyloidogenic Aβ42 in genome. Amyloid formation was accompanied by progressive age-dependent behavioral defects, and life expectancy reduction. Authors did not detect amyloid accumulation and neuron loss as for flies carrying the sequences of less amyloidogenic $A\beta_{40}$ [Finelli et al, 2004; Iijima et al., 2004]. In other work, flies expressing wild-type $A\beta_{42}$ and Arctic mutant $A\beta_{42}$ (Glu22Gly) showed a decline in climbing behavior, increased intracellular Aβ accumulation and diffuse plaques prior to signs of neurodegeneration [Crowther et al., 2005]. Late findings demonstrated that expression of the Arctic mutant significantly enhanced formation of Aβ oligomers and Aβ deposits, together with a decline of locomotor functions when compared with Aβ-art (artificial mutation L17P) [Iijima et al., 2008].

It has been proposed that dysfunction and loss of synapses underlie in the basis of cognitive disturbances at AD [Hardy & Selkoe, 2002; Honer, 2003 Sze et al., 1997; Selkoe, 2002; Terry et al., 1991]. At the analysis of sporadic AD form it has been established that the significant reduction (> 25 %) of synapse density in a frontal and temporal cortex and in hippocampus was observed already in the early stage of disease [Masliah et al., 1994]. Thus loss of synapses is not age-dependent and it is the specific characteristic of AD [Masliah et al., 2001]. Moreover, the degeneration of only insignificant part of synapses is caused by neuron death whereas the appreciable share of synapses is lost by living cells [Coleman & Yao, 2003].

In addition, transgenic models clearly show that synapse loss strictly correlates with cognitive disturbances and precedes formation of neurofibrillary tangles (NFTs) and amyloid deposits [Duyckaerts et al., 2008; Mucke et al., 2000; Oddo et al., 2003]. Now the most researchers suggest that accumulation of soluble toxic Aβ oligomers in neurons lead directly to degeneration of synapses and the neuron loss [Walsh & Selkoe, 2004]. This suggestion, considerably, is based on the data showing correlation between concentration of soluble non-aggregated Aβ in extracts of cortex and hippocampus, reduction of synapses quantity and degree of cognitive disturbances [Lue et al., 1999]. In summary, despite appreciable number of modeling experiments on the transgenic animals [Haass and Selkoe, 2007; LaFerla et al., 2007; Wirths et al., 2004] it is extremely difficult to prove a hypothesis about casuative the role of toxic Aβ oligomer in synaptic dysfunction *in vivo*. Surprisingly, different $A\beta_{42}$ aggregates had distinctive roles in modulation of synaptic functions. While exogenously prepared small $A\beta_{42}$ oligomers or Aβ oligomers secreted from neurons lead to a reduction of neurotransmitter release; larger-sized aggregates, possibly fibrils secreted by muscle cells, enhanced neurotransmitter release and synaptic transmission [Chiang et al., 2009].

The $A\beta_{42}$ expression induced depletion of mitochondria in axons and dendrites and their accumulated in the somata without severe mitochondrial damage or neurodegeneration [Iijima-Ando et al., 2009]. In addition, significant depletion of presynaptic mitochondria occurred before changes in synaptic transmission [Zhao et al., 2010].
Greeve et al. (2004) have taken an alternative approach to generating flies with Aβ deposition. Because BACE activity is very low or not present in *Drosophila* [Carmine-Simmen et al., 2009; Fossgreen et al., 1998;], overexpression of human APP does not lead to secretion of Aβ leading to the interpretation that all phenotypic effects in these transgenic flies should be attributed to the presence of human APP. When human BACE and APP were expressed in combination in fly eyes Aβ was secreted and diffuse amyloid plaques and age-dependent neurodegeneration of photoreceptor cells were observed. The neurodegeneration phenotype was enhanced in the flies expressing dPsn carrying early-onset familial AD mutations. Surprisingly, neurodegeneration was even more pronounced in APP transgenic flies than in APP/BACE double transgenic flies [Greeve et al., 2004]. Our data confirm these results. We did not find differences in age-dependent neurodegeneration in transgenic flies expressing full size APP with BACE or without BACE. However, transgenic expressing APP and BACE had lower levels of the presynaptic protein GFP- synaptobrevin or GFP-synaptotagmin than transgenic expressing APP alone [Sarantseva et al., 2009a, 2009b]. These findings raise the question whether the decline of synaptic proteins levels and/or neurodegeneration are caused by different mechanisms. Alternatively, we suggest that Aβ reflects just a part of a larger pathological process and independently contributes to different neuropathological abnormalities caused by APP overexpression.

3.1 Screening for genetic modifiers

Drosophila represents one of classical tools used to conduct genetic modifiers screens. The main goal of these screens is to identify proteins or pathways that modulate pathological process. One of the most interesting examples is discovery of modifiers of Aβ pathology. Flies expressing $A\beta_{42}$ in retina have been used for detection of Aβ phenotype-modifying mutations in *Drosophila* genome. These flies developed so-called «rough eye» phenotype characterized by disorganization of photoreceptor cells and reduction of the eye size [Finelli et al., 2004]. Modifiers (suppressors and enhancers) of rough eye phenotype were identified from screening the collection of nearly 2,000 *Drosophila* strains carrying in genome inserts of EP transposon. The EP transposon has a GAL4 activated promoter and modulates the gene activity depending on site and orientation insertion [Rorth et al., 1998]. All strains of this collection were individually crossed to the flies expressing $A\beta_{42}$. As a result of screening of phenotypes and the subsequent DNA-analysis 23 modifiers gene have been discovered. They included genes participating in various secretory processes, cholesterol homeostasis, the innate immune pathway, control of transcription and chromatin remodeling. Eight mutations change the total Aβ peptide level, but only one mutation resulted in 70 % decrease of total Aβ level. This mutation revealed insertion in regulatory zone of neprilysin 2 (nep2) gene [Cao et al., 2008; Finelli et al., 2004]. Neprilysin is one of major neuropeptidases of brain of mammals [Iwata et al., 2001, 2005]. Interestingly, epidemiological studies suggest that reduction in Neprilysin levels may contribute to the onset and/or progression of late-onset AD [Hersh & Rodgers, 2008].

Several studies show that normal cellular presenilin functions and the nature of abnormalities caused by PSN1 and PSN2 mutations in familial AD are not restricted by participation of these proteins in γ-secretase complex and required the further investigations [Baki et al., 2004; Bentahir et al., 2006; Singh et al., 2001; Saura et al., 2004; Schwarzman et al., 1999]. For understanding presenilin functions the search of genetic modifiers modulating Psn-dependent phenotype in *Drosophila* wings and notum has been conducted. 177 modifiers, included the proteins regulating intracellular calcium signaling, stress response and protein folding, components of signal transduction, apoptotic factors and proteins of the cellular cycle. Notably, 58 modifiers interacted with APP, including those involved in calcium signaling. These results provide strong evidence for a link between presenilins, APP, and calcium homeostasis, and suggest that these may play an important role in AD pathogenesis [van de Hoef et al., 2009].

4. *Drosophila* model for transthyretin-associated amyloidosis

Transthyretin (TTR), plasma protein primarily synthesized in the liver, choroid plexus and in retinal pigment epithelium, is the basic transporter of thyroxine and retinol-binding protein in mammals [Goodman, D., 1987; Woeber & Ingbar, 1968]. Three human diseases are characterized by extracellular transthyretin deposits - Familial Amyloidotic Polyneuropathy (FAP), Familial Amyloidotic Cardiomyopathy (FAC) and Senile Systemic Amyloidosis (SSA). SSA is the most widespread form of transthyretin associated amyloidosis, in which the lesion of heart, brain, and pancreas is observed [Westermark, et al., 1990]. FAP and FAC are hereditary forms caused by mutations in the transthyretin gene. Now it is known more than 100 human genetic TTR variants differing with unique amino-acid replacement, of which the majority is amyloidogenic [Connors et al., 2003]. TTR forms amyloid through a process that is initiated by tetramer destabilization. This process results in accumulation of monomers, which can misfold and aggregate into fibrillar structures [Wiseman et al., 2005]. TTR is involved in Aβ metabolism, the basic component of amyloid deposits in Alzheimer's disease [Liu & Murphy, 2006; Schwarzman, et al., 1994]. Moreover, binding TTR to Aβ prevented Aβ aggregation and formation of an amyloid both *in vitro* and *in vivo* [S.H. Choi et al, 2007; Buxbaum et al, 2008]. Despite the fact that *Drosophila* does not have distinct TTR homolog, the expression of its two clinical forms TTRV30M [Berg, I. et al, 2009] and TTRL55P and mutant form TTR-A [Pokrzywa et al., 2007], with two amino-acid replacements (TTRV14N/V16E) [Olofsson et al., 2001] led to development of the phenotypes partially reminiscent of the human pathology. Expression of TTRV30M in the nervous system resulted in neurodegeneration, reduced lifespan, climbing ability, whereas the expression of wild type TTR (TTRwt) showed a milder phenotype. Congo red staining of the *Drosophila* brain shows positive amyloid binding in aged TTRV30M flies [Berg, I. et al, 2009]. Similar results have been received at TTRL55P and TTR-A expression: shortened lifespan, locomotive dysfunction, including flight ability [Pokrzywa et al., 2007]. Notably, that the expression of all three TTR forms (TTRL55P, TTR-A and TTRwt) caused the unusual "dragged-wing" phenotype.TTR aggregates possessed different toxicity. So, the most toxic were TTR aggregations separated from hemolymph and fat body of aged TTR-A flies [Pokrzywa et al., 2010].

Drosophila strains expressing TTR can address specific questions in transthyretin biology. For instance, a variety of TTR-binding partners have been identified over the years [Liz et al., 2009]. However, the biological significance of these interactions remains obscure. Use of a tractable genetic system such as *Drosophila* can play a key role for the elucidation of cellular pathways and compartments in which these interactions take place.

5. Modeling prion diseases in *Drospohila*

Prion diseases (transmissible spongiform encephalopaties) are an unusual group of fatal neurodegenerative disease including Gerstmann–Sträussler–Scheinker (GSS) syndrome, familial fatal insomnia (FFI), Creutzfeldt–Jakob disease (CJD) and kuru in human and also scrapie in sheep and goats, bovine spongiform encephalopathy (BSE) in cattle, chronic wasting disease in mule deer and elk, [Prusiner, 1998, Prusiner & Hsiao,1994]. These diseases may present with sporadic, inherited or infectious origins and lead to dementia, motor dysfunction and death [Aguzzi et al., 2008]. The majority of prion diseases cases in humans are classified as sporadic forms and about 10-15 % are the inherited form caused by mutations in *PRNP* gene. Now it is described more than 30 mutations in *PRNP* gene [Mead, 2006]. According to modern considerations, the central pathogenetic event in prion diseases is the conformational conversion of the normal cellular isoform of prion protein (PrP^{C}) into its pathological scarpie isoform (PrP^{Sc}) [Prusiner, 1998]. The precise structural differences between the two PrP isoforms remain to be defined, although it is clear that PrP^{Sc} contains significantly more β-sheet and is more protease-resistant regions. The deposition of PrP^{Sc} in the brain is associated with cerebral damage, including spongiform degeneration and neuronal loss. However, increasing evidence argues against the neurotoxicity of PrP^{Sc}. Significant pathology and/or clinical dysfunction develop with little accumulation of PrP^{Sc} [Flechsig et al., 2000; Manson et al., 1999] and some familial prion diseases are not transmissible, and are not accompanied by the accumulation of protease resistant PrP [Brown et al., 1994; Rodríguez-Martínez et al, 2010; Tateishi & Kitamoto, 1995; Zou et al, 2010]. Thus, it is not clear whether specific conformers are associated with neuronal dysfunction and degeneration [Solomon et al., 2010].

The first attempts to create the model of prion diseases on *Drosophila* were unsuccessful. PrP Syrian hamster (SHaPrP) expression under heat shock promoter Hsp70 did not lead to neuropathology and accumulation of protease-resistent SHaPrP forms [Raeber et al.,1995]. The expression of wild type of the mouse (MoPrP) and human CJD-associated PrP (PG14) [Krasemann et al., 1995] using GAL4-UAS has not also revealed clinical and pathological abnormalities in the flies. Surprisingly, the flies seemed to accumulate very little mutant PrP in the brain compared with the eyes, suggesting that *Drosophila* brain possesses a specific and saturable mechanism that suppresses the accumulation of PG14 [Deleault et al., 2003].

The successes in modeling of prion disease in *Drosophila* was achieved in the expression of wild type mouse prion protein and GSS syndrome-associated mouse prion protein (MoPrP ^{P101L}) in cholinergic and dopaminergic neurons. The $MoPrP^{P101L}$ flies showed severe locomotor dysfunction, decreased lifespan and neuronal vacuolization associated to age-dependent accumulation of misfolded PrP molecules and intracellular PrP aggregates [Gavin et al, 2006]. In addition, $MoPrP^{P101L}$ induced altered synaptic architectures in larval neuromuscular junctions and progressive reduction of a synaptic scaffolding protein, Discs large (DLG), in adult brains [J.K. Choi et al., 2010]. Flies expressing wild type prion protein displayed no phenotype [J.K. Choi et al., 2010; Gavin et al, 2006].

Expression of wild type PrP (SHaPrP) in *Drosophila* neurons caused lifespan reduction, locomotive abnormality and spongiform degeneration of brain neurons. This was a first successful attempt on creation of the sporadic form of prion diseases in *Drosophila*. Notably, PrP underwent conformational changes comparable to those of PrP^{Sc}, however flies did not accumulate proteinase K-resistant PrP, indicating that wild type PrP can induce spongiform degeneration in the absence of its prototypical PrP^{Sc} conformation [Fernandez-Funez et al., 2009].

6. *Drosophila* as a model system for discovery of therapeutic compounds for brain delivery

A major obstacle in the treatment of diseases of the central nervous system is the limited penetration of drugs into the brain. A basic reason for low efficacy of many systemically administered therapeutics is insufficient drug delivery due to the presence of the blood-brain barrier (BBB) [Pardridge, 2005]. The BBB is formed by the complex tight junctions between the endothelial cells of the brain capillaries and their low endocytic activity. This results in capillary walls that behave as a continuous lipid bilayer that prevents the passage of polar and lipid-insoluble substances into the brain [Ballabh et al., 2004; Huber et al., 2001; Reese and Karnovsky, 1967]. The BBB also limits the delivery of protein and peptide-based therapeutics that are highly potent, lack toxicity and may prove extremely efficacious for the treatment of many neurological disorders [Laskowitz et al., 2006].
Limited numbers of investigations of brain delivery of therapeutic compounds described in literature are partially due to the difficulties in evaluating and predicting simultaneously the fate of a compound in a therapeutic intervention and the efficiency with which it crosses the BBB. Current methods such as *in vitro* measurements in cell cultures are insufficient to address problem in modeling of CNS diseases. At the same time present models of neurological diseases using rodents often have serious limitations for repetitive testing of a large number of structural variants of drugs. Therefore, to avoid these difficulties we examined the utility of *Drosophila* and its BBB for neuropharmacological research. Recent studies showing structural and functional similarities between the BBB of *Drosophila* the mammalian BBB suggest that *Drosophila* represents a reasonable model for testing the penetration of drugs and peptide vectors into the CNS [Daneman and Barres, 2005; Genova & Fehon, 2003; Schwabe et al., 2005; Stork et al., 2008; Wu et al., 2004]. We have demonstrated the ability of penetratin (protein transduction domain vector) [Derossi et al., 1994] to carry a cargo (apoE mimetics) across the *Drosophila* BBB into brain cells. These apoE mimetics are peptides derived from the receptor binding region of apoE that mimic the functional anti-inflammatory and neuroprotective effects of the intact apoE protein [Laskowitz et al., 2007; Wang et al., 2007]. Amazingly, penetratin fused with apoE mimetics restored cognitive functions in transgenic *Drosophila*. Moreover, penetratin fused with peptide SH8 (inhibitor of Aβ amyloidosis) [Schwarzman et al., 2005] decreased size of Aβ deposits after abdominal injection in *Drosophila* lines secreting Aβ [Sarantseva et al., 2009a]. These results suggest that *Drosophila* may be a very fruitful model system for the development of CNS drugs and studying drug delivery into the brain.

7. Conclusion

Transgenic *Drosophila* lines reproduce many key signs of Alzheimer's disease, prion diseases, FAP, FAC, SSA. Here it should be noted that although experiments with transgenic *Drosophila* do not faithfully recapitulate all aspects of studied amyloid diseases, they offer real opportunities for studying disease-related pathology. In particular, these models help to explain the contributions of APP and Aβ in familial AD pathogenesis. In general, fly models should be surveyed as the sensitive genetic system, which gives possibility to reveal the cellular processes involved in a pathogenesis of diseases, modifiers of these processes. In a very practical view *Drosophila* strains may be also used to test new therapeutic compounds, which would help resolve a variety of fundamental questions. The discovery of genetic modifiers in *Drosophila* will help to reveal the corresponding human genes and therefore new therapeutic targets.

8. Acknowledgment

This study is supported by the Russian Foundation for Basic Research and by the Program of the Presidium of the Russian Academy of Sciences ''Fundamental Sciences for Medicine''.

9. References

Adams, M.D. & Sekelsky, J.J. (2002). From sequence to phenotype: reverse genetics in *Drosophila melanogaster. Nat Rev Genet,* Vol.3, No.3, (March 2002), pp.189-98, ISSN 1471-0056

Ashley, J., Packard, M., Ataman, B. & Budnik, V. (2005). Fasciclin II signals new synapse formation through amyloid precursor protein and the scaffolding protein dX11/Mint. *J Neurosci,* Vol.25, No.25, (June 2005), pp.5943–5955, ISSN 0270-6474

Aguzzi, A., Baumann, F. & Bremer, J. (2008) The Prion's Elusive Reason for Being. *Annu Rev Neurosci.* Vol.31, pp. 439–477, ISSN 0147-006X

Ballabh, P., Braun, A. Nedergard, M. (2004). The blood–brain barrier: an overview: Structure, regulation, and clinical implications. *Neurobiol. Dis.,* Vol.16, No.13, (June 2004), pp.1-13, ISSN 0261-4189

Baki, L., Shioi, J., Wen, P., Shao, Z., Schwarzman, A., Gama-Sosa, M., Neve & R., Robakis, N.K. (2004). PS1 activates PI3K thus inhibiting GSK-3 activity and tau overphosphorylation: effects of FAD mutations. *EMBO J,* Vol.23, No.13, (July 2004), pp.2586–2596, ISSN 0261-4189

Bellen, H.J., Levis, R.W., Liao, G., He, Y., Carlson, J.W., Tsang, G., Evans-Holm, M., Hiesinger, P.R., Schulze, K.L., Rubin, G.M., Hoskins, R.A. & Spradling, A.C. (2004). The BDGP gene disruption project: single transposon insertions associated with 40% of Drosophila genes. *Genetics, Vol.*167, No.2, (June 2004), pp.761–781, ISSN 0016-6731

Bentahir, M., Nyabi, O.,Verhamme, J.,Tolia, A., Horrer, K., Wiltfang, J., Esselmann, H. & De Strooper, B. (2006). Presenilin clinical mutations can affect c-secretase activity by different mechanisms.*J. Neurochem,* Vol.96, No.3, (February 2006), pp. 732–742, ISSN 0022-3042

Berg, I., Thor, S., & Hammarström, P. (2009). Modeling familial amyloidotic polyneuropathy (Transthyretin V30M) in Drosophila melanogaster. *Neurodegener Dis,* Vol.6, No.3, (May 2009), pp. 127-38, ISSN 1660-2854

Brown, P., Gibbs, C.J., Rodgers-Johnson, P., Asher, D.M., Sulima, M.P., Bacote, A., Goldfarb, L.G., & Gajdusek, D.C. (1994). Human spongiform encephalopathy: the National Institutes of Health series of 300 cases of experimentally transmitted disease. *Ann* Neurol. Vol.35, No.5, (May 1994), pp.513-529, ISSN 0364-5134

Bier, E. (2005). Drosophila, the golden bug, emerges as a tool for human genetics. *Nat Rev Genet*,Vol.6, No.1, (January 2005), pp.9-23, ISSN 1471-0056

Bilen, J. & Bonini, N.M. (2005). Drosophila as a model for human neurodegenerative disease. *Annu Rev Genet*, Vol.39, (December 2005), pp.153-71, ISSN 0066-4197

Brand, A.H. & Perrimon, N. (1993). Targeted gene expression as a means of altering cell fates and generating dominant phenotypes. *Development*, Vol.118, No.2, (January 1999), pp.401–415, ISSN 0950-1991

Buxbaum, J.N., Ye, Z., Reixach, N., Friske, L., Levy, C., Das, P., Golde, T., Masliah, E., Roberts, A.R. & Bartfai, T. (2008). Transthyretin protects Alzheimer's mice from the behavioral and biochemical effects of Abeta toxicity. *Proc. Natl. Acad. Sci. USA*, Vol.105, (February 2008), pp. 2681–2686, ISSN 0027-8424

Cao, W., Song, H.J., Gangi, T., Kelkar, A., Antani, I., Garza, D. & Konsolaki, M. (2008). Identification of novel genes that modify phenotypes induced by Alzheimer's beta-amyloid overexpression in Drosophila. *Genetics*, Vol.178. No.3. (March 2008), pp.1457-7, ISSN 0016-6731

Carmine-Simmen, K., Proctor, T., Tschape, J., Poeck, B., Triphan, T., Strauss, R. & Kretzschmar, D. (2009). Neurotoxic effects induced by the Drosophila amyloid-beta peptide suggest a conserved toxic function. *Neurobiol Dis*. Vol.33, No.2, (February 2009), pp.274–281, ISSN 0969-9961

Chiang, H.C., Iijima, K., Hakker, I. & Zhong, Y. (2009). Distinctive roles of different beta-amyloid 42 aggregates in modulation of synaptic functions. *FASEB* J, Vol.23, No.6, (June 2009), pp. 969–1977, ISSN 0892-6638

Choi, J.K., Jeon, Y.C., Lee, D.W., Oh, J.M., Lee, H.P., Jeong, B.H., Carp, R.I., Koh, Y.H. & Kim, Y.S. (2010). A Drosophila model of GSS syndrome suggests defects in active zones are responsible for pathogenesis of GSS syndrome. *Hum Mol Genet*, Vol.19, No.22, pp. 4474-89, ISSN 0964-6906

Choi, S.H., Leight, S.N., Lee, V.M., Li, T., Wong, P.C., Johnson, J.A. & Saraiva, M.J. (2007) Accelerated Abeta deposition in APPswe/PS1deltaE9 mice with hemizygous deletions of TTR (transthyretin). *J. Neurosci*, Vol.27, No.26, (Jne 2007), pp.7006–7010, ISSN 0020-7454

Coleman, P.D.& Yao, P.J. (2003). Synaptic slaughter in Alzheimer's disease. *Neurobiol. Aging*, Vol.24, N0.8, (December 2003), pp. 1023–1027, ISSN 0197-4580

Connors, L.H., Lim, A., Prokaeva, T., Roskens, V.A. & Costello, C.E. (2003). Tabulation of human transthyretin (TTR) variants. *Amyloid*, Vol.10, No.3, (September 2003), pp.160–184, ISSN 1350-6129

Crowther, D.C., Kinghorn, K.J., Miranda, E., Page, R., Curry, J.A., Duthie, F.A., Gubb, D.C. & Lomas, D.A. (2005). Intraneuronal Abeta, nonamyloid aggregates and neurodegeneration in a Drosophila model of Alzheimer's disease. *Neuroscience*, Vol.132, pp.123–135, ISSN0306-4522

Daneman, R. & Barres, B.A. (2005). The blood-brain barrier lessons from moody flies. *Cell*, Vol.123, No,1, (October 2005), pp.9–12, ISSN 0092-8674

Davis, K. L. & Samuels, S. C. (1998). Dementia and delirium, In: *Pharmacological Management of Neurological and Psychiatric Disorders*. eds Enna S. J. and Coyle J.T., pp. 267–316, McGraw -Hill, ISBN 0070217645, New York

Deleault, N.R., Dolph, P.J., Feany, M.B., Cook, M.E., Nishina, K., Harris, D.A. & Supattapone, S. (2003). Post-transcriptional suppression of pathogenic prion protein expression in *Drosophila* neurons. *J Neurochem*, Vol.85, No.6, (June 2003), pp.1614 -1623, ISSN 0022-3042

Derossi, D., Joliot, A.H., Chassaing, G., Prochiantz, A., 1994. The third helix of the Antennapedia homeodomain translocates through biological membranes. *J. Biol. Chem*, Vol.269, No.14, (April 1994), pp. 10444- 10450, ISSN 0021-9258

Duyckaerts, C., Potier, M.C. & Delatour, B. (2008). Alzheimer disease models and human neuropathology: similarities and differences. *Acta Neuropathol*, Vol.115, No.1, (January 2008), pp.5-38, ISSN 0001-6322

De Strooper, B.D. & Annaert, W. (2001). Presenilins and the intramembrane proteolysis of proteins: facts and fiction. *Nat. Cell Biol*, Vol.3, No.10, (October 2001), pp. 221-25, ISSN 1465-7392

De Strooper, B. & Annaert, W. (2000). Proteolytic processing and cell biological functions of the amyloid precursor protein. *J. Cell Sci*, Vol.113, No.Pt11, (June 2000), pp. 1857-70, ISSN 0021-9533

Elliott, D. & Brand H. (2008). The GAL4 System: A Versatile System for the Expression of Genes, In: *Methods in Molecular Biology: Drosophila: Methods and Protocols*. C. Dahmann, pp. 79-96, Humana Press Inc., ISBN 978-1-58829-817-1, Totowa, NJ.

Enerly, E., Larsson, J. & Lambertsson, A. (2002). Reverse genetics in Drosophila: from sequence to phenotype using UAS-RNAi transgenic flies. *Genesis*, Vol.34, No.1, (October 2002), pp.152-5, ISSN 0016-6731

Fernandez-Funez, P., Casas-Tinto, S., Zhang, Y., Gomez-Velazquez, M., Morales-Garza, M.A., Cepeda-Nieto, A.C., Castilla, J., Soto, C. & Rincon-Limas, D.E. (2009). In vivo generation of neurotoxic prion protein: role for hsp70 in accumulation of misfolded isoforms. *PLoS Genet*, Vol.5, No.6, (June 2009), e1000507, ISSN1553-7390

Finelli, A., Kelkar, A., Song, H.-J., Yang, H. & Konsolaki, M. (2004). A model for studying Alzheimer's AB42-induced toxicity in *Drosophila melanogaster*. *Mol. Cell. Neurosci*, Vol. 26.No.3, (July 2004), pp. 365-375, ISSN 1044-7431

Flechsig, E., Shmerling, D., Hegyi, I., Raeber, A.J., Fischer, M., Cozzio, A., von Mering, C., Aguzzi, A., & Weissmann, C. (2000). Prion protein devoid of the octapeptide repeat region restores susceptibility to scrapie in PrP knockout mice. *Neuron*, Vol.27, No.2, (August 2000), pp.399-408, ISSN 0896-6273

Fortini, M.E., Skupski, M.P., Boguski, M.S. & Hariharan, I.K. (2000). A survey of human disease gene counterparts in the *Drosophila* genome. *J. Cell Biol*, Vol.150, No.2, (July 2000), pp. 23-30, ISSN0021-9525

Fossgreen,A., Bruckner, B., Czech, C., Masters, C.L., Beyreuther, K. & Paro R. (1998). Transgenic Drosophila expressing human amyloid precursor protein show gamma-secretase activityand a blistered-wing phenotype. *Proc Natl Acad Sci USA*, Vol.95, No.23, (November 1998), pp.13703-13708, ISSN 0027-8424

Gavin, B.A., Dolph, M.J., Deleault, N.R., Geoghegan, J.C., Khurana, V., Feany, M.B., Dolph, P.J. & Supattapone, S. (2006). Accelerated accumulation of misfolded prion protein and spongiform degeneration in a Drosophila model of Gerstmann- Straussler-Scheinker syndrome. *J Neurosci*,Vol.26, No.48, (November 2006), pp.12408-14, ISSN 0020-7454

Genova, J.L. & Fehon, R.G. (2003) Neuroglian, Gliotactin, and the Na/K-ATPase are essential for septate junction function in Drosophila. *J. Cell Biol.*, Vol.161, No.5, (June 2003), pp.979-989, ISSN 0021-9525

Goodman, D. (1987). Retinoids and retinol-binding proteins. *Harvey Lect*, Vol.81, pp.111–132, ISSN 0073-0874

Greeve, I., Kretzschmar D., Tschape, J.A., Beyn, A., Brellinger, C., Schweizer, M., Nitsch, R.M. & Reifegerste, R. (2004). Age-dependent neurodegeneration and Alzheimer-amyloid plaque formation in transgenic Drosophila. *J Neurosci,* Vol.24, No. 16, (April 2004), pp.3899–3906, ISSN0020-7454

Gunawardena, S., Goldstein, L.S. (2001). Disruption of axonal transport and neuronal viability by amyloid precursor protein mutations in Drosophila. *Neuron,* Vol.32, No.3, (November 2001), pp.389–401, ISSN0896-6273

Haass, C. &, Selkoe, D.J. (2007). Soluble protein oligomers in neurodegeneration: lessons from the Alzheimer's amyloid beta-peptide. *Nat Rev Mol Cell Biol,* Vol.8, No.2, (February 2007), pp.101-12, ISSN 1471-0072

Han, D. D., Stein, D., & Stevens, L. M. (2000). Investigating the function of follicular subpopulations during *Drosophila* oogenesis through hormone-dependent enhancer-targeted cell ablation. *Development,* Vol.127, No.3, (February 2000), pp. 573–583, ISSN 0950-1991

Hardy, J. & Selkoe, D.J. (2002). The amyloid hypothesis of Alzheimer's disease: progress and problems on the road to therapeutics. *Science,* Vol.297, No. 5580, (July 2002), pp.353–356, ISSN 0193-4511

Hersh, L.B. & Rodgers, D.W. (2008). Neprilysin and amyloid beta peptide degradation. *Curr Alzheimer Res*, Vol.5, No.2, (April 2008), pp.225-31, ISSN 1567-2050

Hirth, F. (2010). Drosophila melanogaster in the study of human neurodegeneration. *CNS Neurol Disord Drug Targets*, Vol. 9. No. 4, (April 2010), pp.504-23, ISSN 1871-5273

Honer, W.G. (2003). Pathology of presynaptic proteins in Alzheimer's disease: more than simple loss of terminals. *Neurobiol Aging*, Vol.24, No.8, (December 2003), pp.1047-62, ISSN 0197-4580

Huber, J.D., Egleton, R.D.& Davis, T.P. (2001). Molecular physiology and pathophysiology of tight junctions in the blood-brain barrier. *Trends Neurosci.*, Vol.24, No.1, (December 2001), ISSN 719 –725.

Huet, F., Lu, J.T., Myrick, K.V., Baugh, L.R., Crosby, M.A. & Gelbart, W.M. (2002). A deletion-generator compound element allows deletion saturation analysis for genomewide phenotypic annotation. *Proc Natl Acad Sci U S A*. Vol. 99, No.15. (July 2002), pp.9948-53, ISSN 0027-8424

Iijima, K., Liu, H.-P., Chiang, A.-S., Hearn, S., Konsolaki, M. & Zhong Y. (2004). Dissecting the pathological effects of human Aβ40 and Aβ42 in *Drosophila*: A potential model for Alzheimer's disease. *PNAS,* Vol.101, No.17, (April 2004), pp.6623–6628, ISSN 0027-8424

Iijima, K., Chiang, H.C., Hearn, S.A., Hakker, I., Gatt, A., Shenton, C., Granger, L., Leung, A., Iijima-Ando, K. & Zhong, Y. (2008). Abeta42 mutants with different aggregation profiles induce distinct pathologies in Drosophila. *PLoS ONE,* Vol.3, No.2, (February 2008), e1703, ISSN 1932-6203

Iijima-Ando, K., Hearn, S.A., Shenton, C., Gatt, A., Zhao, L. & Iijima, K. (2009). Mitochondrial Mislocalization Underlies Ab42-Induced Neuronal Dysfunction in a Drosophila Model of Alzheimer's Disease. *PLoS ONE,* Vol.4, No.12. (Devember 2009), e8310, ISSN 1932-6203

Iijima-Ando, K.& Iijima, K. (2010). Transgenic Drosophila models of Alzheimer's disease and tauopathies. *Brain Struct Funct.*, Vol.214, No.2-3, (March 2010), pp.245-62, ISSN 1863-2653

Iwata, N., Tsubuki, S., Takaki, Y., Shirotani, K., Lu, B., Gerard, N.P., Gerard, C., Hama, E., Lee, H.J. & Saido, T.C. (2001). Metabolic regulation of brain Ah by neprilysin. *Science*, Vol.292, No. 292(5521), (May 2001), pp. 1550- 1552, ISSN 0193-4511

Iwata, N., Higuchi, M. & Saido, T. (2005). Metabolism of amyloid-β peptide and Alzheimer's disease *Pharmacology & Therapeutics*, Vol.108, No. , pp. 129 - 148. ISSN

Kazazian, H.H. (2004). Mobile elements: drivers of genome evolution. *Science*, Vol.303. No.303(5664), (March 2004), pp.1626-1632, ISSN 0193-4511

Krasemann, S., Zerr, I., Weber, T., Poser, S., Kretzschmar, H., Hunsmann, G. & Bodemer W. (1995). Prion disease associated with a novel nine octapeptide repeat insertion in the PRNP gene. *Brain Res. Mol. Brain Res*, Vol.34, No.1, (December 1995), pp.173-176, ISSN 0169-328X

LaFerla, F.M., Green, K.N. & Oddo S (2007). Intracellular amyloid-beta in Alzheimer's disease. *Nat Rev Neurosci*, Vol.8, No.7, (July 2007), pp.499 -509, ISSN 1471-003X

Laskowitz, D.T., Fillit, H., Yeung, N., Toku, K., & Vitek, M.P. (2006). Apolipoprotein E-derived peptides reduce CNS inflammation: implications for therapy of neurological disease. *Acta Neurol Scand Suppl*, Vol.185, pp.15-20, ISSN 0065-1427

Laskowitz, D.T. & Vitek, M.P. (2007). Apolipoprotein E and neurological disease: therapeutic potential and pharmacogenomic interactions. *Pharmacogenomics*, Vol.8, No.8, (August 2007) pp.959-969, ISSN 1462-2416

Liz, M.A., Fleming, C.E., Nunes, A.F., Almeida, M.R., Mar, F.M., Choe, Y., Craik, C.S., Powers, J.C., Bogyo, M. & Sousa, M.M. (2009) Substrate specificity of transthyretin: identification of natural substrates in the nervous system. *Biochem J*, Vol.419, No.2, (April 2009), pp.467-74, ISSN 0264-6021

Liu, L. & Murphy, R.M. (2006) Kinetics of inhibition of beta-amyloid aggregation by transthyretin. *Biochemistry*, Vol.45, No. 51, (December 2006), pp. 15702-15709, ISSN 0006-2960

Lu, B. & Vogel, H. (2009). Drosophila models of neurodegenerative diseases. *Annu Rev Pathol*, Vol.4, pp. 315-42, ISSN 1553-4006

Lue, L.F., Kuo, Y.M., Roher, A.E., Brachova, L., Shen, Y., Sue, L., Beach, T., Kurth, J.H., Rydel, R.E., Rogers. J. (1999). Soluble amyloid beta peptide concentration as a predictor of synaptic change in Alzheimer's disease. *Amer. J. Pathol.* Vol. 155, No.3, (September 1999), pp. 853-862, ISSN 0002-9440

Luo, L.Q., Martin-Morris, L.E. & White, K. (1990). Identification, secretion, and neural expression of APPL, a *Drosophila* protein similar to human amyloid protein precursor. *J. Neurosci*, Vol.10, No.12, (December 1990), pp. 3849-61, ISSN 0020-7454

Luo, L., Tully, T. & White, K. (1992). Human amyloid precursor protein ameliorates behavioral deficit of flies deleted for *Appl* gene. *Neuron*, Vol. 9, No.4, (October 1992), pp. 595- 605, ISSN 0896-6273

Manson, J.C., Jamieson, E., Baybutt, H., Tuzi, N.L., Barron, R., McConnell, I., Somerville, R., Ironside, J., Will, R., Sy, M.S., Melton, D.W., Hope, J. & Bostock, C. (1999). A single amino acid alteration (101L) introduced into murine PrP dramatically alters incubation time of transmissible spongiform encephalopathy. *EMBO J*, Vol.18, No.23, (December 1999), pp.6855-6864, ISSN 0261-4189

Marsh, J.L. & Thompson LM. (2006). Drosophila in the study of neurodegenerative disease. *Neuron*, Vol.52, No.1, (October 2006), pp.169-78, ISSN 0896-6273

Masliah, E., Mallory, M., Hansen, L., DeTeresa, R., Alford, M. & Terry, R. (1994). Synaptic and neuritic alterations during the progression of Alzheimer's Disease. *Neuroscie. Let*, Vol.174. No.1, (June 1994), pp. 67-72, ISSN 0306-4522

Masliah, E., Mallory, M., Alford, M., DeTeresa, R., Hansen, L.A., McKeel, Jr, D.W. & Morris, J.C. (2001). Altered expression of synaptic proteins occurs early during progression of Alzheimer's disease. *Neurology*, Vol.56, No.1, (January 2001), pp.127–129, ISSN 0028-3878

Matsumoto, K., Toh-e, A., & Oshima, Y. (1978). Genetic control of galactokinase synthesis in *Saccharomyces cerevisiae*: evidence for constitutive expression of the positive regulatory gene gal4. *J. Bacteriol*, Vol.134, No.2, (May 1978), pp.446–457, ISSN 0021-9193

McGuire, S. E., Le, P. T., Osborn, A. J., Matsumoto, K., and Davis, R. L. (2003). Spatiotemporal rescue of memory dysfunction in *Drosophila*. *Science*, Vol.302, No.5651, (December 2003), pp.1765–1768, ISSN 0193-4511

Mead, S. (2006). Prion disease genetics. *Eur. J. Hum. Genet*, Vol.14, No. 3, (March 2006),pp.273-281, ISSN 1018-4813

Metaxakis, A., Oehler, S., Klinakis, A. & Savakis, C. (2005). Minos as a genetic and genomic tool in Drosophila melanogaster. *Genetics*, Vol.171, No.12, (October 2005), pp.571-81, ISSN 0016-6731

Moloney, A., Sattelle, D.B.,.Lomas, D.A. & Crowther, D.C. (2010). Alzheimer's disease: insights from Drosophila melanogaster models. *Trends Biochem Sci*, Vol.35, No.4, (April 2010), pp. 228-35, ISSN 0968-0004

Mucke, L., Masliah, E., Yu, G.Q., Mallory, M., Rockenstein, E.M., Tatsuno, G., Hu, K., Kholodenko, D., Johnson-Wood, K. & McConlogue, L. (2000). High-level neuronal expression of A_1-42 in wild-type human amyloid protein precursor transgenic mice: synaptotoxicity without plaque formation. *J Neurosci*, Vol.20, pp.4050–4058, ISSN0020-7454

Myrick, K.V., Huet, F., Mohr, S.E., Alvarez-García, I., Lu, J.T., Smith, M.A., Crosby, M.A. & Gelbart, W.M. (2009). Large-scale functional annotation and expanded implementations of the P{wHy} hybrid transposon in the Drosophila melanogaster genome. *Genetics*, Vol. 182, No. 3, (July 2009), pp.653-60, ISSN 0016-6731

Nicholson, L., Singh, G.K., Osterwalder, T., Roman, G.W., Davis, R.L.& Keshishian, H. (2008). Spatial and temporal control of gene expression in Drosophila using the inducible GeneSwitch GAL4 system. I. Screen for larval nervous system drivers. *Genetics*, Vol.178, No.1, (January 2008), pp.215-34, ISSN 0016-6731

Oddo, S., Caccamo, A., Shepherd, J.D., Murphy, M.P., Golde, T.E., Kayed, R., Metherate, R., Mattson, M.P., Akbari, Y. & LaFerla, F.M. (2003). Tripletransgenic model of Alzheimer's disease with plaques and tangles: intracellular Abeta and synaptic dysfunction. *Neuron*, Vol.39, No.3, (June 2003), pp.409–421, ISSN 0896-6273

Olofsson, A., Ippel, H.J., Baranov, V., Horstedt, P., Wijmenga, S. & Lundgren, E. (2001). Capture of a dimeric intermediate during transthyretin amyloid formation. *J. Biol. Chem.*, Vol.276, No.4, (October 2001), pp. 39592–39599, ISSN 0021-9258

Osterwalder, T.,Yoon, K. S., White, B. H. & Keshishian, H. (2001). A conditional tissue-specific transgene expression system using inducible GAL4. *Proc. Natl. Acad. Sci. USA,* Vol.98, No.22, (October 2001), pp.596–601, ISSN 0027-8424

Pardridge, W.M. (2005). The blood-brain barrier: bottleneck in brain drug development. *NeuroRx,* Vol.2, No.1, (January 2005), pp.3–14, ISSN 1545-5343

Pokrzywa, M., Dacklin, I., Hultmark, D. & Lundgren, E. (2007). Misfolded transthyretin causes behavioral changes in a *Drosophila* model for transthyretin-associated amyloidosis. *Eur J Neurosci,* Vol.26, No.4, (August 2007), pp. 913-24, ISSN 0953-816X

Pokrzywa, M., Dacklin, I., Vestling, M., Hultmark, D., Lundgren, E.& Cantera, R. (2010). Uptake of Aggregating Transthyretin by Fat Body in a Drosophila Model for TTR-Associated Amyloidosis. *PLoS ONE,* Vol.5, No.12., (December 2010), e14343. ISSN 1932-6203

Prusiner, S. B. (1998). Prions. *PNAS,* Vol.95, No.23, (November 1998), pp.13363–13383, ISSN0027-8424

Prusiner, S.B. (1998). The prion diseases. *Brain Pathol,* Vol.8, No.3, (July 1998), pp.499-513, ISSN 1015-6305

Prusiner, S.B. & Hsiao, K.K. (1994). Human prion diseases. *Ann Neurol,* Vol.35, No.4, (April 1994), pp. 385-95, ISSN 0364-5134

Raeber, A.J., Muramoto, T., Kornberg, T.B. & Prusiner, S.B. (1995). Expression and targeting of Syrian hamster prion protein induced by heat shock in transgenic *Drosophila melanogaster. Mech Dev,* Vol. No.2-3, (June 1995), pp.317-27, ISSN 0925-4773

Reese, T.S. & Karnovsky, M.J. (1967) Fine structural localization of a blood-brain barrier to exogenous peroxidase. *J Cell Biol.,* Vol.34, No.1, (July 1967), pp.207–217, ISSN 0021-9525

Reiter, L.T., Potocki, L., Chien, S., Gribskov, M.& Bier, E. (2001). A systematic analysis of human disease-associated gene sequences in *Drosophila melanogaster. Genome Res,* Vol. 11, No.6, (June 2001), pp.1114–25, ISSN 1088-9051

Rodríguez-Martínez, A.B., Garrido, J.M., Zarranz, J.J., Arteagoitia, J.M., de Pancorbo, M.M., Atarés, B., Bilbao, M.J., Ferrer, I., Juste, R.A. (2010). A novel form of human disease with a protease-sensitive prion protein and heterozygosity methionine/valine at codon 129: Case report. *BMC Neurol,* Vol. 10, No. 99, (October 2010), ISSN 1471-2377

Roman, G., Endo, K., Zong, L., and Davis, R. L. (2001). P[Switch], a system for spatial and temporal control of gene expression in *Drosophila melanogaster. Proc. Natl. Acad. Sci. USA,* Vol.98, No.12, pp.602–607, ISSN 0027-8424

Rørth, P. (1996).A modular misexpression screen in *Drosophila* detecting tissue-specific phenotypes. *Proc Natl Acad Sci U S A,* Vol. 93. No.22, (October 1996), pp.12418-22, ISSN 0027-8424

Rørth, P., Szabo, K., Bailey, A., Laverty, T., Rehm, J., Rubin, G.M., Weigmann, K., Milán, M., Benes, V., Ansorge, W. & Cohen, S.M. (1998). Systematic gain-of-function genetics in Drosophila. *Development,* Vol.125, No.6, (March 1998), pp.1049–1057, ISSN 0950-1991

Rosen, D.R., Martin-Morris, L., Luo, L. & White, K. A. (1989). *Drosophila* gene encoding a protein resembling the human b-amyloid protein precursor. *Proc Natl Acad Sci USA,* Vol.86, No.7, (April 1989), pp. 2478 –2482, ISSN 0027-8424

Rubin, G.M. & Spradling, A.C. (1982). Genetic transformation of Drosophila with transposable element vectors. *Science*, Vol. 218, No.4570, (October 1982), pp.348-53, ISSN 0193-4511

Sang, T.K., Jackson, G.R. (2005). Drosophila models of neurodegenerative disease. *NeuroRx.* Vol. 2, No. 3, (July 2010), pp.438-46, ISSN 1545-5343

Sarantseva, S., Timoshenko, S., Bolshakova, O., Karaseva, E., Rodin, D., Schwarzman, A.L. & Vitek, M.P. (2009a). Apolipoprotein E-mimetics inhibit neurodegeneration and restore cognitive functions in a transgenic Drosophila model of Alzheimer's disease. *PLoS One,* Vol.4, No.12, (December 2009), e8191, ISSN1932-6203

Sarantseva, S., Bolshakova, O., Timoshenko, S., Vitek, M.P.& Schwarzman, A.L. (2009b). Overexpression of human amyloid precursor protein causes neurodegeneration and loss of synaptic proteins in transgenic *Drosophila*. In: Hanin I., Fisher A., pp.245-248, Medimont, ISBN 978-88-7587-528-2, Prague, Czech Republic

Saura, C., Choi, S.-Y., Beglopoulos, V., Malkani, S., Zhang, D., Rao, B.S.S., Chattarji, S., Kelleher, R., Kandel, E., Duff, K. Kirkwood A, Shen J. (2004). Loss of presenilin function causes impairments of memory and synaptic plasticity followed by age-dependent neurodegeneration. *Neuron,* Vol.42, No.1, (April 2004), pp.23–36, ISSN 0896-6273

Schwabe, T., Bainton, R.J., Fetter, R.D., Heberlein, U. & Gaul, U. (2005). GPCR signaling is required for blood-brain barrier formation in Drosophila. *Cell,* Vol.123, No.7, (October 2005), pp.133–144, ISSN0092-8674

Schwarzman, A.L., Gregori, L., Vitek, M.P., Lyubski, S., Strittmatter, W.J., Enghilde, J.J., Bhasin, R., Silverman, J., Weisgraber, K.H. & Coyle, P.K. (1994). Transthyretin sequesters amyloid beta protein and prevents amyloid formation. *Proc.Natl.Acad.Sci.USA*. Vol.91, No.18, (August 1994), pp.8368-8372, ISSN0027-8424

Schwarzman, A.L., Singh, N., Tsiper, M., Gregori, L., Dranovsky, A., Vitek, M., Glabe, C., St.George-Hyslop, P. & Goldgaber, D. (1999). Endogenous presenilin 1 redistributes to the lamellipodia upon adhesion of Jurkat cells to a collagen matrix. *Proc.Natl. Acad.Sci.USA*, Vol.96, No.14, (July 1999), pp. 7932-7937, ISSN 0027-8424

Schwarzman, A.L., Tsiper, M., Gregori, L., Goldgaber, D., Fracowiak, J., Mazur-Kolecka, B., Taraskina, A., Pchelina, S. & Vitek, M.P. (2005). Selection of peptides binding to the amyloid Ab-protein reveals potential inhibitors of amyloid formation. *Amyloid,* Vol.12, No.4, (December 2005), pp.1–11, ISSN 1350-6129

Selkoe, D.J. (1998). The cell biology of β-amyloid precursor protein and presenilin in Alzheimer's disease. *Trends Cell Biol,* Vol.8, No.11, (November 1998), pp. 447–53, ISSN 0962-8924

Selkoe, D.J. (1999). Translating cell biology into therapeutic advances in Alzheimer's disease. *Nature*. Vol.399, pp. 23–31, No. 6738 Suppl, (June 1999), ISSN 0028-0836

Selkoe, D.J. (2002). Alzheimer's disease is a synaptic failure. *Science,* Vol.298, No.5594, (October 2002) pp.789 –791, ISSN 0193-4511

Singh, N., Tsiper, M., Romanov, V., Dranovsky, A.,Talalayeva, Y., Colflesh, D., Rudamen, G., Vitek, M.P.Shen , J., Yang, X., Goldgaber, D. & Schwarzman, A.L. (2001). The role of Alzheimer's disease-related presenilin 1 in intercellular adhesion. *Exp.Cell.Res*, Vol.263, No.1. (February 2001), pp.1-13, ISSN 0014-4827

Sipe, J.D., Benson, M.D., Buxbaum, J.N., Ikeda, S., Merlini, G., Saraiva, M.J. & Westermark, P. (2010). Amyloid fibril protein nomenclature: 2010 recommendations from the nomenclature committee of the International Society of Amyloidosis. *Amyloid,* Vol.17, No.13-14, (September 2010), pp.101-4, ISSN 1350-6129

Smith, D., Wohlgemuth, J., Calvi, B. R. Franklin I, Gelbart WM. (1993). *hobo* enhancer trapping mutagenesis in *Drosophila* reveals an insertion specificity different from *P* elements. *Genetics,* Vol. 135, No.4, (December 1993), pp. 1063–1076, ISSN 0016-6731

Solomon, I.H., Schepker, J.A. & Harris, D.A. (2010). Prion neurotoxicity: insights from prion protein mutants. *Curr Issues Mol Biol,* Vol.12, No.2, pp.51-61, ISSN 1467-3037

Staudt, N., Molitor, A., Somogyi. K., Mata, J., Curado, S., Eulenberg, K., Meise, M., Siegmund, T., Häder, T., Hilfiker, A., Brönner, G., Ephrussi, A., Rørth, P., Cohen, S.M,, Fellert, S., Chung, H.R., Piepenburg, O., Schäfer, U., Jäckle, H. & Vorbrüggen, G. (2005). Gain-of-function screen for genes that affect Drosophila muscle pattern formation. *PLoS Genet,* Vol.1, No.4, (October 2005), e55, ISSN 1553-7390

Stork, T., Engelen, D., Krudewig, A., Silies, M., Bainton, R.J.& Klämbt, C. (2008). Organization and function of the blood-brain barrier in Drosophila. *J Neurosci,* Vol.28, No.3, (January 2008), pp.587-97, ISSN 0270-6474

Sze, C.I., Troncosom J,C,, Kawas, C., Mouton, P., Price, D.L. & Martin, L.J. (1997). Loss of the presynaptic vesicle protein synaptophysin in hippocampus correlates with cognitive decline in Alzheimer disease. *J Neuropathol Exp Neurol,* Vol.56, No.8, (August 1997), pp.933–944, ISSN 0022-3069

Tateishi, J. & Kitamoto, T.(1995). Inherited prion diseases and transmission to rodents. *Brain Pathol,* Vol.5, No.1, (January 1995), pp.53-9, ISSN 1015-6305

Terry, R.D., Masliah, E., Salmon, D.P., Butters, N., DeTeresa, R., Hill, R., Hansen, L.A. &, Katzman, R. (1991). Physical basis of cognitive alterations in Alzheimer's disease: synapse loss is the major correlate of cognitive impairment. *Ann Neurol,* Vol.30, No.4, (October 1991), pp.572–580, ISSN 0364-5134

Torroja, L., Luo, L. & White, K. (1996). APPL, the *Drosophila* member of the APP-family, exhibits differential trafficking and processing in CNS neurons. *J Neurosci,* Vol.16, No.15, (August 1996), pp. 4638–4650, ISSN0020-7454

Torroja L, Chu H, Kotovsky I, White K (1999a) Neuronal overexpression of APPL, the Drosophila homologue of the amyloid precursor protein (APP), disrupts axonal transport. *Curr Biol,* Vol.9, No.9, (May 1999), pp.489–492, ISSN 0960-9822

Torroja, L., Packard, M., Gorczyca, M., White, K. & Budnik, V. (1999b). The Drosophila beta-amyloid precursor protein homolog promotes synapse differentiation at the neuromuscular junction. *J Neurosci,* Vol.19, No.18, (September 1999), pp.7793–7803, ISSN 0020-7454

van de Hoef, D.L., Hughes, J., Livne-Bar, I., Garza, D., Konsolaki, M.& Boulianne, G.L. (2009). Identifying genes that interact with Drosophila presenilin and amyloid precursor protein. *Genesis,* Vol. 47, No.4, (April 2009), pp. 246-60, ISSN 1526-954X

Wang, H., Durham, L., Dawson, H., Song, P., Warner, D.S., Sullivan, P.M., Vitek, M.P. & Laskowitz, D.T. (2007). An apolipoprotein E-based therapeutic improves outcome and reduce Alzheimer's disease pathology following closed head injury: evidence of pharmacogenomic interaction. *Neuroscience,* Vol.144, No.4, (February 2007), pp.1324–33, ISSN 0306-4522

Walsh, D.M. & Selkoe, D.J. (2004). Deciphering the molecular basis of memory failure in Alzheimer's disease. *Neuron,* Vol.44, No.1, (September 2004), pp.181-193, ISSN 0896-6273

Westermark, P., Sletten, K., Johansson, B. & Cornwell, G.G. 3rd. (1990). Fibril in senile systemic amyloidosis is derived from normal transthyretin. *Proc Natl Acad Sci U S A*, Vol.87, No.7, (April 1990), pp. 2843-5, ISSN 0027-8424

Westermark, P., Benson, M.D., Buxbaum, J.N., Cohen AS, Frangione B, Ikeda S, Masters CL, Merlini G, Saraiva MJ, Sipe JD. (2007). A primer of amyloid nomenclature. *Amyloid*, Vol.14, No.3, (September 2007), pp.179–183, ISSN 1350-6129

Wirths, O., Multhaup, G. & Bayer, T.A. (2004). A modified beta-amyloid hypothesis: intraneuronal accumulation of the beta-amyloid peptide—the first step of a fatal cascade. *J Neurochem*, Vol.91, No.3, (November 2004), pp.513–520, ISSN 0022-3042

Wiseman, R.L., Powers, E.T. & Kelly, J.W. (2005). Partitioning conformational intermediates between competing refolding and aggregation pathways: insights into transthyretin amyloid disease. *Biochemistry*, Vol. 44, No.50, (December 2005), pp.16612–16623, ISSN 0006-2960

Woeber, K. A. & Ingbar, S. H. (1968). The contribution of thyroxinebinding prealbumin to the binding of thyroxine in human serum, as assessed by immunoadsorption. *J. Clin. Invest*, Vol.47, No.7, (July 1968), pp.1710–1721, ISSN 0021-9738

Wu, V.M., Schulte, J., Hirschi, A., Tepass, U. & Beitel, G.J. (2004). Sinuous is a Drosophila claudin required for septate junction organization and epithelial tube size control. *J. Cell Biol.*, Vol.164, No.2, (January 2004), pp.313–323, ISSN 0021-9525

Yagi, Y., Tomita, S., Nakamura, M. & Suzuki, T. (2000). Overexpression of human amyloid precursor protein in Drosophila. *Mol. Cell. Biol. Res. Commun*, Vol.4, No.1, (July 2000), pp. 43–49, ISSN 1522-4724

Ye, Y. & Fortini, M.E. (1998). Characterization of *Drosophila* presenilin and its colocalization with Notch during development. *Mech. Dev*, Vol.79, No.1, (December 1998), pp.199–211, ISSN 0925-4773

Zhao, X.L., Wang, W.A., Tan, J.X., Huang, J.K., Zhang, X., Zhang, B.Z., Wang, Y.H., YangCheng, H.Y., Zhu, H.L., Sun, X.J., Huang, F.D. (2010). Expression of beta-amyloid induced age-dependent presynaptic and axonal changes in Drosophila. *J Neurosci*, Vol.20, No.4, (January 2010), pp.1512-22, ISSN0020-7454

Zou, W.Q., Puoti, G., Xiao, X., Yuan, J., Qing, L., Cali, I., Shimoji, M., Langeveld, J.P., Castellani, R., Notari, S., Crain, B., Schmidt, R.E., Ge schwind, M., Dearmond, S.J., Cairns, N.J., Dickson, D., Honig, L., Torres, J.M., Mastrianni, J., Capellari, S., Giaccone, G., Belay, E.D., Schonberger, L.B., Cohen, M., Perry, G., Kong, Q., Parchi, P., Tagliavini, F. & Gambetti, P. (2010). Variably protease-sensitive prionopathy: a new sporadic disease of the prion protein. *Ann Neurol*. Vol. 68, No.2, (August 2010), pp.162-72, ISSN 0364-5134